Resistance to Targeted Anti-Cancer Therapeutics

Volume 12

Series Editor:
Benjamin Bonavida

More information about this series at http://www.springer.com/series/11727

Olivier Micheau
Editor

TRAIL, Fas Ligand, TNF and TLR3 in Cancer

Springer

Editor
Olivier Micheau
INSERM, LNC UMR 1231
Dijon, France

ISSN 2196-5501 ISSN 2196-551X (electronic)
Resistance to Targeted Anti-Cancer Therapeutics
ISBN 978-3-319-56804-1 ISBN 978-3-319-56805-8 (eBook)
DOI 10.1007/978-3-319-56805-8

Library of Congress Control Number: 2017943866

Printed on acid-free paper

This Springer imprint is published by Springer Nature
The registered company is Springer International Publishing AG
The registered company address is: Gewerbestrasse 11, 6330 Cham, Switzerland

Preface

Receptors and ligands of the TNF superfamily, with the exception of a few members, are transmembrane glycoproteins. They display pleiotropic functions. Several receptors of the family are able to induce apoptosis or cell death. Their cognate ligands are instrumental to immune cells, allowing eradication of unwanted, virally infected or transformed cells. Among these, TRAIL has early on attracted a major interest in oncology, owing to its ability to selectively trigger tumor cell killing while sparing normal cells. TRAIL induces cell death through binding to its two agonist receptors, namely TRAIL-R1 and TRAIL-R2. Its use in the clinic, however, despite clear clinical evidence of antitumoral activity, has remained limited due to a plethora of molecular mechanisms leading to cell resistance as well as to our poor understanding of the biological function and regulation of its receptors. Therapeutic strategies or options to exploit TRAIL or its derivatives in oncology should benefit from a deeper understanding of the signal transduction pathways induced by each TRAIL agonist receptor or beyond. The reader will find in this book chapters describing our current understanding of the molecular mechanisms leading to cell death or tumor cell resistance to TRAIL-induced killing, and beyond to receptors of the TNF family or unrelated receptors, such as Fas/CD95 or TLR3, respectively. Nonapoptotic signaling capabilities of these receptors will also be presented with a special emphasis on Fas/CD95, as increasing body of evidence demonstrates that some of these receptors may also exhibit atypical immune functions and even prometastatic activities. The pleiotropic signaling capabilities of transmembrane receptors and ligands cannot be dissociated from their biochemical context. They are surrounded by lipids and undergo post-translational modifications. We will discuss, in the light of the most recent discoveries, how partitioning, sphingolipids, and glycosylation of TNF receptors or ligands are likely to alter or contribute to their signal transduction capabilities. Last, in silico modeling of these complex systems will be presented, as these simulations are likely to be useful to understand how cellular protein, lipid, or sugar heterogeneities are likely to affect the therapeutic efficacy of TRAIL or TRAIL derivatives.

I would like to thank personally each of the authors for their effort and thoughtful contribution. This timely and comprehensive volume addresses the most advanced knowledge of TNF signaling with a special emphasis on TRAIL. With its strong focus on therapy and innovative concepts, this book will serve as a reference in the field for a wide audience of readers comprising researchers, medical professionals, students, and biotech and pharmaceutical companies.

Dijon, France Olivier Micheau

Contents

Contributors

Nathalie Andrieu-Abadie INSERM UMR 1037, CRCT, Toulouse, France

Equipe Labellisée Ligue Contre Le Cancer, Toulouse, France

Bassam Badran Université Libanaise, Ecole Doctorale de Sciences et Technologies, Campus Universitaire de Rafic Hariri, Hadath, Lebanon

Grégory Batt Inria Saclay – Ile-de-France, Palaiseau, France

François Bertaux INRIA Paris, Paris, France

Department of Mathematics, Imperial College London, London, UK

Inria Saclay – Ile-de-France, Palaiseau, France

Fatima Bilal INSERM UMR 1037, CRCT, Toulouse, France

Equipe Labellisée Ligue Contre Le Cancer, Toulouse, France

Université Libanaise, Ecole Doctorale de Sciences et Technologies, Campus Universitaire de Rafic Hariri, Hadath, Lebanon

Université Toulouse III—Paul Sabatier, Toulouse, France

Ahmad Daher Université Libanaise, Ecole Doctorale de Sciences et Technologies, Campus Universitaire de Rafic Hariri, Hadath, Lebanon

Lubna Danish Institute of Cell Biology and Immunology, University of Stuttgart, Stuttgart, Germany

Dirk Drasdo INRIA Paris, Paris, France

Laurence Dubrez Université de Bourgogne Franche-Comté, LNC UMR1231, Dijon, France

Institut National de la Santé et de la Recherche Médicale (Inserm), LNC UMR1231, Dijon, France

Jürgen Eberle Department of Dermatology and Allergy, Skin Cancer Center Charité, Charité-Universitätsmedizin Berlin, Berlin, Germany

Wafik El-Deiry Laboratory of Translational Oncology and Experimental Cancer Therapeutics, Department of Hematology/Oncology and Molecular Therapeutics Program, Fox Chase Cancer Center, Philadelphia, PA, USA

Yann Estornes Centre de Recherche en Cancérologie de Lyon, UMR INSERM 1052—CNRS 5286, Centre Léon Bérard Batiment Cheney D, Lyon, France

Simone Fulda Institute for Experimental Cancer Research in Pediatrics, Goethe--University Frankfurt, Frankfurt, Germany

German Cancer Consortium (DKTK), Heidelberg, Germany

German Cancer Research Center (DKFZ), Heidelberg, Germany

Consuelo Gajate Laboratory of Cell Death and Cancer Therapy, Department of Cellular and Molecular Medicine, Centro de Investigaciones Biológicas, Consejo Superior de Investigaciones Científicas (CSIC), Madrid, Spain

Christina Leah Kline Laboratory of Translational Oncology and Experimental Cancer Therapeutics, Department of Hematology/Oncology and Molecular Therapeutics Program, Fox Chase Cancer Center, Philadelphia, PA, USA

Serge Lebecque Centre de Recherche en Cancérologie de Lyon, UMR INSERM 1052—CNRS 5286, Centre Léon Bérard Batiment Cheney D, Lyon, France

Université Claude Bernard Lyon 1, Lyon, France

Hospices Civils de Lyon, Centre Hospitalier Lyon Sud, Pierre Bénite, France

Patrick Legembre Centre Eugène Marquis, INSERM U1242-COSS Equipe, Labellisée Ligue Contre Le Cancer, Rue Bataille Flandres Dunkerque, Rennes, France

Université de Rennes-1, Rennes, France

Thierry Levade INSERM UMR 1037, CRCT, Toulouse, France

Equipe Labellisée Ligue Contre Le Cancer, Toulouse, France

Université Toulouse III—Paul Sabatier, Toulouse, France

Laboratoire de Biochimie, Institut Fédératif de Biologie, CHU Purpan, Toulouse, France

Olivier Micheau Université de Bourgogne Franche-Comté, LNC UMR1231, Dijon, France

Institut National de la Santé et de la Recherche Médicale (Inserm), LNC UMR1231, Dijon, France

FCS Bourgogne Franche-Comté, Laboratoire d'Excellence LipSTIC, Dijon, France

UFR Science de santé, Inserm LNC UMR1231, Dijon, cedex, France

Andrea Mohr Cancer and Stem Cell Biology Group, School of Biological Sciences, University of Essex, Colchester, UK

Faustino Mollinedo Laboratory of Cell Death and Cancer Therapy, Department of Cellular and Molecular Medicine, Centro de Investigaciones Biológicas, Consejo Superior de Investigaciones Científicas (CSIC), Madrid, Spain

Michaël Pérès INSERM UMR 1037, CRCT, Toulouse, France

Equipe Labellisée Ligue Contre Le Cancer, Toulouse, France

Amanda Poissonnier Centre Eugène Marquis, INSERM U1242-COSS Equipe, Labellisée Ligue Contre Le Cancer, Rue Bataille Flandres Dunkerque, Rennes, France

Université de Rennes-1, Rennes, France

Nadine Pollak Institute of Cell Biology and Immunology, University of Stuttgart, Stuttgart, Germany

Vivek M. Rangnekar Graduate Center for Toxicology and Cancer Biology, University of Kentucky, Lexington, KY, USA

Department of Radiation Medicine, University of Kentucky, Lexington, KY, USA

Department of Microbiology, Immunology and Molecular Genetics, University of Kentucky, Lexington, KY, USA

Lucille Parker Markey Cancer Center, University of Kentucky, Lexington, KY, USA

Toufic Renno Centre de Recherche en Cancérologie de Lyon, UMR INSERM 1052—CNRS 5286, Centre Léon Bérard Batiment Cheney D, Lyon, France

Peter Scheurich Institute of Cell Biology and Immunology, University of Stuttgart, Stuttgart, Germany

Bruno Ségui INSERM UMR 1037, CRCT, Toulouse, France

Equipe Labellisée Ligue Contre Le Cancer, Toulouse, France

Université Toulouse III—Paul Sabatier, Toulouse, France

James Sledziona Graduate Center for Toxicology and Cancer Biology, University of Kentucky, Lexington, KY, USA

Daniela Stöhr Institute of Cell Biology and Immunology, University of Stuttgart, Stuttgart, Germany

Jessica Wagner Laboratory of Translational Oncology and Experimental Cancer Therapeutics, Department of Hematology/Oncology and Molecular Therapeutics Program, Fox Chase Cancer Center, Philadelphia, PA, USA

Ralf Zwacka Cancer and Stem Cell Biology Group, School of Biological Sciences, University of Essex, Colchester, UK

About the Editor

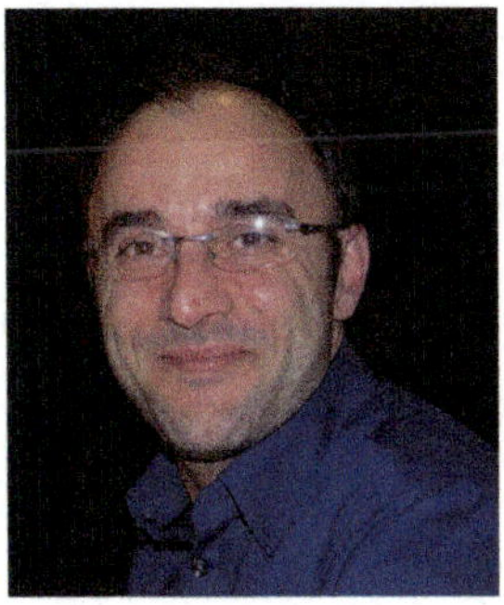

Olivier Micheau is a research director of the INSERM (French National Institute of Health), UMR1231. He received his PhD in Biochemistry and Molecular and Cellular Biology in 1999 from the University of Burgundy, France. He next moved as a postdoctoral fellow to Jurg Tschopp's laboratory in Epalinges, Switzerland, from 1999 to 2003, where he elucidated the molecular mechanisms underlying TNFR1's dual signaling ability. He described for the first time TNFR1 cytosolic proapoptotic complex II. In 2003 he joined the INSERM unit U517 headed by Professor E. Solary in Dijon, France, as an INSERM researcher. Member of several scientific councils, including INSERM CSS3 (2012–2016) and ARC, a French Charity (since 2015), he is also Associate Editor of the British Journal of Pharmacology since 2012. His scientific interest focuses on TRAIL receptor signaling and its use in cancer therapy.

Chapter 1
Resistance to TRAIL Pathway-Targeted Therapeutics in Cancer

Jessica Wagner, Christina Leah Kline, and Wafik El-Deiry

Abstract As cancer therapies become more widely used, there is an increased rate of drug resistance in the population. Drug resistance has become one of the major causes of cancer treatment failure. There has been an increased use of combinational therapies in the clinic with the hopes of getting around therapeutic resistance to mono-agent chemotherapy. Unfortunately, combinational therapies present increased risks of toxicity. In developing new therapies, a key goal is to understand mechanisms of resistance and create agents that target or bypass resistance mechanisms. Tumor necrosis factor-related apoptosis-inducing ligand (TRAIL) is a potent and specific inducer of apoptosis in cancer cells. With little effect in normal cells, TRAIL-based therapies have become an attractive option for development. Unfortunately, a significant portion of tumor cells is relatively resistant to TRAIL, or becomes TRAIL-resistant after exposure to TRAIL-based therapies. Understanding and targeting these resistance mechanisms may help realize the therapeutic potential of the TRAIL pathway.

Keywords Tumor necrosis factor (TNF)-related apoptosis-inducing ligand (TRAIL) • Death receptors • Apoptosis • Resistance • Cancer therapy

1.1 Mechanisms of TRAIL-Induced Apoptosis

1.1.1 TRAIL Ligand and TRAIL Receptors

Cell death via apoptosis can be triggered by either intrinsic or extrinsic stimuli. The intrinsic pathway, commonly activated within the mitochondria, can be induced through stresses inside the cell, such as stress and oncogene activation. Alternatively, the extrinsic pathway is triggered by ligands binding to specific transmembrane

J. Wagner • C.L. Kline • W. El-Deiry (✉)
Laboratory of Translational Oncology and Experimental Cancer Therapeutics, Department of Hematology/Oncology and Molecular Therapeutics Program, Fox Chase Cancer Center, Philadelphia, PA, USA
e-mail: wafik.eldeiry@gmail.com

O. Micheau (ed.), *TRAIL, Fas Ligand, TNF and TLR3 in Cancer*, Resistance to Targeted Anti-Cancer Therapeutics, DOI 10.1007/978-3-319-56805-8_1

receptors, consequently activating caspases and cell death [1–3]. The tumor necrosis factor-related apoptosis-inducing ligand (TRAIL) is a member of the tumor necrosis factor (TNF) family of proteins that activate the extrinsic pathway. The protein TRAIL is 20 kDa and is encoded by five exons on chromosome 3 [4, 5]. TRAIL was first cloned based on the sequence homology of its extracellular domain with the CD95L ligand and TNFα. Its extracellular carboxyl terminal portion is proteolytically cleaved (such as by cathepsin E), to form its biologically active soluble form [6–8]. Unlike TNF-α, which elicits severe toxicity after systemic exposure, TRAIL typically and selectively induces apoptosis in cancer cells, leaving the normal cells viable [9–12].

The mechanism by which the TRAIL ligand induces apoptosis involves binding to its prospective receptors: death receptor 4 (DR4), death receptor 5 (DR5), decoy receptor 1 (DcR1/TRID), decoy receptor 2 (DcR2/TRUNDD), and osteoprotegerin [13, 14]. The two active receptors which induce apoptosis, DR4 and DR5, are type I transmembrane proteins with a sequence homology of 58% and a death domain capable of recruiting adaptor proteins to trigger cell death through caspase activation [14–16]. While TRAIL requires both DR4 and DR5 for optimal cellular apoptosis in certain cancer cells, several cancer types that contain similar amounts of both receptors being present on the cell surface appear to have one receptor acting as the primary receptor required for cell death [17–19]. Additionally, DR4 and DR5 antagonistic antibodies revealed that DR4 or DR5 is selectively more important in a cell type-specific manner [20].

DR4 and DR5 gene expression is regulated by transcription factors CHOP, AP-1, NF-kB, and FOXO3A. While all of these factors impact both death receptors, transcription factors selective for either death receptor do exist. For example, DR5 can be uniquely induced by ELK-1 while DR4 can be repressed by GLI-3 [21–26].

1.1.2 Engagement of the Extrinsic Pathway of Apoptosis

The binding of TRAIL to its receptors induces receptor trimerization and conformational change (Fig. 1.1). The latter event exposes the intracellular death domains of the receptor, thereby facilitating the formation of the death-inducing signalling complex (DISC). The DISC formed by TRAIL consists of the death receptors, the adaptor protein Fas-associated death domain protein (FADD) which interacts with the death domain of the receptors, and procaspase-8 or -10 which interacts with FADD via the death effector domains [15, 27–29]. The localization of procaspase-8 and procaspase-10 to the DISC promotes caspase dimerization, subsequent activation, and autocatalytic cleavage into both large (18 or 20 kDa, respectively) and small (10 kDa) fragments [27, 28, 30, 31]. The resulting large and small fragments interact to form an active protease, subsequently cleaving the effector caspases: caspases-3, 6, and 7, resulting in apoptosis [32].

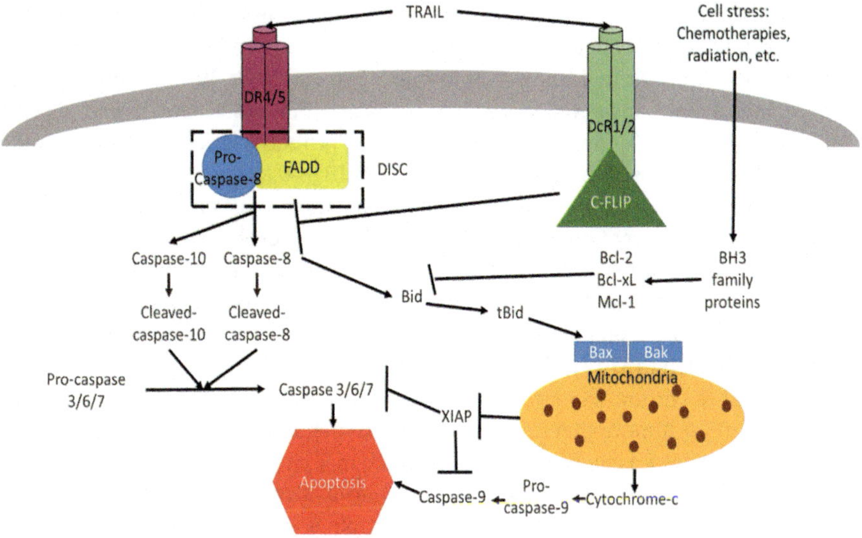

Fig. 1.1 Signalling pathways of TRAIL-induced apoptosis

1.1.3 Engagement of the Intrinsic Pathway of Apoptosis

The activation of cleaved caspase-8 by TRAIL can also activate and amplify the intrinsic apoptotic pathway through the mitochondria by cleaving the activator BH3-only protein Bid [3, 32]. The truncated Bid interacts and induces the oligomerization of Bax and Bak proteins at the mitochondrial membrane (Fig. 1.1), promoting the formation of the mitochondrial outer membrane pore and subsequent release of cytochrome c [33]. Cytochrome c binds to the apoptosis protease activating factor 1 (Apaf1) and results in a secondary activation of caspase-9 and effector caspases from the mitochondria [34, 35]. Activation of the intrinsic pathway through TRAIL also requires the inactivation of intracellular apoptosis inhibitors such as the X-linked inhibitor of apoptosis protein (XIAP), a protein that directly inhibits caspase activity [36].

Taken together, the TRAIL pathway is critical to inducing apoptosis via the extrinsic pathway but is capable of activating the intrinsic pathway via Bid cleavage and inactivation of apoptosis inhibitors such as XIAP.

1.2 TRAIL's Impact on Metastasis

The complex process of metastasis begins when a small portion of cells successfully detach and migrate from the primary tumor, invade into the surrounding stroma, intravasate into the circulation, and colonize on distant organ sites. For metastasis to ensue, cells must survive in an anchorage-independent manner [37, 38]. Typically, when normal cells detach, they undergo anoikis, a form of induced apoptosis that is primarily activated through the death receptor pathway [38, 39]. However, malignant cells that are considered metastatic in nature can resist anoikis and survive detachment in an anchorage-independent fashion, primarily through expressing the death receptor caspase-activation inhibitor c-FLIP [40, 41]. Since a majority of cancer-related deaths are associated to metastasis, there exists a need for therapies to address both primary tumor and metastatic disease preventions [42].

Studies have established that TRAIL suppresses metastasis in the liver of melanoma cancer patients. A death receptor knockout mouse model demonstrated that death receptors play a suppressive role in cancer metastasis while the primary tumor remains unaffected [43, 44]. Further, a significant loss of DR5 expression has been found in both the primary tumors that metastasize and their metastatic lesions compared to primary tumors that do not exhibit any metastatic progression [45]. One study identified DR5 as the key receptor in death receptor anti-metastatic signalling. DR5 agonist antibodies attenuated long-term survival of metastatic cancer in vivo, and were found to reduce the growth of lymph nodes and lung metastases in MDA-MB-231 xenograft models [46].

While DR5 and TRAIL's impact on metastases have been well documented, there remains contrasting evidence of a correlation between overexpression of DR5 and tumor aggressiveness. In this regard, TRAIL has been shown to strongly induce pro-inflammatory cytokines and enhanced invasion in pancreatic cancer cells and liver metastases [47, 48]. This strong contradiction has confounded researchers. One possible hypothesis that has been widely considered and is currently being researched is that in primary tumors that express DR5/FADD, there is increased apoptosis, preventing metastases. However, in primary tumors that overcome anoikis and metastasize, the primary tumor and metastatic tumor cells upregulate pro-metastatic signalling pathways including increasing DR5 levels [49]. Further research is ongoing to either support or refute this hypothesis.

1.3 Development of TRAIL Pathway-Targeted Therapeutics

The first publication that indicated the relevance of the TRAIL ligand to cancer research demonstrated that TRAIL selectively induces apoptosis in malignant cells while sparing normal cells. Further studies have been performed using recombinant TRAIL or agonistic human monoclonal antibodies against DR4 and DR5 [50]. These early reports indicated that a histidine-tagged or FLAG-tagged TRAIL induces apoptosis in some normal cells including hepatocytes and astrocytes [51, 52]. However, non-tagged and recombinant TRAIL did not exert any toxic effects in normal-cells in vitro or in vivo, indicating that under normal natural conditions TRAIL does not induce apoptosis in normal healthy cells [34, 53]. The role of TRAIL has since been well established to include different cell types and mechanisms of action. Acting as an immune effector molecule, TRAIL is expressed on the surface of activated immune cells including natural killer cells, CD4+ T cells, macrophages, and dendritic cells [54]. The ligand has been found to play a critical role in T-cell homeostasis and NK-mediated killing of oncogenically transformed cells [55, 56].

1.3.1 Optimization of TRAIL Delivery

Given the ability of TRAIL to target cancer cells and leave normal cells unharmed, efforts to optimize TRAIL administration have been made. The efficacy of the TRAIL ligand has been limited by suboptimal delivery and short protein half-life. To improve the pharmacokinetic profile of soluble TRAIL, an N-terminal PEGylated TRAIL has been developed and is currently being pursued in the clinic [22, 57]. Cell-based delivery of TRAIL, in particular, via mesenchymal stem cells (MSCs), has also been found to be promising. MSCs have been transduced to express a secreted form of recombinant TRAIL or TRAIL variants (that target only one of the death receptors). These provide an on-site sustained release of TRAIL, effectively inhibiting tumor growth [58, 59] and eradicating metastasis [167]. TRAIL has also been conjugated with nanoliposomes and E-selectin (ES). The ES/TRAIL liposomes bind to leukocytes under conditions of shear flow via selectin ligands on the leukocyte surface [60, 61]. The leukocytes serve as carriers of TRAIL and have been shown to kill circulating tumor cells in vivo [62] and in lymphoma and leukemia patients [63, 64]. All of these methods of TRAIL delivery are still being optimized but have shown extraordinary promise in delivering TRAIL into the body and tumor cells while overcoming the clinical barriers that soluble TRAIL exhibited.

1.3.2 TRAIL Receptor Antibodies

An alternative strategy to exploit the TRAIL pro-apoptotic pathway is the use of TRAIL receptor antibodies. These death receptor antibodies stimulate the TRAIL-apoptotic pathway independently of TRAIL induction and have been found efficacious either as monotherapies or in combination [65, 66]. There are ongoing Phase II trials that evaluate the combinational therapies of TRAIL receptor agonists with various FDA-approved therapies [67, 68]. Several of the DR5 antibody based therapies that are being tested in clinical trials have shown promise as therapeutic agents, and are discussed below. However, unlike DR5, DR4-targeted therapies have been lacking in recent years, with only one anti-DR4 product in clinical trials. Mapatumumab (HGS1012), a human agonistic monoclonal antibody that is specific to DR4, has been evaluated as a safe mono-agent and safe in combination with several chemotherapies including carboplatin, paclitaxel, and gemcitabine. Although the trials are still ongoing, mapatumumab has shown promising efficacy. However, in the TRAIL-resistant NSCLC, mapatumumab showed no clinical benefit in combination with paclitaxel or carboplatin [69–72]. Nevertheless, the development of potential DR4-based therapies such as mapatumumab does warrant further exploration since evidence that TRAIL induces apoptosis exclusively through DR4 in certain cancers including ovarian, melanoma, and chronic lymphocytic leukemia exists [73, 74]. Single agents that act as dual DR4/DR5 agonists have also become an area of interest for many researchers. Given the variability of DR4 and DR5 receptor levels in tissue types or mutations in individual receptors within specific tumor cells, these agonists are expected to have a broader spectrum of efficacy than receptor-specific agonists. The first major dual DR4/DR5 agonist demonstrated a greater potency and increased caspase-3 levels in cells and xenografts than a combination of DR4 and DR5 agonists [75].

1.3.3 Small Molecules to Induce TRAIL and Upregulate DR5

ONC201, a novel first-in-class anticancer therapy currently in development is known to upregulate endogenous TRAIL levels in both bulk tumor and stem cells through dual inactivation of the kinases Akt and ERK in a p53-independent manner. Due to the nature of endogenous upregulation, ONC201 successfully overcomes the limitations of TRAIL-based therapies discussed above. Importantly, ONC201 also upregulates DR5 levels as discussed below, causing both an increase in the ligand and receptor of the death receptor pathway [76–78].

Unfortunately, many cancer types are resistant to TRAIL-induced cytotoxicity and are, therefore, not susceptible to TRAIL-based therapies or DR4/5 monoclonal antibodies [19, 79]. The rest of this chapter discusses the mechanisms behind resistance to TRAIL pathway-targeted therapeutics, and the strategies that are being developed to obviate these resistance mechanisms.

1.4 Mechanisms of Resistance to TRAIL Pathway-Targeted Therapeutics

1.4.1 Aberration in Death Receptor Expression

Intrinsic TRAIL resistance has been associated with either dysfunctional DR4 and/or DR5 (DR4/DR5) at the cell surface or aberrant surface localization of the receptors [80, 81]. Inhibition of death receptor activation can occur as a result of mutations within the TRAIL receptors, loss of receptor expression through homozygous deletion or gene silencing, and death receptor sequestration [82, 83]. The genes for DR4 and DR5 reside on chromosome 8p. Loss of heterozygosity on chromosome 8p is common in cancer [84, 85]. The *DR4* gene promoter can also be hypermethylated, resulting in downregulation of expression [86–88]. Mutations in the *DR4* and *DR5* genes, particularly in the region coding for the death domain or in the ligand-binding region of DR4, have been detected in a number of cancers [82, 89–91]. A number of point mutations in the *DR5* gene result in a DR5 protein that does not have a functional death domain. The mutant protein exerts a dominant-negative effect, competing with functional DR4 for TRAIL ligand and, therefore, downregulating TRAIL-induced apoptosis [92].

TRAIL resistance may not be brought about by genetic defects in receptor expression but by aberrations in surface receptor protein expression. C-Met, a transmembrane tyrosine kinase sequesters DR5, consequently, preventing DISC formation. Knockdown of the c-Met protein sensitizes TRAIL-resistant brain tumor cells to the TRAIL-based therapies [93, 94]. Surface levels of the receptor can also be affected by receptor glycosylation. DR4 and DR5 can undergo N-linked or O-linked glycosylation in a cell-dependent manner. Receptor O-glycosylation, although found in several tumor cell lines, occurs at a higher rate in TRAIL-sensitive tumor cells. A recent study determined that mRNA expression of *GALNT14*, a gene that encodes for an initiating enzyme of O-glycosylation, is upregulated in TRAIL-sensitive pancreatic, non-small cell lung, and melanoma cell lines [10].

Alterations in the localization of death receptors can affect TRAIL sensitivity. DR5 can be localized in the nucleus rather than in the plasma membrane. Two functional nuclear localization signal (NLS) sequences have been identified in DR5. Importin β1 interacts with DR5 potentially at the NLS sites and shuttles DR5 after DR5 synthesis, from the ER to the nucleus. Consequently, DR5 surface expression and sensitivity to TRAIL is reduced. Knocking down importin β1 is sufficient to improve response to TRAIL in TRAIL-resistant cell lines [95]. DR4 and DR5 have also been found in autophagosomes. TRAIL-resistant cells have been observed to have higher basal autophagic rates. Inhibition of autophagy has been shown to be sufficient in increasing localization of DR4 to the membrane and subsequent formation of a functional DISC [96]. Surface levels of the receptor can also be downregulated by receptor endocytosis. Increased clathrin-dependent endocytosis pathways have been found in TRAIL-resistant tumor cells. DR4 contains a dileucine-based sorting signal (EAQC^{337}LL) that may be recognized by the clathrin-mediated endocytosis machinery [81, 97].

1.4.2 Strategies to Address Low Surface Levels of Death Receptors

Histone deacetylase inhibitors (HDAC) have been effectively used to induce TRAIL sensitivity by reversing the epigenetic silencing of expression of death receptors and procaspase-8 [98–100]. The use of HDAC inhibitors in combination is being pursued in the clinic and will be discussed further below. A related strategy is the use of DNA methyltransferase inhibitors like decitabine. This class of compounds has induced expression of DR4 and caspase-8 [86, 101]. The small molecule ONC201 also increases the level of death receptors through the integrated stress response (ISR) involving the transcription factor ATF4 and transactivator CHOP, and may aid tumors in overcoming their low death receptor level status [77]. Furthermore, the restoration of surface expression of DR4 and DR5 has been achieved by introducing endocytosis inhibitors which successfully restored cellular sensitivity to TRAIL [81].

1.4.3 Expression of TRAIL Decoy Receptors

In many TRAIL-resistant tumor cells, there is an upregulation of TRAIL decoy receptors. These decoy receptors TRAIL-R3 (DcR1), TRAIL-R4 (DcR2), and the soluble receptor OPG lack the functional death domain on DR4 and DR5. Therefore, they cannot signal for apoptosis when bound to the TRAIL ligand. Due to their similar selectivity to TRAIL as both DR4 and DR5, these decoy receptors are considered to be competitive inhibitors that regulate TRAIL-induced apoptosis in tumor cells [102–104]. Soluble OPG, however, has a lower binding affinity to TRAIL as other death receptors and is therefore not considered a competitive inhibitor of the TRAIL pathway [105].

The presence of the decoy receptors DcR1 and DcR2 correlates with TRAIL resistance in some cancer cells. However, these expression levels do not wholly explain the lack of response of many cancer cells to antibodies specifically targeting DR4 or DR5 [3]. For example, MCF7 breast cancer cells, which are relatively resistant to TRAIL, express both functional DR4 and DR5 on the cell surface and only minimally express decoy receptors [81, 106].

1.4.4 Dysfunction in the DISC and FADD

DISC formation is critical to TRAIL-induced apoptosis. Defects in the mobilization of procasepase-8 to the DISC and procaspase-8 activation have been associated with TRAIL resistance. A whole genome study found that 7% of patients (including patients with head and neck squamous cell carcinoma, hepatocellular carcinoma, and colorectal carcinoma) carry a mutation in their *caspase-8* gene. These mutations encode for mutant procaspase-8 that fails to undergo processing in response to TRAIL, and therefore serves as markers of resistance to death ligands [107–109].

Another mechanism of TRAIL resistance is mediated by the FLICE-inhibitory protein (c-FLIP). C-FLIP has a high degree of homology to caspase-8 and caspase-10, specifically containing two death effector domains. These domains enable c-FLIP to compete with procaspase-8 and procaspase-10 for binding to FADD. Because c-FLIP, however, lacks enzymatic activity due to a substitution of several amino acids in the catalytic domain, it cannot cleave effector caspases and induce apoptosis. Elevated expression of c-FLIP has been associated with TRAIL resistance in cancer cells [110–113]. Downregulating c-FLIP has been shown to sensitize colorectal cancer to both death receptor ligand-induced and chemotherapy-induced cell death [114, 115]. Furthermore, knockdown of c-FLIP in human lung carcinoma cells reversed resistance to agonistic antibodies against DR5 [116].

1.4.5 Perturbation in Downstream Pro-apoptotic Signals

Caspase signalling and activation can be negatively regulated through the anti-apoptotic Bcl-2 family proteins and inhibitor of apoptosis proteins (IAP) [117, 118]. The anti-apoptotic XIAP protein inhibits the activation of caspase-3 by inhibiting caspase-3 cleavage, effectively blocking apoptosis and increasing resistance to TRAIL. In TRAIL-resistant pancreatic cancer cell lines, XIAP is expressed at high levels. When XIAP is downregulated or its function inhibited within the cells by XIAP inhibitors and cells are then treated with TRAIL, the resulting synergy suppressed tumor growth in vitro and in vivo [119–121]. Silencing of XIAP and treatment with TRAIL-based therapies have been shown to block metastatic growth in mouse models [122]. Other IAP inhibitors have been under development.

1.4.6 Strategies to Address Aberrations in Downstream Pathways of Apoptosis

Given the key role of IAPs in TRAIL resistance, strategies to combine TRAIL with agents that downregulate IAPs have been developed. YM-155, a small molecule suppressant of the IAP survivin has been shown to reverse TRAIL resistance of TRAIL-resistant gliomas [123, 124]. Smac mimetics, small molecules that mimic the endogenous IAP inhibitor protein Smac, increase susceptibility to TRAIL not only through IAP inhibition but also through Bcl-2 cleavage (by caspase-3) [125, 126].

Alternatively, small molecules to downregulate the expression of anti-apoptotic Bcl-2 family members have been identified. Bay 61-3606, a small molecule sensitizer to TRAIL, reduces the levels of Mcl-1 not only by inhibiting *Mcl-1* gene transcription but also by promoting ubiquitin-dependent Mcl-1 degradation [117, 127]. In addition to small molecules targeting a specific Bcl-2 family member, compounds that can inhibit multiple Bcl-2 family proteins have also been effective TRAIL sensitizers [128]. Some Bcl2/Bcl-XL small molecule inhibitors have been approved for clinical use against certain forms of cancer.

The expression of IAPs and anti-apoptotic Bcl-2 family of proteins can be activated by NFκB [129]. The challenge is that TRAIL itself can induce NFκB. Thus, a viable strategy is to combine an NFκB inhibitor with TRAIL. In earlier years, compounds that may impede a number of pathways, including NFκB signalling, have been combined with TRAIL. More recently, however, targeted NFκB therapies have been developed. Given that NFκB is activated by the complex of IκB kinase (IKK) and NFκB essential modulator (NEMO), compounds that bind to IKK and NEMO have been used to downregulate NFκB signalling. The IKK inhibitor BMS-34541 has been successfully combined with TRAIL in TRAIL-resistant-neuroblastoma [130]. The mechanisms behind the efficacy of small molecule inhibitors of NFκB are cell type-specific. In neuroblastoma cells, BMS-34541 promotes susceptibility to TRAIL by downregulating the levels of the anti-apoptotic Bcl-2 protein Mcl-1 (an NFκB transcriptional target). NEMO-binding peptides have been used in combination with TRAIL in pancreatic and colorectal cancer cells [24, 130–132].

1.4.7 Resistance of Normal Cells

The mechanisms behind the resistance of normal cells to TRAIL are similar to the mechanisms of resistance that have been observed in TRAIL-resistant tumors. Caspase-8 expression has been found to be significantly diminished in fibroblasts. Furthermore, the requisite ubiquitination of caspase-8 for TRAIL-induced apoptosis is lacking in normal cells, in primary keratinocytes, natural killer and CD8(+) T cells [133–135]. Normal cells possess multiple resistance mechanisms, rather than just having one [136–138]. For instance, human fibroblasts overexpress c-FLIP and XIAP, thereby inhibiting TRAIL-induced apoptosis at the level of the DISC and the downstream pathways of apoptosis [136]. Increased TRAIL decoy receptor expression is a classical feature of some normal cells.

1.5 Complex Nature of TRAIL Resistance

1.5.1 Multiple Resistance Mechanisms

While all of the mechanisms listed above play a role in TRAIL resistance, none of the factors have been shown to be consistently correlated across multiple cancer types [10]. In fact, many cancer cells employ multiple resistance mechanisms to escape TRAIL signalling. In HL60 human leukemia cells, TRAIL resistance was associated with decreased cell surface expression of DR4 and loss of the pro-caspase 8 protein due to the novel mutation Leu22Phe [19].

1.5.2 Acquisition of Resistance

In the highly TRAIL-sensitive breast cancer cell line MDA-MB-231, acquired resistance due to long-term exposure to subtoxic doses of TRAIL has been attributed to diminished cell surface expression of DR4 and DR5 along with sustained activation of c-Flip [139]. Acquisition of TRAIL resistance has been also been observed in colon, leukemia, ovarian, and melanoma cancer cell lines exposed to high levels of TRAIL [19, 80, 140, 141].

1.6 Addressing Resistance to TRAIL Pathway-Targeted Therapeutics in the Clinic

1.6.1 Single Agent

Monoclonal DR5/TRAIL receptor agonist antibodies such as AMG 655, dulanermin, lexatumumab, and apomab have been evaluated in clinical trials [70, 142–145]. Although favorable responses have been observed in certain cancer types such as lung adenocarcinoma and follicular lymphoma, response in a large patient population has been rare [71]. Nevertheless, some patients respond well. There has been very limited toxicity with a few patients exhibiting transaminitis, a side effect that was easily reversible [143]. Therefore, the potential of DR5 agonists can be maximized by identifying those patients who would successfully respond to these treatments. Because of the safety of DR5 agonists as single agents, their efficacy can be boosted by combining them with other therapies.

The small molecule ONC201 underwent a successful Phase I clinical trial and demonstrated an acceptable safety profile, pharmacokinetic and pharmacodynamic profile, and compelling initial efficacy. Given its low toxicity and demonstrated efficacy in in vivo studies in multiple solid and hematological malignancies, ONC201 has entered into several clinical trials. Trials in advanced solid tumors (Rutgers Cancer Institute), Leukemia and lymphoma (MD Anderson Cancer Center), glioblastoma (Massachusetts General Hospital/Dana-Farber Cancer Institute), and a clinical trial evaluating administration schedules in solid tumors and multiple myeloma (Fox Chase Cancer Center) have opened to patient enrollment.

1.6.2 Combinational

One rationale for combining TRAIL pathway-targeted therapies with chemotherapeutic agents is to sensitize TRAIL-resistant cancers. Pancreatic cancer cells, although intrinsically resistant to TRAIL, can be inhibited by combining tigatuzumab (a human agonistic monoclonal DR5 antibody) and gemcitabine, a first-line agent for pancreatic ductal adenocarcinomas [146, 147]. Furthermore, since pancreatic stem cells express DR5 and gemcitabine is effective in reducing the primary tumor size but not efficacious against stem cells, the combinational therapy demonstrated superb antitumor results [148, 149]. Clinicians later found in early phase II trials that this combination is very effective in treating TRAIL-resistant metastatic pancreatic cells [150].

Chemotherapeutic agents and radiotherapies have been shown to heighten TRAIL sensitivity. Thus, combining these chemotherapeutics or radiotherapies can be more efficacious than administering TRAIL alone [151]. Therapies that induce the tumor suppressor p53 have been shown to cause an upregulation of DR4 and DR5 expression [152, 153]. Therefore, these therapies are being investigated in combination with TRAIL-based therapies [154–156].

FDA-approved proteasome inhibitor bortezomib promotes apoptosis by preventing ubiquitin-mediated degradation of pro-apoptotic proteins. Bortezomib treatment has been shown to upregulate p53 and DR5 expression levels. Moreover, it also downregulates c-FLIP expression [157, 158]. Bortezomib enhances TRAIL efficacy through recruitment of caspase 8 and FADD into the DISC [159]. The combination of TRAIL and bortezomib has shown promise as a therapeutic for TRAIL-resistant breast, colon, and kidney tumors in vivo [159, 160]. Sorafenib, a protein tyrosine kinase inhibitor, is also able to sensitize tumor cells to TRAIL-mediated apoptosis in vitro by shifting cells from an anti-apoptotic state to a pro-apoptotic state. This occurs through several mechanisms including proteolytic degradation of c-FLIP and decrease in expression of Mcl-1 [117, 161]. However, despite promising results of synergy existing between sorafenib and the DR4 agonist mapatumumab, a phase II study demonstrated no increased efficacy in hepatocellular carcinomas when in combination, differing from the in vitro studies previously performed. One possible reason for the difference in results could be variability of DR4 expression in hepatocellular carcinomas [162, 163].

As discussed previously, certain histone deacetylases (HDACs) inhibitors have been shown to enhance the apoptotic effects of TRAIL in TRAIL-sensitive sells, and sensitize TRAIL-resistant breast cancer cell lines in vitro. HDAC inhibitors epigenetically alter gene expression through increased histone acetylation, thereby increasing gene transcription and upregulating DR5 expression in tumor cells [98]. Furthermore, HDAC inhibitors enhance the apoptosis-inducing potential of TRAIL in multiple cell lines and synergize with TRAIL, through engaging the mitochondrial pathway of apoptosis in the MDA-MB-468 xenograft model [99]. By activating the mitochondrial pathway of apoptosis, HDAC inhibitors increase caspase activation and decrease expression of the anti-apoptotic molecules such as Bcl-2 [91, 164]. The benefits of HDAC blockade in enhancing the therapeutic potential of TRAIL makes HDAC inhibitor-TRAIL combinations a promising avenue for clinical studies.

Overall, combinational therapies aim to increase TRAIL susceptibility or decrease TRAIL resistance. However, although successful in vitro or in vivo, these combinational or monotherapies have yet to successfully pass clinical trials. Nevertheless, clinical research on novel monotherapies or combinational therapies is still ongoing. Also, based on the results of mapatumumab and sorafenib in hepatocellular carcinomas, clinicians and researchers should be aware of mechanisms that can affect response, such as death receptor expression levels in individual tumors. Therefore, it is prudent to develop: (a) biomarker studies of patient tumors to determine a patient's susceptibility to death receptor agonists, (b) therapies that increase TRAIL susceptibility, and (c) therapies that can help overcome inherent

Table 1.1 TRAIL-based therapies and soluble TRAIL delivery strategies in development

Molecule/therapeutic	Target	Comments
His-TRAIL (rhTRAIL variant)	DR4/DR5/Dc receptors	High toxicity [51]
Flag-TRAIL	DR4/DR5/Dc receptors	High toxicity [165]
Non-tagged rhTRAIL	DR4/DR5/Dc receptors	High toxicity [50]
TRA-8 (agonist)	DR5	Nontoxic in Phase I [66]
AMG-655 (agonist)	DR5	Nontoxic and antitumor efficacy in Phase I [145]
Lexatumuab (agonist)	DR5	Phase I/II showed safe as monotherapy and in combination [166]
Apomab (agonist)	DR5	Currently in Phase II [29]
Mapatumumab	DR4	Phase I showed nontoxic, phase Ib showed promise in combination [71, 72]
ONC201	DR5/TRAIL	Has shown efficacy in bulk tumors and stem cells in vivo. Phase showed non-toxic and promising PK and efficacy. Currently in several Phase I/II for several bulk tumor tissue types and hematological malignancies [76–78]
Stem-cell based TRAIL delivery	TRAIL	Has shown some efficacy in in vivo studies [59, 167]
PEG-TRAIL	TRAIL	Increased half-life, successful efficacy in vivo [57]
TRAIL-loaded nanoliposomes or leukocytes	TRAIL	Sustained TRAIL release, tumor killing, and CTC apoptosis [62]
TRAIL nanoparticle delivery	TRAIL	Increased antitumor activity and demonstrated tumor killing [168]

TRAIL resistance. Preclinical data have demonstrated that adjusting cells' susceptibility/resistance to TRAIL could be beneficial to inhibiting tumor growth and metastases (Tables 1.1 and 1.2).

1.7 Conclusion

The ability of TRAIL to induce apoptosis selectively in tumors and to inhibit metastases compels us to continue to seek to understand and address the mechanisms behind TRAIL resistance. The use of TRAIL as a monotherapy has faced complications, and there is a large drive in the field to overcome the shortcomings of soluble TRAIL in the clinic or utilizing DR4/5 agonists. Researchers have found that by manipulating the endogenous properties or regulation of the DISC/FADD complex, caspase-8, IAPs, c-FLIP, and Bcl-2 family proteins, sensitivity to TRAIL can be increased. Although combining TRAIL with agents that can obviate TRAIL

Table 1.2 Combination of TRAIL-based therapies and FDA-approved therapies in the clinic

Molecule/therapeutic	Target	Mechanism
Tunicamycin	ER stress	Increases DR5 via the unfolded protein response [169]
Oligomycin	ER stress	Disrupts the extrinsic apoptotic pathway [170]
Bortezomib	Proteasome pathway	Decreases FLIP, activation of both the extrinsic and intrinsic apoptotic pathway [171, 172]
MG132	Proteasome pathway	
HDAC inhibitor (MS-275, SAHA)	Autophagy	Activation of downstream caspase-3 which activates both apoptotic pathways [98, 173]
HDAC inhibitor LGP1	Epigenetic modulation	Activate the DR5 gene through p53-independent mechanism
5-FU	DNA damaging agents	Downregulate c-FLIP, increase TRAIL receptors [174]
Cisplatin	DNA damaging agents	
Sorafenib	Kinase inhibitor	Decrease Mcl-1 [175, 176]
Flavopiridol	Kinase inhibitor	Increase TRAIL receptor, decrease c-FLIP and Bcl-xL [177]

resistance has been efficacious in vitro and in vivo, success in the clinic remains yet to be seen. Biomarker development and genetic sequencing can potentially be leveraged to identify patient responders to TRAIL monotherapy, patient-specific resistance mechanisms, and concomitant TRAIL pathway therapeutic combinations.

References

1. Hall MA, Cleveland JL (2007) Clearing the TRAIL for cancer therapy. Cancer Cell 12(1):4–6
2. Ashkenazi A (2008) Targeting the extrinsic apoptosis pathway in cancer. Cytokine Growth Factor Rev 19(3–4):325–331. doi:10.1016/j.cytogfr.2008.04.001
3. Takeda K, Stagg J, Yagita H, Okumura K, Smyth MJ (2007) Targeting death-inducing receptors in cancer therapy. Oncogene 26(25):3745–3757. doi:10.1038/sj.onc.1210374
4. Snell V, Clodi K, Zhao S, Goodwin R, Thomas EK, Morris SW, Kadin ME, Cabanillas F, Andreeff M, Younes A (1997) Activity of TNF-related apoptosis-inducing ligand (TRAIL) in haematological malignancies. Br J Haematol 99(3):618–624
5. Jeremias I, Herr I, Boehler T, Debatin KM (1998) TRAIL/Apo-2-ligand-induced apoptosis in human T cells. Eur J Immunol 28(1):143–152. doi:10.1002/(SICI)1521-4141(199801)28:01<143::AID-IMMU143>3.0.CO;2-3
6. Mariani SM, Krammer PH (1998) Surface expression of TRAIL/Apo-2 ligand in activated mouse T and B cells. Eur J Immunol 28(5):1492–1498. doi:10.1002/(SICI)1521-4141(199805)28:05<1492::AID-IMMU1492>3.0.CO;2-X
7. Monleón I, Martínez-Lorenzo MJ, Monteagudo L, Lasierra P, Taulés M, Iturralde M, Piñeiro A, Larrad L, Alava MA, Naval J, Anel A (2001) Differential secretion of Fas ligand- or APO2 ligand/TNF-related apoptosis-inducing ligand-carrying microvesicles during activation-induced death of human T cells. J Immunol 167(12):6736–6744

8. Kawakubo T, Okamoto K, Iwata J, Shin M, Okamoto Y, Yasukochi A, Nakayama KI, Kadowaki T, Tsukuba T, Yamamoto K (2007) Cathepsin E prevents tumor growth and metastasis by catalyzing the proteolytic release of soluble TRAIL from tumor cell surface. Cancer Res 67(22):10869–10878. doi:10.1158/0008-5472.CAN-07-2048
9. Castro Alves C, Terziyska N, Grunert M, Gündisch S, Graubner U, Quintanilla-Martinez L, Jeremias I (2012) Leukemia-initiating cells of patient-derived acute lymphoblastic leukemia xenografts are sensitive toward TRAIL. Blood 119(18):4224–4227. doi:10.1182/blood-2011-08-370114
10. Wagner KW, Punnoose EA, Januario T, Lawrence DA, Pitti RM, Lancaster K, Lee D, von Goetz M, Yee SF, Totpal K, Huw L, Katta V, Cavet G, Hymowitz SG, Amler L, Ashkenazi A (2007) Death-receptor O-glycosylation controls tumor-cell sensitivity to the proapoptotic ligand Apo2L/TRAIL. Nat Med 13(9):1070–1077. doi:10.1038/nm1627. nm1627 [pii]
11. Lawrence D, Shahrokh Z, Marsters S, Achilles K, Shih D, Mounho B, Hillan K, Totpal K, DeForge L, Schow P, Hooley J, Sherwood S, Pai R, Leung S, Khan L, Gliniak B, Bussiere J, Smith CA, Strom SS, Kelley S, Fox JA, Thomas D, Ashkenazi A (2001) Differential hepatocyte toxicity of recombinant Apo2L/TRAIL versions. Nat Med 7(4):383–385
12. Oikonomou E, Kothonidis K, Taoufik E, Probert E, Zografos G, Nasioulas G, Andera L, Pintzas A (2007) Newly established tumourigenic primary human colon cancer cell lines are sensitive to TRAIL-induced apoptosis in vitro and in vivo. Br J Cancer 97(1):73–84. doi:10.1038/sj.bjc.6603835
13. Wu GS, Burns TF, McDonald ER, Jiang W, Meng R, Krantz ID, Kao G, Gan DD, Zhou JY, Muschel R, Hamilton SR, Spinner NB, Markowitz S, Wu G, el-Deiry WS (1997) KILLER/DR5 is a DNA damage-inducible p53-regulated death receptor gene. Nat Genet 17(2):141–143. doi:10.1038/ng1097-141
14. Carlo-Stella C, Lavazza C, Locatelli A, Viganò L, Gianni AM, Gianni L (2007) Targeting TRAIL agonistic receptors for cancer therapy. Clin Cancer Res 13(8):2313–2317. doi:10.1158/1078-0432.CCR-06-2774
15. Falschlehner C, Emmerich CH, Gerlach B, Walczak H (2007) TRAIL signalling: decisions between life and death. Int J Biochem Cell Biol 39(7–8):1462–1475
16. Corazza N, Kassahn D, Jakob S, Badmann A, Brunner T (2009) TRAIL-induced apoptosis: between tumor therapy and immunopathology. Ann N Y Acad Sci 1171:50–58. doi:10.1111/j.1749-6632.2009.04905.x
17. Schneider P, Thome M, Burns K, Bodmer JL, Hofmann K, Kataoka T, Holler N, Tschopp J (1997) TRAIL receptors 1 (DR4) and 2 (DR5) signal FADD-dependent apoptosis and activate NF-kappaB. Immunity 7(6):831–836
18. Kelley RF, Totpal K, Lindstrom SH, Mathieu M, Billeci K, Deforge L, Pai R, Hymowitz SG, Ashkenazi A (2005) Receptor-selective mutants of apoptosis-inducing ligand 2/tumor necrosis factor-related apoptosis-inducing ligand reveal a greater contribution of death receptor (DR) 5 than DR4 to apoptosis signaling. J Biol Chem 280(3):2205–2212. doi:10.1074/jbc.M410660200
19. Cheng J, Hylander BL, Baer MR, Chen X, Repasky EA (2006) Multiple mechanisms underlie resistance of leukemia cells to Apo2 Ligand/TRAIL. Mol Cancer Ther 5(7):1844–1853
20. van Geelen CM, Pennarun B, Le PT, de Vries EG, de Jong S (2011) Modulation of TRAIL resistance in colon carcinoma cells: different contributions of DR4 and DR5. BMC Cancer 11:39. doi:10.1186/1471-2407-11-39
21. Yoshida T, Maeda A, Tani N, Sakai T (2001) Promoter structure and transcription initiation sites of the human death receptor 5/TRAIL-R2 gene. FEBS Lett 507(3):381–385
22. Oh Y, Park O, Swierczewska M, Hamilton JP, Park JS, Kim TH, Lim SM, Eom H, Jo DG, Lee CE, Kechrid R, Mastorakos P, Zhang C, Hahn SK, Jeon OC, Byun Y, Kim K, Hanes J, Lee KC, Pomper MG, Gao B, Lee S (2015) Systemic PEGylated TRAIL treatment ameliorates liver cirrhosis in rats by eliminating activated hepatic stellate cells. Hepatology 64(1):209–223. doi:10.1002/hep.28432

23. Guan B, Yue P, Lotan R, Sun SY (2002) Evidence that the human death receptor 4 is regulated by activator protein 1. Oncogene 21(20):3121–3129. doi:10.1038/sj.onc.1205430
24. Ravi R, Bedi GC, Engstrom LW, Zeng Q, Mookerjee B, Gélinas C, Fuchs EJ, Bedi A (2001) Regulation of death receptor expression and TRAIL/Apo2L-induced apoptosis by NF-kappaB. Nat Cell Biol 3(4):409–416. doi:10.1038/35070096
25. Shoeb M, Ramana KV, Srivastava SK (2013) Aldose reductase inhibition enhances TRAIL-induced human colon cancer cell apoptosis through AKT/FOXO3a-dependent upregulation of death receptors. Free Radic Biol Med 63:280–290. doi:10.1016/j.freeradbiomed.2013.05.039
26. Kurita S, Mott JL, Almada LL, Bronk SF, Werneburg NW, Sun SY, Roberts LR, Fernandez-Zapico ME, Gores GJ (2010) GLI3-dependent repression of DR4 mediates hedgehog antagonism of TRAIL-induced apoptosis. Oncogene 29(34):4848–4858. doi:10.1038/onc.2010.235
27. Muzio M, Stockwell BR, Stennicke HR, Salvesen GS, Dixit VM (1998) An induced proximity model for caspase-8 activation. J Biol Chem 273(5):2926–2930
28. Sprick MR, Rieser E, Stahl H, Grosse-Wilde A, Weigand MA, Walczak H (2002) Caspase-10 is recruited to and activated at the native TRAIL and CD95 death-inducing signalling complexes in a FADD-dependent manner but can not functionally substitute caspase-8. EMBO J 21(17):4520–4530
29. Ashkenazi A, Dixit VM (1998) Death receptors: signaling and modulation. Science 281(5381):1305–1308
30. Scott FL, Stec B, Pop C, Dobaczewska MK, Lee JJ, Monosov E, Robinson H, Salvesen GS, Schwarzenbacher R, Riedl SJ (2009) The Fas-FADD death domain complex structure unravels signalling by receptor clustering. Nature 457(7232):1019–1022. doi:10.1038/nature07606. nature07606 [pii]
31. Wachmann K, Pop C, van Raam BJ, Drag M, Mace PD, Snipas SJ, Zmasek C, Schwarzenbacher R, Salvesen GS, Riedl SJ (2010) Activation and specificity of human caspase-10. Biochemistry 49(38):8307–8315. doi:10.1021/bi100968m
32. Li H, Zhu H, Xu CJ, Yuan J (1998) Cleavage of BID by caspase 8 mediates the mitochondrial damage in the Fas pathway of apoptosis. Cell 94(4):491–501
33. Luo X, Budihardjo I, Zou H, Slaughter C, Wang X (1998) Bid, a Bcl2 interacting protein, mediates cytochrome c release from mitochondria in response to activation of cell surface death receptors. Cell 94(4):481–490
34. Walczak H, Miller RE, Ariail K, Gliniak B, Griffith TS, Kubin M, Chin W, Jones J, Woodward A, Le T, Smith C, Smolak P, Goodwin RG, Rauch CT, Schuh JC, Lynch DH (1999) Tumoricidal activity of tumor necrosis factor-related apoptosis-inducing ligand in vivo. Nat Med 5(2):157–163
35. Zhang L, Zhang X, Barrisford GW, Olumi AF (2007) Lexatumumab (TRAIL-receptor 2 mAb) induces expression of DR5 and promotes apoptosis in primary and metastatic renal cell carcinoma in a mouse orthotopic model. Cancer Lett 251(1):146–157
36. Holoch PA, Griffith TS (2009) TNF-related apoptosis-inducing ligand (TRAIL): a new path to anti-cancer therapies. Eur J Pharmacol 625(1–3):63–72. doi:10.1016/j.ejphar.2009.06.066
37. Nguyen DX, Bos PD, Massagué J (2009) Metastasis: from dissemination to organ-specific colonization. Nat Rev Cancer 9(4):274–284. doi:10.1038/nrc2622
38. Eccles SA, Welch DR (2007) Metastasis: recent discoveries and novel treatment strategies. Lancet 369(9574):1742–1757. doi:10.1016/S0140-6736(07)60781-8
39. Simpson CD, Anyiwe K, Schimmer AD (2008) Anoikis resistance and tumor metastasis. Cancer Lett 272(2):177–185. doi:10.1016/j.canlet.2008.05.029
40. Zhou XD, Yu JP, Liu J, Luo HS, Chen HX, Yu HG (2004) Overexpression of cellular FLICE-inhibitory protein (FLIP) in gastric adenocarcinoma. Clin Sci 106(4):397–405
41. Jönsson G, Paulie S, Grandien A (2003) High level of cFLIP correlates with resistance to death receptor-induced apoptosis in bladder carcinoma cells. Anticancer Res 23(2B):1213–1218
42. Weigelt B, Peterse JL, van't Veer LJ (2005) Breast cancer metastasis: markers and models. Nat Rev Cancer 5(8):591–602. doi:10.1038/nrc1670

43. Grosse-Wilde A, Voloshanenko O, Bailey SL, Longton GM, Schaefer U, Csernok AI, Schütz G, Greiner EF, Kemp CJ, Walczak H (2008) TRAIL-R deficiency in mice enhances lymph node metastasis without affecting primary tumor development. J Clin Invest 118(1):100–110. doi:10.1172/JCI33061
44. Laguinge LM, Samara RN, Wang W, El-Deiry WS, Corner G, Augenlicht L, Mishra L, Jessup JM (2008) DR5 receptor mediates anoikis in human colorectal carcinoma cell lines. Cancer Res 68(3):909–917. doi:10.1158/0008-5472.CAN-06-1806
45. Elrod HA, Fan S, Muller S, Chen GZ, Pan L, Tighiouart M, Shin DM, Khuri FR, Sun SY (2010) Analysis of death receptor 5 and caspase-8 expression in primary and metastatic head and neck squamous cell carcinoma and their prognostic impact. PLoS One 5(8):e12178. doi:10.1371/journal.pone.0012178
46. Malin D, Chen F, Schiller C, Koblinski J, Cryns VL (2011) Enhanced metastasis suppression by targeting TRAIL receptor 2 in a murine model of triple-negative breast cancer. Clin Cancer Res 17(15):5005–5015. doi:10.1158/1078-0432.CCR-11-0099
47. Trauzold A, Siegmund D, Schniewind B, Sipos B, Egberts J, Zorenkov D, Emme D, Röder C, Kalthoff H, Wajant H (2006) TRAIL promotes metastasis of human pancreatic ductal adenocarcinoma. Oncogene 25(56):7434–7439. doi:10.1038/sj.onc.1209719
48. Hoogwater FJ, Nijkamp MW, Smakman N, Steller EJ, Emmink BL, Westendorp BF, Raats DA, Sprick MR, Schaefer U, Van Houdt WJ, De Bruijn MT, Schackmann RC, Derksen PW, Medema JP, Walczak H, Borel Rinkes IH, Kranenburg O (2010) Oncogenic K-Ras turns death receptors into metastasis-promoting receptors in human and mouse colorectal cancer cells. Gastroenterology 138(7):2357–2367. doi:10.1053/j.gastro.2010.02.046
49. Sun SY (2011) Understanding the role of the death receptor 5/FADD/caspase-8 death signaling in cancer metastasis. Mol Cell Pharmacol 3(1):31–34
50. Ashkenazi A, Pai RC, Fong S, Leung S, Lawrence DA, Marsters SA, Blackie C, Chang L, McMurtrey AE, Hebert A, DeForge L, Koumenis IL, Lewis D, Harris L, Bussiere J, Koeppen H, Shahrokh Z, Schwall RH (1999) Safety and antitumor activity of recombinant soluble Apo2 ligand. J Clin Invest 104(2):155–162
51. Jo M, Kim TH, Seol DW, Esplen JE, Dorko K, Billiar TR, Strom SC (2000) Apoptosis induced in normal human hepatocytes by tumor necrosis factor-related apoptosis-inducing ligand. Nat Med 6(5):564–567
52. Nitsch R, Bechmann I, Deisz RA, Haas D, Lehmann TN, Wendling U, Zipp F (2000) Human brain-cell death induced by tumour-necrosis-factor-related apoptosis-inducing ligand (TRAIL). Lancet 356(9232):827–828. doi:10.1016/S0140-6736(00)02659-3
53. Srivastava RK (2001) TRAIL/Apo-2L: mechanisms and clinical applications in cancer. Neoplasia 3(6):535–546. doi:10.1038/sj/neo/7900203
54. Kayagaki N, Yamaguchi N, Nakayama M, Kawasaki A, Akiba H, Okumura K, Yagita H (1999) Involvement of TNF-related apoptosis-inducing ligand in human CD4+ T cell-mediated cytotoxicity. J Immunol 162(5):2639–2647
55. Hayakawa Y, Screpanti V, Yagita H, Grandien A, Ljunggren HG, Smyth MJ, Chambers BJ (2004) NK cell TRAIL eliminates immature dendritic cells in vivo and limits dendritic cell vaccination efficacy. J Immunol 172(1):123–129
56. Janssen EM, Droin NM, Lemmens EE, Pinkoski MJ, Bensinger SJ, Ehst BD, Griffith TS, Green DR, Schoenberger SP (2005) CD4+ T-cell help controls CD8+ T-cell memory via TRAIL-mediated activation-induced cell death. Nature 434(7029):88–93
57. Kim TH, Youn YS, Jiang HH, Lee S, Chen X, Lee KC (2011) PEGylated TNF-related apoptosis-inducing ligand (TRAIL) analogues: pharmacokinetics and antitumor effects. Bioconjug Chem 22(8):1631–1637. doi:10.1021/bc200187k
58. Kim SM, Lim JY, Park SI, Jeong CH, Oh JH, Jeong M, Oh W, Park SH, Sung YC, Jeun SS (2008) Gene therapy using TRAIL-secreting human umbilical cord blood-derived mesenchymal stem cells against intracranial glioma. Cancer Res 68(23):9614–9623. doi:10.1158/0008-5472.CAN-08-0451

59. Sasportas LS, Kasmieh R, Wakimoto H, Hingtgen S, van de Water JA, Mohapatra G, Figueiredo JL, Martuza RL, Weissleder R, Shah K (2009) Assessment of therapeutic efficacy and fate of engineered human mesenchymal stem cells for cancer therapy. Proc Natl Acad Sci U S A 106(12):4822–4827. doi:10.1073/pnas.0806647106
60. Läubli H, Borsig L (2010) Selectins promote tumor metastasis. Semin Cancer Biol 20(3):169–177. doi:10.1016/j.semcancer.2010.04.005
61. Seifert O, Pollak N, Nusser A, Steiniger F, Rüger R, Pfizenmaier K, Kontermann RE (2014) Immuno-LipoTRAIL: targeted delivery of TRAIL-functionalized liposomal nanoparticles. Bioconjug Chem 25(5):879–887. doi:10.1021/bc400517j
62. Mitchell MJ, Wayne E, Rana K, Schaffer CB, King MR (2014) TRAIL-coated leukocytes that kill cancer cells in the circulation. Proc Natl Acad Sci U S A 111(3):930–935. doi:10.1073/pnas.1316312111
63. De Miguel D, Gallego-Lleyda A, Anel A, Martinez-Lostao L (2015) Liposome-bound TRAIL induces superior DR5 clustering and enhanced DISC recruitment in histiocytic lymphoma U937 cells. Leuk Res 39(6):657–666. doi:10.1016/j.leukres.2015.03.019
64. De Miguel D, Gallego-Lleyda A, Galan-Malo P, Rodriguez-Vigil C, Marzo I, Anel A, Martinez-Lostao L (2015) Immunotherapy with liposome-bound TRAIL overcomes partial protection to soluble TRAIL-induced apoptosis offered by down-regulation of Bim in leukemic cells. Clin Transl Oncol 17(8):657–667. doi:10.1007/s12094-015-1295-x
65. Buchsbaum DJ, Zhou T, Grizzle WE, Oliver PG, Hammond CJ, Zhang S, Carpenter M, LoBuglio AF (2003) Antitumor efficacy of TRA-8 anti-DR5 monoclonal antibody alone or in combination with chemotherapy and/or radiation therapy in a human breast cancer model. Clin Cancer Res 9(10 Pt 1):3731–3741
66. Ichikawa K, Liu W, Zhao L, Wang Z, Liu D, Ohtsuka T, Zhang H, Mountz JD, Koopman WJ, Kimberly RP, Zhou T (2001) Tumoricidal activity of a novel anti-human DR5 monoclonal antibody without hepatocyte cytotoxicity. Nat Med 7(8):954–960
67. Soria JC, Márk Z, Zatloukal P, Szima B, Albert I, Juhász E, Pujol JL, Kozielski J, Baker N, Smethurst D, Hei YJ, Ashkenazi A, Stern H, Amler L, Pan Y, Blackhall F (2011) Randomized phase II study of dulanermin in combination with paclitaxel, carboplatin, and bevacizumab in advanced non-small-cell lung cancer. J Clin Oncol 29(33):4442–4451. doi:10.1200/JCO.2011.37.2623
68. Thorburn A, Behbakht K, Ford H (2008) TRAIL receptor-targeted therapeutics: resistance mechanisms and strategies to avoid them. Drug Resist Updat 11(1–2):17–24. doi:10.1016/j.drup.2008.02.001
69. von Pawel J, Harvey JH, Spigel DR, Dediu M, Reck M, Cebotaru CL, Humphreys RC, Gribbin MJ, Fox NL, Camidge DR (2014) Phase II trial of mapatumumab, a fully human agonist monoclonal antibody to tumor necrosis factor-related apoptosis-inducing ligand receptor 1 (TRAIL-R1), in combination with paclitaxel and carboplatin in patients with advanced non-small-cell lung cancer. Clin Lung Cancer 15(3):188–196 e182. doi:10.1016/j.cllc.2013.12.005
70. Tolcher AW, Mita M, Meropol NJ, von Mehren M, Patnaik A, Padavic K, Hill M, Mays T, McCoy T, Fox NL, Halpern W, Corey A, Cohen RB (2007) Phase I pharmacokinetic and biologic correlative study of mapatumumab, a fully human monoclonal antibody with agonist activity to tumor necrosis factor-related apoptosis-inducing ligand receptor-1. J Clin Oncol 25(11):1390–1395
71. Hotte SJ, Hirte HW, Chen EX, Siu LL, Le LH, Corey A, Iacobucci A, MacLean M, Lo L, Fox NL, Oza AM (2008) A phase 1 study of mapatumumab (fully human monoclonal antibody to TRAIL-R1) in patients with advanced solid malignancies. Clin Cancer Res 14(11):3450–3455. doi:10.1158/1078-0432.CCR-07-1416. 14/11/3450 [pii]
72. Trarbach T, Moehler M, Heinemann V, Köhne CH, Przyborek M, Schulz C, Sneller V, Gallant G, Kanzler S (2010) Phase II trial of mapatumumab, a fully human agonistic monoclonal antibody that targets and activates the tumour necrosis factor apoptosis-inducing ligand receptor-1

(TRAIL-R1), in patients with refractory colorectal cancer. Br J Cancer 102(3):506–512. doi:10.1038/sj.bjc.6605507
73. Horak P, Pils D, Haller G, Pribill I, Roessler M, Tomek S, Horvat R, Zeillinger R, Zielinski C, Krainer M (2005) Contribution of epigenetic silencing of tumor necrosis factor-related apoptosis inducing ligand receptor 1 (DR4) to TRAIL resistance and ovarian cancer. Mol Cancer Res 3(6):335–343
74. MacFarlane M, Kohlhaas SL, Sutcliffe MJ, Dyer MJ, Cohen GM (2005) TRAIL receptor-selective mutants signal to apoptosis via TRAIL-R1 in primary lymphoid malignancies. Cancer Res 65(24):11265–11270. doi:10.1158/0008-5472.CAN-05-2801
75. Milutinovic S, Kashyap AK, Yanagi T, Wimer C, Zhou S, O'Neil R, Kurtzman AL, Faynboym A, Xu L, Hannum CH, Diaz PW, Matsuzawa S, Horowitz M, Horowitz L, Bhatt RR, Reed JC (2016) Dual agonist surrobody simultaneously activates death receptors DR4 and DR5 to induce cancer cell death. Mol Cancer Ther 15(1):114–124. doi:10.1158/1535-7163.MCT-15-0400
76. Allen JE, Krigsfeld G, Mayes PA, Patel L, Dicker DT, Patel AS, Dolloff NG, Messaris E, Scata KA, Wang W, Zhou JY, Wu GS, El-Deiry WS (2013) Dual inactivation of Akt and ERK by TIC10 signals Foxo3a nuclear translocation, TRAIL gene induction, and potent antitumor effects. Sci Transl Med 5(171):171ra117. doi:10.1126/scitranslmed.3004828
77. Kline CL, Van den Heuvel AP, Allen JE, Prabhu VV, Dicker DT, El-Deiry WS (2016) ONC201 kills solid tumor cells by triggering an integrated stress response dependent on ATF4 activation by specific eIF2α kinases. Sci Signal 9(415):ra18. doi:10.1126/scisignal.aac4374
78. Prabhu VV, Allen JE, Dicker DT, El-Deiry WS (2015) Small-molecule ONC201/TIC10 targets chemotherapy-resistant colorectal cancer stem-like cells in an Akt/Foxo3a/TRAIL-dependent manner. Cancer Res 75(7):1423–1432. doi:10.1158/0008-5472.CAN-13-3451
79. Di Pietro R, Zauli G (2004) Emerging non-apoptotic functions of tumor necrosis factor-related apoptosis-inducing ligand (TRAIL)/Apo2L. J Cell Physiol 201(3):331–340. doi:10.1002/jcp.20099
80. Jin Z, McDonald ER, Dicker DT, El-Deiry WS (2004) Deficient tumor necrosis factor-related apoptosis-inducing ligand (TRAIL) death receptor transport to the cell surface in human colon cancer cells selected for resistance to TRAIL-induced apoptosis. J Biol Chem 279(34):35829–35839. doi:10.1074/jbc.M405538200
81. Zhang Y, Zhang B (2008) TRAIL resistance of breast cancer cells is associated with constitutive endocytosis of death receptors 4 and 5. Mol Cancer Res 6(12):1861–1871. doi:10.1158/1541-7786.MCR-08-0313
82. Lee SH, Shin MS, Kim HS, Lee HK, Park WS, Kim SY, Lee JH, Han SY, Park JY, Oh RR, Kang CS, Kim KM, Jang JJ, Nam SW, Lee JY, Yoo NJ (2001) Somatic mutations of TRAIL-receptor 1 and TRAIL-receptor 2 genes in non-Hodgkin's lymphoma. Oncogene 20(3):399–403
83. Ozören N, Fisher MJ, Kim K, Liu CX, Genin A, Shifman Y, Dicker DT, Spinner NB, Lisitsyn NA, El-Deiry WS (2000) Homozygous deletion of the death receptor DR4 gene in a nasopharyngeal cancer cell line is associated with TRAIL resistance. Int J Oncol 16(5):917–925
84. Emi M, Fujiwara Y, Nakajima T, Tsuchiya E, Tsuda H, Hirohashi S, Maeda Y, Tsuruta K, Miyaki M, Nakamura Y (1992) Frequent loss of heterozygosity for loci on chromosome 8p in hepatocellular carcinoma, colorectal cancer, and lung cancer. Cancer Res 52(19):5368–5372
85. Wistuba II, Behrens C, Virmani AK, Milchgrub S, Syed S, Lam S, Mackay B, Minna JD, Gazdar AF (1999) Allelic losses at chromosome 8p21-23 are early and frequent events in the pathogenesis of lung cancer. Cancer Res 59(8):1973–1979
86. Hopkins-Donaldson S, Ziegler A, Kurtz S, Bigosch C, Kandioler D, Ludwig C, Zangemeister-Wittke U, Stahel R (2003) Silencing of death receptor and caspase-8 expression in small cell lung carcinoma cell lines and tumors by DNA methylation. Cell Death Differ 10(3):356–364
87. Horak P, Pils D, Kaider A, Pinter A, Elandt K, Sax C, Zielinski CC, Horvat R, Zeillinger R, Reinthaller A, Krainer M (2005) Perturbation of the tumor necrosis factor--related apoptosis-inducing ligand cascade in ovarian cancer: overexpression of FLIPL and deregulation of the

functional receptors DR4 and DR5. Clin Cancer Res 11(24 Pt 1):8585–8591. doi:10.1158/1078-0432.CCR-05-1276
88. Elias A, Siegelin MD, Steinmüller A, von Deimling A, Lass U, Korn B, Mueller W (2009) Epigenetic silencing of death receptor 4 mediates tumor necrosis factor-related apoptosis-inducing ligand resistance in gliomas. Clin Cancer Res 15(17):5457–5465. doi:10.1158/1078-0432.CCR-09-1125
89. Dechant C, Schauenberg P, Antoni CE, Kraetsch HG, Kalden JR, Manger B (2004) [Longterm outcome of TNF blockade in adult-onset Still's disease]. Dtsch Med Wochenschr 129(23):1308–1312. doi:10.1055/s-2004-826865
90. Fulda S (2009) Caspase-8 in cancer biology and therapy. Cancer Lett 281(2):128–133. doi:10.1016/j.canlet.2008.11.023
91. Fulda S (2008) Modulation of TRAIL-induced apoptosis by HDAC inhibitors. Curr Cancer Drug Targets 8(2):132–140
92. Bin L, Thorburn J, Thomas LR, Clark PE, Humphreys R, Thorburn A (2007) Tumor-derived mutations in the TRAIL receptor DR5 inhibit TRAIL signaling through the DR4 receptor by competing for ligand binding. J Biol Chem 282(38):28189–28194. doi:10.1074/jbc.M704210200. M704210200 [pii]
93. Du W, Uslar L, Sevala S, Shah K (2014) Targeting c-met receptor overcomes TRAIL-resistance in brain tumors. PLoS One 9(4):e95490. doi:10.1371/journal.pone.0095490
94. Abounader R, Reznik T, Colantuoni C, Martinez-Murillo F, Rosen EM, Laterra J (2004) Regulation of c-Met-dependent gene expression by PTEN. Oncogene 23(57):9173–9182. doi:10.1038/sj.onc.1208146
95. Kojima Y, Nakayama M, Nishina T, Nakano H, Koyanagi M, Takeda K, Okumura K, Yagita H (2011) Importin β≤1 protein-mediated nuclear localization of death receptor 5 (DR5) limits DR5/tumor necrosis factor (TNF)-related apoptosis-inducing ligand (TRAIL)-induced cell death of human tumor cells. J Biol Chem 286(50):43383–43393. doi:10.1074/jbc.M111.309377
96. Di X, Zhang G, Zhang Y, Takeda K, Rivera Rosado LA, Zhang B (2013) Accumulation of autophagosomes in breast cancer cells induces TRAIL resistance through downregulation of surface expression of death receptors 4 and 5. Oncotarget 4(9):1349–1364. doi:10.18632/oncotarget.1174
97. Austin CD, Lawrence DA, Peden AA, Varfolomeev EE, Totpal K, De Mazière AM, Klumperman J, Arnott D, Pham V, Scheller RH, Ashkenazi A (2006) Death-receptor activation halts clathrin-dependent endocytosis. Proc Natl Acad Sci U S A 103(27):10283–10288. doi:10.1073/pnas.0604044103
98. Singh TR, Shankar S, Srivastava RK (2005) HDAC inhibitors enhance the apoptosis-inducing potential of TRAIL in breast carcinoma. Oncogene 24(29):4609–4623. doi:10.1038/sj.onc.1208585
99. Srivastava RK, Kurzrock R, Shankar S (2010) MS-275 sensitizes TRAIL-resistant breast cancer cells, inhibits angiogenesis and metastasis, and reverses epithelial-mesenchymal transition in vivo. Mol Cancer Ther 9(12):3254–3266. doi:10.1158/1535-7163.MCT-10-0582
100. Venza I, Visalli M, Oteri R, Teti D, Venza M (2014) Class I-specific histone deacetylase inhibitor MS-275 overrides TRAIL-resistance in melanoma cells by downregulating c-FLIP. Int Immunopharmacol 21(2):439–446. doi:10.1016/j.intimp.2014.05.024
101. Eramo A, Pallini R, Lotti F, Sette G, Patti M, Bartucci M, Ricci-Vitiani L, Signore M, Stassi G, Larocca LM, Crinò L, Peschle C, De Maria R (2005) Inhibition of DNA methylation sensitizes glioblastoma for tumor necrosis factor-related apoptosis-inducing ligand-mediated destruction. Cancer Res 65(24):11469–11477. doi:10.1158/0008-5472.CAN-05-1724
102. Degli-Esposti MA, Dougall WC, Smolak PJ, Waugh JY, Smith CA, Goodwin RG (1997) The novel receptor TRAIL-R4 induces NF-kappaB and protects against TRAIL-mediated apoptosis, yet retains an incomplete death domain. Immunity 7(6):813–820
103. Held J, Schulze-Osthoff K (2001) Potential and caveats of TRAIL in cancer therapy. Drug Resist Updat 4(4):243–252. doi:10.1054/drup.2001.0208

104. Pan G, Ni J, Wei YF, Yu G, Gentz R, Dixit VM (1997) An antagonist decoy receptor and a death domain-containing receptor for TRAIL. Science 277(5327):815–818
105. Emery JG, McDonnell P, Burke MB, Deen KC, Lyn S, Silverman C, Dul E, Appelbaum ER, Eichman C, DiPrinzio R, Dodds RA, James IE, Rosenberg M, Lee JC, Young PR (1998) Osteoprotegerin is a receptor for the cytotoxic ligand TRAIL. J Biol Chem 273(23):14363–14367
106. Kurokawa H, Nishio K, Fukumoto H, Tomonari A, Suzuki T, Saijo N (1999) Alteration of caspase-3 (CPP32/Yama/apopain) in wild-type MCF-7, breast cancer cells. Oncol Rep 6(1):33–37
107. Li C, Egloff AM, Sen M, Grandis JR, Johnson DE (2014) Caspase-8 mutations in head and neck cancer confer resistance to death receptor-mediated apoptosis and enhance migration, invasion, and tumor growth. Mol Oncol 8(7):1220–1230. doi:10.1016/j.molonc.2014.03.018
108. Agrawal N, Frederick MJ, Pickering CR, Bettegowda C, Chang K, Li RJ, Fakhry C, Xie TX, Zhang J, Wang J, Zhang N, El-Naggar AK, Jasser SA, Weinstein JN, Treviño L, Drummond JA, Muzny DM, Wu Y, Wood LD, Hruban RH, Westra WH, Koch WM, Califano JA, Gibbs RA, Sidransky D, Vogelstein B, Velculescu VE, Papadopoulos N, Wheeler DA, Kinzler KW, Myers JN (2011) Exome sequencing of head and neck squamous cell carcinoma reveals inactivating mutations in NOTCH1. Science 333(6046):1154–1157. doi:10.1126/science.1206923
109. Kim HS, Lee JW, Soung YH, Park WS, Kim SY, Lee JH, Park JY, Cho YG, Kim CJ, Jeong SW, Nam SW, Kim SH, Lee JY, Yoo NJ, Lee SH (2003) Inactivating mutations of caspase-8 gene in colorectal carcinomas. Gastroenterology 125(3):708–715
110. Tschopp J, Irmler M, Thome M (1998) Inhibition of fas death signals by FLIPs. Curr Opin Immunol 10(5):552–558
111. Krueger A, Schmitz I, Baumann S, Krammer PH, Kirchhoff S (2001) Cellular FLICE-inhibitory protein splice variants inhibit different steps of caspase-8 activation at the CD95 death-inducing signaling complex. J Biol Chem 276(23):20633–20640
112. Bagnoli M, Canevari S, Mezzanzanica D (2010) Cellular FLICE-inhibitory protein (c-FLIP) signalling: a key regulator of receptor-mediated apoptosis in physiologic context and in cancer. Int J Biochem Cell Biol 42(2):210–213. doi:10.1016/j.biocel.2009.11.015. S1357-2725(09)00345-8 [pii]
113. Irmler M, Thome M, Hahne M, Schneider P, Hofmann K, Steiner V, Bodmer JL, Schröter M, Burns K, Mattmann C, Rimoldi D, French LE, Tschopp J (1997) Inhibition of death receptor signals by cellular FLIP. Nature 388(6638):190–195. doi:10.1038/40657
114. McCourt C, Maxwell P, Mazzucchelli R, Montironi R, Scarpelli M, Salto-Tellez M, O'Sullivan JM, Longley DB, Waugh DJ (2012) Elevation of c-FLIP in castrate-resistant prostate cancer antagonizes therapeutic response to androgen receptor-targeted therapy. Clin Cancer Res 18(14):3822–3833. doi:10.1158/1078-0432.CCR-11-3277
115. Wilson TR, McLaughlin KM, McEwan M, Sakai H, Rogers KM, Redmond KM, Johnston PG, Longley DB (2007) c-FLIP: a key regulator of colorectal cancer cell death. Cancer Res 67(12):5754–5762. doi:10.1158/0008-5472.CAN-06-3585. 67/12/5754 [pii]
116. Chen F, Guo J, Zhang Y, Zhao Y, Zhou N, Liu S, Liu Y, Zheng D (2009) Knockdown of c-FLIP(L) enhanced AD5-10 anti-death receptor 5 monoclonal antibody-induced apoptosis in human lung cancer cells. Cancer Sci 100(5):940–947. doi:10.1111/j.1349-7006.2009.01119.x
117. Kim SH, Ricci MS, El-Deiry WS (2008) Mcl-1: a gateway to TRAIL sensitization. Cancer Res 68(7):2062–2064. doi:10.1158/0008-5472.CAN-07-6278
118. Deveraux QL, Roy N, Stennicke HR, Van Arsdale T, Zhou Q, Srinivasula SM, Alnemri ES, Salvesen GS, Reed JC (1998) IAPs block apoptotic events induced by caspase-8 and cytochrome c by direct inhibition of distinct caspases. EMBO J 17(8):2215–2223. doi:10.1093/emboj/17.8.2215
119. Giagkousiklidis S, Vellanki SH, Debatin KM, Fulda S (2007) Sensitization of pancreatic carcinoma cells for gamma-irradiation-induced apoptosis by XIAP inhibition. Oncogene 26(49):7006–7016. doi:10.1038/sj.onc.1210502

120. Vogler M, Dürr K, Jovanovic M, Debatin KM, Fulda S (2007) Regulation of TRAIL-induced apoptosis by XIAP in pancreatic carcinoma cells. Oncogene 26(2):248–257. doi:10.1038/sj.onc.1209776
121. Vogler M, Walczak H, Stadel D, Haas TL, Genze F, Jovanovic M, Gschwend JE, Simmet T, Debatin KM, Fulda S (2008) Targeting XIAP bypasses Bcl-2-mediated resistance to TRAIL and cooperates with TRAIL to suppress pancreatic cancer growth in vitro and in vivo. Cancer Res 68(19):7956–7965. doi:10.1158/0008-5472.CAN-08-1296
122. Mohr A, Albarenque SM, Deedigan L, Yu R, Reidy M, Fulda S, Zwacka RM (2010) Targeting of XIAP combined with systemic mesenchymal stem cell-mediated delivery of sTRAIL ligand inhibits metastatic growth of pancreatic carcinoma cells. Stem Cells 28(11):2109–2120. doi:10.1002/stem.533
123. Nakahara T, Kita A, Yamanaka K, Mori M, Amino N, Takeuchi M, Tominaga F, Hatakeyama S, Kinoyama I, Matsuhisa A, Kudoh M, Sasamata M (2007) YM155, a novel small-molecule survivin suppressant, induces regression of established human hormone-refractory prostate tumor xenografts. Cancer Res 67(17):8014–8021. doi:10.1158/0008-5472.CAN-07-1343
124. Premkumar DR, Jane EP, Foster KA, Pollack IF (2013) Survivin inhibitor YM-155 sensitizes tumor necrosis factor- related apoptosis-inducing ligand-resistant glioma cells to apoptosis through Mcl-1 downregulation and by engaging the mitochondrial death pathway. J Pharmacol Exp Ther 346(2):201–210. doi:10.1124/jpet.113.204743
125. Allensworth JL, Sauer SJ, Lyerly HK, Morse MA, Devi GR (2013) Smac mimetic Birinapant induces apoptosis and enhances TRAIL potency in inflammatory breast cancer cells in an IAP-dependent and TNF-α-independent mechanism. Breast Cancer Res Treat 137(2):359–371. doi:10.1007/s10549-012-2352-6
126. Fakler M, Loeder S, Vogler M, Schneider K, Jeremias I, Debatin KM, Fulda S (2009) Small molecule XIAP inhibitors cooperate with TRAIL to induce apoptosis in childhood acute leukemia cells and overcome Bcl-2-mediated resistance. Blood 113(8):1710–1722. doi:10.1182/blood-2007-09-114314
127. Kim SY, Park SE, Shim SM, Park S, Kim KK, Jeong SY, Choi EK, Hwang JJ, Jin DH, Chung CD, Kim I (2015) Bay 61-3606 sensitizes TRAIL-induced apoptosis by downregulating Mcl-1 in breast cancer cells. PLoS One 10(12):e0146073. doi:10.1371/journal.pone.0146073
128. Hetschko H, Voss V, Horn S, Seifert V, Prehn JH, Kogel D (2008) Pharmacological inhibition of Bcl-2 family members reactivates TRAIL-induced apoptosis in malignant glioma. J Neuro-Oncol 86(3):265–272. doi:10.1007/s11060-007-9472-6
129. Kucharczak J, Simmons MJ, Fan Y, Gélinas C (2003) To be, or not to be: NF-kappaB is the answer--role of Rel/NF-kappaB in the regulation of apoptosis. Oncogene 22(56):8961–8982. doi:10.1038/sj.onc.1207230
130. Ammann JU, Haag C, Kasperczyk H, Debatin KM, Fulda S (2009) Sensitization of neuroblastoma cells for TRAIL-induced apoptosis by NF-kappaB inhibition. Int J Cancer 124(6):1301–1311. doi:10.1002/ijc.24068
131. Thomas RP, Farrow BJ, Kim S, May MJ, Hellmich MR, Evers BM (2002) Selective targeting of the nuclear factor-kappaB pathway enhances tumor necrosis factor-related apoptosis-inducing ligand-mediated pancreatic cancer cell death. Surgery 132(2):127–134
132. Ravi R, Bedi A (2002) Requirement of BAX for TRAIL/Apo2L-induced apoptosis of colorectal cancers: synergism with sulindac-mediated inhibition of Bcl-x(L). Cancer Res 62(6):1583–1587
133. Crowder RN, Dicker DT, El-Deiry WS (2016) The deubiquitinase inhibitor PR-619 sensitizes normal human fibroblasts to tumor necrosis factor-related apoptosis-inducing ligand (TRAIL)-mediated cell death. J Biol Chem 291(11):5960–5970. doi:10.1074/jbc.M115.713545
134. Leverkus M, Neumann M, Mengling T, Rauch CT, Bröcker EB, Krammer PH, Walczak H (2000) Regulation of tumor necrosis factor-related apoptosis-inducing ligand sensitivity in primary and transformed human keratinocytes. Cancer Res 60(3):553–559

135. Mirandola P, Ponti C, Gobbi G, Sponzilli I, Vaccarezza M, Cocco L, Zauli G, Secchiero P, Manzoli FA, Vitale M (2004) Activated human NK and CD8+ T cells express both TNF-related apoptosis-inducing ligand (TRAIL) and TRAIL receptors but are resistant to TRAIL-mediated cytotoxicity. Blood 104(8):2418–2424
136. van Dijk M, Halpin-McCormick A, Sessler T, Samali A, Szegezdi E (2013) Resistance to TRAIL in non-transformed cells is due to multiple redundant pathways. Cell Death Dis 4:e702. doi:10.1038/cddis.2013.214
137. Song JJ, An JY, Kwon YT, Lee YJ (2007) Evidence for two modes of development of acquired tumor necrosis factor-related apoptosis-inducing ligand resistance. Involvement of Bcl-xL. J Biol Chem 282(1):319–328. doi:10.1074/jbc.M608065200
138. Song JH, Bellail A, Tse MC, Yong VW, Hao C (2006) Human astrocytes are resistant to Fas ligand and tumor necrosis factor-related apoptosis-inducing ligand-induced apoptosis. J Neurosci 26(12):3299–3308
139. Yoshida T, Zhang Y, Rivera Rosado LA, Zhang B (2009) Repeated treatment with subtoxic doses of TRAIL induces resistance to apoptosis through its death receptors in MDA-MB-231 breast cancer cells. Mol Cancer Res 7(11):1835–1844. doi:10.1158/1541-7786.MCR-09-0244
140. Lane D, Côté M, Grondin R, Couture MC, Piché A (2006) Acquired resistance to TRAIL-induced apoptosis in human ovarian cancer cells is conferred by increased turnover of mature caspase-3. Mol Cancer Ther 5(3):509–521. doi:10.1158/1535-7163.MCT-05-0362
141. Zhang XD, Wu JJ, Gillespie S, Borrow J, Hersey P (2006) Human melanoma cells selected for resistance to apoptosis by prolonged exposure to tumor necrosis factor-related apoptosis-inducing ligand are more vulnerable to necrotic cell death induced by cisplatin. Clin Cancer Res 12(4):1355–1364. doi:10.1158/1078-0432.CCR-05-2084
142. Herbst RS, Eckhardt SG, Kurzrock R, Ebbinghaus S, O'Dwyer PJ, Gordon MS, Novotny W, Goldwasser MA, Tohnya TM, Lum BL, Ashkenazi A, Jubb AM, Mendelson DS (2010) Phase I dose-escalation study of recombinant human Apo2L/TRAIL, a dual proapoptotic receptor agonist, in patients with advanced cancer. J Clin Oncol 28(17):2839–2846. doi:10.1200/JCO.2009.25.1991. JCO.2009.25.1991 [pii]
143. Camidge DR (2008) Apomab: an agonist monoclonal antibody directed against death receptor 5/TRAIL-receptor 2 for use in the treatment of solid tumors. Expert Opin Biol Ther 8(8):1167–1176. doi:10.1517/14712598.8.8.1167
144. Wakelee HA, Patnaik A, Sikic BI, Mita M, Fox NL, Miceli R, Ullrich SJ, Fisher GA, Tolcher AW (2010) Phase I and pharmacokinetic study of lexatumumab (HGS-ETR2) given every 2 weeks in patients with advanced solid tumors. Ann Oncol 21 (2):376–381. doi:10.1093/annonc/mdp292. mdp292 [pii]
145. Kindler HL, Richards DA, Garbo LE, Garon EB, Stephenson JJ, Rocha-Lima CM, Safran H, Chan D, Kocs DM, Galimi F, McGreivy J, Bray SL, Hei Y, Feigal EG, Loh E, Fuchs CS (2012) A randomized, placebo-controlled phase 2 study of ganitumab (AMG 479) or conatumumab (AMG 655) in combination with gemcitabine in patients with metastatic pancreatic cancer. Ann Oncol 23(11):2834–2842. doi:10.1093/annonc/mds142
146. Burris HA, Moore MJ, Andersen J, Green MR, Rothenberg ML, Modiano MR, Cripps MC, Portenoy RK, Storniolo AM, Tarassoff P, Nelson R, Dorr FA, Stephens CD, Von Hoff DD (1997) Improvements in survival and clinical benefit with gemcitabine as first-line therapy for patients with advanced pancreas cancer: a randomized trial. J Clin Oncol 15(6):2403–2413
147. Ozawa F, Friess H, Kleeff J, Xu ZW, Zimmermann A, Sheikh MS, Büchler MW (2001) Effects and expression of TRAIL and its apoptosis-promoting receptors in human pancreatic cancer. Cancer Lett 163(1):71–81
148. Rajeshkumar NV, Rasheed ZA, García-García E, López-Ríos F, Fujiwara K, Matsui WH, Hidalgo M (2010) A combination of DR5 agonistic monoclonal antibody with gemcitabine targets pancreatic cancer stem cells and results in long-term disease control in human pancreatic cancer model. Mol Cancer Ther 9(9):2582–2592. doi:10.1158/1535-7163.MCT-10-0370

149. Kaplan-Lefko PJ, Graves JD, Zoog SJ, Pan Y, Wall J, Branstetter DG, Moriguchi J, Coxon A, Huard JN, Xu R, Peach ML, Juan G, Kaufman S, Chen Q, Bianchi A, Kordich JJ, Ma M, Foltz IN, Gliniak BC (2010) Conatumumab, a fully human agonist antibody to death receptor 5, induces apoptosis via caspase activation in multiple tumor types. Cancer Biol Ther 9(8):618–631
150. Forero-Torres A, Infante JR, Waterhouse D, Wong L, Vickers S, Arrowsmith E, He AR, Hart L, Trent D, Wade J, Jin X, Wang Q, Austin T, Rosen M, Beckman R, von Roemeling R, Greenberg J, Saleh M (2013) Phase 2, multicenter, open-label study of tigatuzumab (CS-1008), a humanized monoclonal antibody targeting death receptor 5, in combination with gemcitabine in chemotherapy-naive patients with unresectable or metastatic pancreatic cancer. Cancer Med 2(6):925–932. doi:10.1002/cam4.137
151. Gliniak B, Le T (1999) Tumor necrosis factor-related apoptosis-inducing ligand's antitumor activity in vivo is enhanced by the chemotherapeutic agent CPT-11. Cancer Res 59(24):6153–6158
152. Liu Y, Meyer C, Xu C, Weng H, Hellerbrand C, ten Dijke P, Dooley S (2013) Animal models of chronic liver diseases. Am J Physiol Gastrointest Liver Physiol 304(5):G449–G468. doi:10.1152/ajpgi.00199.2012
153. Takimoto R, El-Deiry WS (2000) Wild-type p53 transactivates the KILLER/DR5 gene through an intronic sequence-specific DNA-binding site. Oncogene 19(14):1735–1743. doi:10.1038/sj.onc.1203489
154. Keane MM, Ettenberg SA, Nau MM, Russell EK, Lipkowitz S (1999) Chemotherapy augments TRAIL-induced apoptosis in breast cell lines. Cancer Res 59(3):734–741
155. Nimmanapalli R, Perkins CL, Orlando M, O'Bryan E, Nguyen D, Bhalla KN (2001) Pretreatment with paclitaxel enhances apo-2 ligand/tumor necrosis factor-related apoptosis-inducing ligand-induced apoptosis of prostate cancer cells by inducing death receptors 4 and 5 protein levels. Cancer Res 61(2):759–763
156. Mizutani Y, Yoshida O, Miki T, Bonavida B (1999) Synergistic cytotoxicity and apoptosis by Apo-2 ligand and adriamycin against bladder cancer cells. Clin Cancer Res 5(9):2605–2612
157. Bonvini P, Zorzi E, Basso G, Rosolen A (2007) Bortezomib-mediated 26S proteasome inhibition causes cell-cycle arrest and induces apoptosis in CD-30+ anaplastic large cell lymphoma. Leukemia 21(4):838–842. doi:10.1038/sj.leu.2404528
158. Sayers TJ, Brooks AD, Koh CY, Ma W, Seki N, Raziuddin A, Blazar BR, Zhang X, Elliott PJ, Murphy WJ (2003) The proteasome inhibitor PS-341 sensitizes neoplastic cells to TRAIL-mediated apoptosis by reducing levels of c-FLIP. Blood 102(1):303–310
159. Seki N, Toh U, Sayers TJ, Fujii T, Miyagi M, Akagi Y, Kusukawa J, Kage M, Shirouzu K, Yamana H (2010) Bortezomib sensitizes human esophageal squamous cell carcinoma cells to TRAIL-mediated apoptosis via activation of both extrinsic and intrinsic apoptosis pathways. Mol Cancer Ther 9(6):1842–1851. doi:10.1158/1535-7163.MCT-09-0918
160. Brooks AD, Ramirez T, Toh U, Onksen J, Elliott PJ, Murphy WJ, Sayers TJ (2005) The proteasome inhibitor bortezomib (Velcade) sensitizes some human tumor cells to Apo2L/TRAIL-mediated apoptosis. Ann N Y Acad Sci 1059:160–167. doi:10.1196/annals.1339.042
161. Llobet D, Eritja N, Yeramian A, Pallares J, Sorolla A, Domingo M, Santacana M, Gonzalez-Tallada FJ, Matias-Guiu X, Dolcet X (2010) The multikinase inhibitor Sorafenib induces apoptosis and sensitises endometrial cancer cells to TRAIL by different mechanisms. Eur J Cancer 46(4):836–850. doi:10.1016/j.ejca.2009.12.025
162. Kriegl L, Jung A, Engel J, Jackstadt R, Gerbes AL, Gallmeier E, Reiche JA, Hermeking H, Rizzani A, Bruns CJ, Kolligs FT, Kirchner T, Göke B, De Toni EN (2010) Expression, cellular distribution, and prognostic relevance of TRAIL receptors in hepatocellular carcinoma. Clin Cancer Res 16(22):5529–5538. doi:10.1158/1078-0432.CCR-09-3403
163. Ciuleanu T, Bazin I, Lungulescu D, Miron L, Bondarenko I, Deptala A, Rodriguez-Torres M, Giantonio B, Fox NL, Wissel P, Egger J, Ding M, Kalyani RN, Humphreys R, Gribbin M, Sun W (2016) A randomized, double-blind, placebo-controlled phase II study to assess the

efficacy and safety of mapatumumab with sorafenib in patients with advanced hepatocellular carcinoma. Ann Oncol 27(4):680–687. doi:10.1093/annonc/mdw004
164. Fulda S, Debatin KM (2005) Resveratrol-mediated sensitisation to TRAIL-induced apoptosis depends on death receptor and mitochondrial signalling. Eur J Cancer 41(5):786–798. doi:10.1016/j.ejca.2004.12.020
165. Schneider P, Holler N, Bodmer JL, Hahne M, Frei K, Fontana A, Tschopp J (1998) Conversion of membrane-bound Fas(CD95) ligand to its soluble form is associated with downregulation of its proapoptotic activity and loss of liver toxicity. J Exp Med 187(8):1205–1213
166. Plummer R, Attard G, Pacey S, Li L, Razak A, Perrett R, Barrett M, Judson I, Kaye S, Fox NL, Halpern W, Corey A, Calvert H, de Bono J (2007) Phase 1 and pharmacokinetic study of lexatumumab in patients with advanced cancers. Clin Cancer Res 13(20):6187–6194. doi:10.1158/1078-0432.CCR-07-0950. 13/20/6187 [pii]
167. Loebinger MR, Eddaoudi A, Davies D, Janes SM (2009) Mesenchymal stem cell delivery of TRAIL can eliminate metastatic cancer. Cancer Res 69(10):4134–4142. doi:10.1158/0008-5472.CAN-08-4698
168. Perlstein B, Finniss SA, Miller C, Okhrimenko H, Kazimirsky G, Cazacu S, Lee HK, Lemke N, Brodie S, Umansky F, Rempel SA, Rosenblum M, Mikklesen T, Margel S, Brodie C (2013) TRAIL conjugated to nanoparticles exhibits increased anti-tumor activities in glioma cells and glioma stem cells in vitro and in vivo. Neuro-Oncology 15(1):29–40. doi:10.1093/neuonc/nos248
169. Jiang CC, Chen LH, Gillespie S, Kiejda KA, Mhaidat N, Wang YF, Thorne R, Zhang XD, Hersey P (2007) Tunicamycin sensitizes human melanoma cells to tumor necrosis factor-related apoptosis-inducing ligand-induced apoptosis by up-regulation of TRAIL-R2 via the unfolded protein response. Cancer Res 67(12):5880–5888. doi:10.1158/0008-5472.CAN-07-0213
170. He L, Jang JH, Choi HG, Lee SM, Nan MH, Jeong SJ, Dong Z, Kwon YT, Lee KS, Lee KW, Chung JK, Ahn JS, Kim BY (2013) Oligomycin a enhances apoptotic effect of TRAIL through CHOP-mediated death receptor 5 expression. Mol Carcinog 52(2):85–93. doi:10.1002/mc.21831
171. Jane EP, Premkumar DR, Pollack IF (2011) Bortezomib sensitizes malignant human glioma cells to TRAIL, mediated by inhibition of the NF-{kappa}B signaling pathway. Mol Cancer Ther 10(1):198–208. doi:10.1158/1535-7163.MCT-10-0725
172. Li X, Huang T, Jiang G, Gong W, Qian H, Zou C (2013) Proteasome inhibitor MG132 enhances TRAIL-induced apoptosis and inhibits invasion of human osteosarcoma OS732 cells. Biochem Biophys Res Commun 439(2):179–186. doi:10.1016/j.bbrc.2013.08.066
173. Nakata S, Yoshida T, Horinaka M, Shiraishi T, Wakada M, Sakai T (2004) Histone deacetylase inhibitors upregulate death receptor 5/TRAIL-R2 and sensitize apoptosis induced by TRAIL/APO2-L in human malignant tumor cells. Oncogene 23(37):6261–6271
174. Newsom-Davis T, Prieske S, Walczak H (2009) Is TRAIL the holy grail of cancer therapy? Apoptosis 14(4):607–623. doi:10.1007/s10495-009-0321-2
175. Abdulghani J, Allen JE, Dicker DT, Liu YY, Goldenberg D, Smith CD, Humphreys R, El-Deiry WS (2013) Sorafenib sensitizes solid tumors to Apo2L/TRAIL and Apo2L/TRAIL receptor agonist antibodies by the Jak2-Stat3-Mcl1 axis. PLoS One 8(9):e75414. doi:10.1371/journal.pone.0075414
176. Hamed HA, Yamaguchi Y, Fisher PB, Grant S, Dent P (2013) Sorafenib and HDAC inhibitors synergize with TRAIL to kill tumor cells. J Cell Physiol 228(10):1996–2005. doi:10.1002/jcp.24362
177. Miyashita K, Shiraki K, Fuke H, Inoue T, Yamanaka Y, Yamaguchi Y, Yamamoto N, Ito K, Sugimoto K, Nakano T (2006) The cyclin-dependent kinase inhibitor flavopiridol sensitizes human hepatocellular carcinoma cells to TRAIL-induced apoptosis. Int J Mol Med 18(2):249–256

Chapter 2
TRAIL-R3/R4 and Inhibition of TRAIL Signalling in Cancer

Lubna Danish, Daniela Stöhr, Peter Scheurich, and Nadine Pollak

Abstract The tumour necrosis factor (TNF) ligand family member TNF-related apoptosis-inducing ligand (TRAIL) induces apoptosis predominantly in tumour cells, but not in normal tissues, representing therefore an attractive candidate for cancer therapy. The human TRAIL/TRAIL receptor system is very complex, four different membrane receptors bind the ligand. Two of these receptors, TRAIL-R1 and TRAIL-R2, transmit apoptotic but also non-apoptotic signals, whereas the other two, TRAIL-R3 and TRAIL-R4, act as inhibitors. Most tumour cells co-express several TRAIL receptors, allowing receptor interference. Several molecular mechanisms have been proposed by which TRAIL-R3 and TRAIL-R4 may counteract pro-apoptotic TRAIL signalling at the plasma membrane level, but possibly also intracellularly. A detailed understanding of the role of the individual TRAIL receptors and their interplay will be advantageous for the development of new TRAIL receptor agonists for cancer therapy. In fact, new TRAIL formulations will be needed since first clinical studies with soluble TRAIL or receptor agonistic antibodies showed only limited success. This review summarizes the complex TRAIL/TRAIL receptor system and the mechanisms by which TRAIL-R3 and TRAIL-R4 may interfere with TRAIL-mediated apoptosis induction. In addition, we discuss the prognostic and predictive value of TRAIL receptor expression in patients' tumour material.

Keywords Apoptosis • Death receptor • Decoy receptor • Membrane receptor • Signalling complex • TNFSF • TNFRSF • TRAIL • TRAIL receptor

2.1 Introduction

Human cytokines belonging to the tumour necrosis factor (TNF) ligand family and their cognate TNF receptors regulate a multitude of biological processes. Their functions are crucial in the regulation of immune responses, such as co-stimulatory

---

Lubna Danish and Daniela Stöhr contributed equally to this work.

L. Danish • D. Stöhr • P. Scheurich • N. Pollak (✉)
Institute of Cell Biology and Immunology, University of Stuttgart,
Allmandring 31, 70569 Stuttgart, Germany
e-mail: nadine.pollak@izi.uni-stuttgart.de

O. Micheau (ed.), *TRAIL, Fas Ligand, TNF and TLR3 in Cancer*, Resistance to Targeted Anti-Cancer Therapeutics, DOI 10.1007/978-3-319-56805-8_2

signalling or cell death induction in potentially harmful cells [1]. Accordingly, many of these cytokines and their receptors are interesting candidates as therapeutic agents or targets [2]. TNF superfamily ligands as well as their receptors are structurally related. Most ligand members are initially expressed as homotrimeric type I transmembrane proteins. In addition, soluble forms of the ligands can be generated by proteolytic cleavage or alternative splicing with significant consequences on bioactivity of these molecules, being typically higher in the membrane-presented mode [3]. Ligand bioactivity is exerted by binding and activating the corresponding partner(s) within the TNF receptor family. Typically, TNF receptors are expressed as type II transmembrane proteins and contain one to six cysteine-rich domains (CRDs) in their extracellular part. These CRDs have been demonstrated to not only harbour the ligand interaction site but additionally a homophilic interaction site called the pre-ligand binding assembly domain (PLAD).

Induction of apoptosis, a form of programmed cell death, is attributed to a subgroup within the TNF receptor members, the death receptors like TNF-R1, Fas (CD95), TRAIL-R1 and TRAIL-R2. In particular, the TRAIL system has gained enormous attraction since its apoptotic capacity is restricted to cancer cells whereas normal cells are insensitive to TRAIL [4]. Remarkably, the TRAIL receptor system is of particular complexity. Four specific membrane-expressed TRAIL receptors are capable to bind the ligand. Two of them, TRAIL-R1 and TRAIL-R2, are characterized by an intracellular death domain (DD) and are thus known as death receptors transmitting the apoptotic TRAIL-induced signal. TRAIL-R3 is membrane-anchored by a glycosylphosphatidylinositol (GPI) moiety and presumably not capable of intracellular signalling at all while TRAIL-R4 features a truncated DD with restricted signalling capacity. TRAIL-R3 and TRAIL-R4 are often referred to as decoy or regulatory receptors since they interfere with TRAIL-induced apoptosis induction. Intracellularly located TRAIL receptors have been detected more recently and proposed to be functional, representing a further level of complexity within the TRAIL signalling system. In particular, nuclear TRAIL-R2 has been proposed to enhance the malignancy of tumour cells [5].

In this chapter, we will introduce the TRAIL signalling system strongly focusing on the interference of TRAIL-R3 and TRAIL-R4 with TRAIL death receptors and the value of TRAIL receptor expression in different types of cancer as prognostic factor since this might determine the successful application of TRAIL-based therapeutics.

2.2 The TRAIL Signalling System

2.2.1 Structure of TRAIL

The ligand TRAIL, also called Apo2 ligand (Apo2L), TNF superfamily member 10 (TNFSF10), TNF ligand 2 (TL2), CD253 or TNF ligand gene 6A (TNLG6A), was first described in the late nineties by two independent groups [6, 7]. TRAIL was soon shown to represent a potential anti-tumour agent, while physiologically playing a role in the regulation of the innate and adaptive immune responses. The gene coding for human TRAIL consists of five exons and is located on chromosome 3. The molecule TRAIL shows 23% sequence homology to the death receptor ligand member FasL and 19% identity with TNF [6]. Until now, three splice variants of the full-length protein (TRAIL α) are known. These are TRAIL β, lacking exon 3, TRAIL γ, lacking exons 2 and 3, and TRAIL δ, lacking exons 3 and 4 [8]. All these latter molecules are depleted in their receptor interaction domain and are thus thought to be unable of receptor activation. They have been rather suggested to compete with TRAIL α for translation, in this way regulating TRAIL signalling [9, 10]. TRAIL transcripts are found in many different tissues such as liver, lung, colon, brain, heart, testis and kidney, but also in different cells of the haematopoietic system where TRAIL expression is inducible [6, 11]. When expressed on the surface of human cells, TRAIL is a type II transmembrane glycoprotein with a short amino-terminal cytoplasmic and a long extracellular carboxyl-terminal domain composed of two anti-parallel β-sheets [6, 7]. Similar to other TNF superfamily members, the extracellular domains (ECD) of TRAIL protomers associate at hydrophobic interfaces to form compact homotrimers. Unique for TRAIL is a zinc-binding site at the trimer interface which is indispensable for the structure and stability of the trimer, hence also for its bioactivity [12]. Limited proteolysis of membrane-bound TRAIL by cysteine proteases has been suggested as a mechanism to generate the soluble form of the ligand [13]. However, soluble TRAIL is capable to induce apoptosis predominantly via TRAIL-R1 whereas full activation of TRAIL-R2 is achieved only by membrane-integrated TRAIL [14].

2.2.2 *Structure and Function of TRAIL Receptors*

As mentioned above the TRAIL/TRAIL receptor system is relatively complex, comprising altogether six receptor molecules, of which four are membrane-bound and two are soluble (Fig. 2.1). Among the membrane-bound receptors, TRAIL-R1, also called death receptor 4 (DR4) or TNFR superfamily member 10 A (TNFRSF10A), was the first to be discovered in 1997 by a group around Dixit while searching the human genome database for sequences with homology to the TNF receptor 1 [15]. A second receptor, TRAIL-R2, DR5, TNFRSF10B, Apo2, TRAIL receptor inducer of cell killing 2 (TRICK2), or KILLER was discovered independently by several groups [16–22]. The receptors are encoded by two genes located on chromosome 8p and are expressed as type I transmembrane proteins with one partial and two complete CRDs in their extracellular portion and a DD in their cytoplasmic region. TRAIL-R1 and TRAIL-R2 both exist in two splice variants including full-length TRAIL-R1 comprising 468 amino acids and its splice variant (bDR4) lacking 168 amino acids within the extracellular ligand-binding region [23] as well as long DR5 (DR5(L)) containing 440 amino acids and short DR5 (DR5(S)) lacking 29 amino acids within the ECD and the predicted transmembrane domain [17].

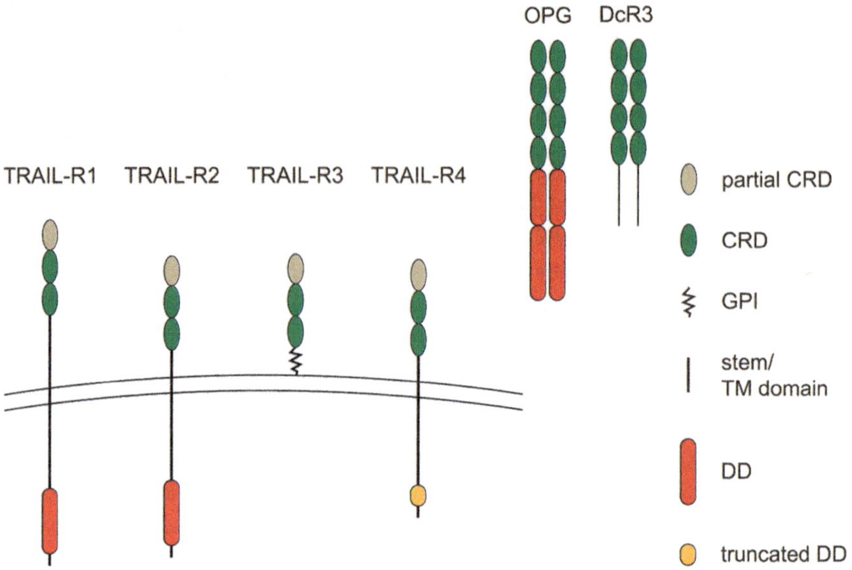

Fig. 2.1 Schematic representation of the structural features of human TRAIL receptors. The extracellular parts of TRAIL-R1 to TRAIL-R4 consist of cysteine-rich domains (CRDs, *grey and green*), a structural feature of receptors belonging to the TNF receptor superfamily. The first CRD, a partial one, mediates homophilic interactions between pre-ligand binding assembly domains (PLAD-PLAD) while the membrane proximal CRD2 and CRD3 form the ligand interaction site. The death receptors TRAIL-R1 and TRAIL-R2 are characterized by a functional death domain (DD, *red*) in their intracellular part, this domain is truncated for TRAIL-R4. TRAIL-R3 completely lacks an intracellular domain, it is linked to the membrane via a glycosylphosphatidylinositol (GPI) anchor. Splice variants for TRAIL-R1, TRAIL-R2 and TRAIL-R4 are reported, here only the longer protein variants are depicted (see text for detail). In addition to the four membrane receptors two soluble receptors have been suggested to be capable of TRAIL binding, namely OPG and DcR3. Both secreted receptors form disulfide-linked dimers. OPG consists of four CRDs and two DD-related domains while DcR3 is composed of four CRDs followed by a heparin-binding domain at its C-terminus

Interestingly, chimpanzees and humans have two death-inducing TRAIL receptors, whereas all other vertebrates solely display one. Since TRAIL-R1 shows only about 50% sequence identity with TRAIL-R2, one could speculate of different functions for these two receptor molecules. It is clear that both TRAIL death receptors can induce apoptosis in tumour cells, however, divergent reports exist regarding their contribution in cells co-expressing both receptors [24]. Moreover, recent reports show that both receptors can be also found in the cytoplasm and the nucleus of different cell lines in addition to their localization at the cell surface [25]. The mechanism of action of intracellular receptors is mainly undefined, but data suggest a proliferative role for nuclear TRAIL-R2 rather than a pro-apoptotic function [5]. Furthermore, a novel apoptosis-counteracting function for membrane-bound TRAIL-R2 in *KRAS* mutated tumour cells has been revealed. Here, TRAIL binding promotes migration and invasion via a DD-independent signalling pathway [26].

In addition to TRAIL-R1 and TRAIL-R2 two more receptors have been discovered in the late nineties referred to as TRAIL-R3, Decoy Receptor 1 (DcR1), TNFRSF10C, TRAIL Receptor without an Intracellular Domain (TRID), CD263 or Lymphocyte Inhibitor of TRAIL (LIT) [16, 18, 20, 27, 28] and TRAIL-R4, also named DcR2, TNFRSF10D, CD264, or TRAIL Receptor with a truncated Death Domain (TRUNDD) [29–31]. As already suggested by the names, these two molecules are most likely incapable of apoptotic signalling since TRAIL-R3 completely lacks any transmembrane and intracellular domain, whereas TRAIL-R4 has only a truncated DD. Similar to TRAIL-R1 and TRAIL-R2, TRAIL-R3 and TRAIL-R4 display one partial and two complete CRDs in their extracellular parts (Fig. 2.1).

TRAIL-R3 is not a transmembrane protein but is rather anchored in the cell membrane via a GPI moiety. It consists of 259 amino acids and in contrast to the other membrane-bound TRAIL receptors no splice variant has yet been identified. Signalling of TRAIL-R3 has so far not been studied intensively. However, the complete absence of a transmembrane and an intracellular domain indicates the lack of classical signalling capabilities, although signalling via its GPI anchor cannot be excluded [32].

Two splice variants have been identified for TRAIL-R4, TRAIL-R4-α and TRAIL-R-β, with 386 and 348 amino acids, respectively, the latter lacking the first complete CRD [33]. As TRAIL-R4 contains only an incomplete DD it is suggested to be not capable to transmit an apoptotic signal upon TRAIL binding. However, it is still under debate whether TRAIL-R4 transmits non-apoptotic signals (see below). The role of TRAIL-R3 and TRAIL-R4 as inhibitory receptors rendering cells resistant against TRAIL-mediated apoptosis is discussed in more detail later in this chapter.

Besides the membrane-integrated receptors TRAIL-R1 to TRAIL-R4, two soluble members of the TNF receptor family have been reported to be capable of binding TRAIL, namely osteoprotegerin (OPG, TNFRSF11B) and decoy receptor 3 (DcR3, TNFRSF6B) (Fig. 2.1). OPG is secreted by osteoblasts and regulates osteoclast differentiation based on its ability to block receptor activator of nuclear factor "kappa-light-chain-enhancer" of activated B-cells ligand (RANKL)-stimulated osteoclast formation [34]. OPG was shown to bind to TRAIL, although with very low affinity, thereby also acting as a decoy receptor in TRAIL signalling [35]. Recent studies indicate that OPG might be involved in the pathogenesis of cardiovascular disease, in the development of both type 1 and type 2 diabetes, in endothelia cell biology and in kidney diseases, but the role of TRAIL binding in these processes is still undefined [36].

The *DcR3* gene is frequently amplified in tumour cells and the protein is overexpressed in various cancer cells [37, 38]. Ligands of DcR3 beside TRAIL also include FasL, TNF-like molecule 1A (TL1A), and LIGHT [37, 39, 40]. The interaction between DcR3 and TRAIL was demonstrated only recently in pancreatic cells, revealing a lower affinity as compared to that of LIGHT [41]. In these cells the apoptotic response to either TRAIL or FasL was enhanced when DcR3 levels were decreased [41, 42]. In summary, OPG and DcR3 might play a role in cancer progression, but whether these molecules do this by interference with the TRAIL signalling system remains to be investigated.

2.2.3 *TRAIL Receptor Signalling*

2.2.3.1 Apoptotic Signalling

The term apoptosis was introduced by Kerr and colleagues in 1972 [43] and describes a tightly regulated process of cell death with distinct morphological changes such as cell shrinkage, membrane blebbing and fragmentation of the nucleus. In contrast to unregulated cell death, necrosis, where loss of membrane integrity leads to the release of damage-associated molecular patterns (DAMPs) causing an inflammatory response, apoptosis is a rather immunological silent form of cell death since apoptotic cells become phagocytosed by immune cells to prevent activation of the immune system [44]. In the human body each day around ten billion of malignant and infected but also overaged and redundant cells die by apoptosis [45]. Interestingly, apoptosis not only occurs in the adult body but takes part also in embryogenesis, being involved for example in the development of limbs and modelling of the nervous system. Apoptosis can be triggered either by binding of death ligands like TNF, FasL or TRAIL to their cognate cell surface receptors resulting in the execution of the so-called extrinsic apoptotic pathway. Alternatively, intracellular stimuli such as DNA damage or oxidative stress induce apoptosis via activation of the intrinsic pathway of this signalling network. Depending on the cell type TRAIL-mediated apoptosis either involves solely the extrinsic pathway or includes both pathways. In type I cells, binding of TRAIL, TRAIL-fusion proteins or agonistic antibodies specific for TRAIL-R1 or TRAIL-R2, often referred to as pro-apoptotic receptor agonists (PARAs), initially triggers receptor clustering, thereby forming the death-inducing signalling complex (DISC), comprising Fas-associated protein with death domain (FADD), procaspase –8/–10 and cellular FLICE-like inhibitory protein (cFLIP). Essential for DISC formation are homophilic interactions of the DDs of the TRAIL receptors with those of FADD and, in addition, death effector domain (DED) interactions between FADD and the initiator procaspases. During DISC assembly procaspase –8/–10 oligomerizes and gets activated through proximity-induced formation of procaspase dimers and autoproteolysis, allowing the activated initiator caspases to further cleave and activate effector procaspases –3/–6/–7 to finally dismantle the cell. In type II cells the very same signalling pathway becomes activated by stimulation of TRAIL-R1 and/or TRAIL-R2, but remains at the level of only a very weak activation of initiator caspases not sufficient for strong effector caspase activation. Accordingly, these cells need amplification of the apoptotic signal by the mitochondrial intrinsic pathway to successfully trigger apoptosis. To this, receptor-activated caspase-8 cleaves truncated BH3 interacting domain death agonist (Bid), a pro-apoptotic B-cell lymphoma 2 (Bcl-2) family member, to form truncated Bid (tBid) which then translocates to the mitochondria to become an integral membrane protein triggering the polymerization of proapoptotic Bcl-2 family members Bax and/or Bak in the mitochondrial outer membrane. This leads to release of the pro-apoptotic factors cytochrome c, apoptosis inducing factor (AIF) and second mitochondria derived activator of apoptosis (Smac) into the cytoplasm. In the presence of dATP, cytochrome c induces formation of the apoptosome, comprising also procaspase-9 and the apoptotic protease activating factor-1 (Apaf-1). Activated caspase-9 subsequently cleaves and activates effector procaspases to allow execution of the apoptotic program [46, 47].

2.2.3.2 Necroptotic Signalling

More recently it was shown that members of the TNF superfamily such as TRAIL, but also various toxic stimuli, can induce another form of programmed cell death referred to as necroptosis. In this signalling pathway TRAIL binding to TRAIL-R1/R2 leads to the recruitment of receptor-interacting kinase 1 (RIP1), as well as cellular inhibitors of apoptosis proteins, cIAP1 and cIAP2, into the signalling complex, resulting in RIP1 polyubiquitination. Polyubiquinated RIP1 subsequently binds FADD and procaspase-8 forming a complex called ripoptosome in which procaspase-8 becomes activated and is also capable to execute the apoptotic program. However, in the case of inhibited caspase-8 activity, RIP1 can alternatively bind RIP3 to form the so-called necroptosome leading to auto-phosphorylation and activation of RIP3 and further recruitment and oligomerization of mixed lineage kinase domain-like (MLKL). Disruption of the cell membrane, causing a necrotic type of cell death is finally induced when MLKL oligomers are inserted into the membrane.

As mentioned before necrosis but also necroptosis can lead to the release of DAMPs and as a consequence to an extensive inflammatory response in the human body. Concerning tumour development these released immunostimulatory molecules can have two sides. On the one hand it was shown that production of DAMPs during necroptosis can help to eliminate cancer cells by activating natural killer (NK) cells and cytotoxic T cells, on the other hand these molecules can also have a tumour promoting function facilitating tumour angiogenesis as well as invasion and metastasis. In any case, necroptosis seems to represent a backup mechanism in the human body to eliminate infected, damaged or malignant cells which are for any reason resistant against apoptotic cell death [44, 48].

2.2.3.3 Non-cytotoxic Signalling

In TRAIL-resistant cells, ligation of TRAIL-R1 and/or TRAIL-R2 not only initiates apoptotic signals, but also stimulates cellular survival via activation of the transcription factor nuclear factor "kappa-light-chain-enhancer" of activated B-cells (NF-kB), as well as the mitogen-activated protein kinases (MAPKs) and the phosphoinositide-3-kinase/Akt (PI3K/Akt) pathways [49]. Concerning the molecular mechanism of this pro-survival signalling, the formation of a secondary signalling complex including FADD, procaspase-8, RIP1, TNFR-associated factor 2 (TRAF2) and the inhibitor of kB kinase (IKKγ) was proposed [50]. However, more recent publications suggest an RIP1-independent process [51] or a subdivided mechanism [52]. Beside TRAIL-R1 and TRAIL-R2, TRAIL-R4 was also suggested to be capable of intracellular pro-survival NF-kB and Akt signalling, as discussed further in more detail below.

Interestingly, beside the differential expression levels of intracellular proteins also the localization of TRAIL receptors at the plasma membrane was proposed to determine the formation of differential signalling complexes. It was shown that activation of aggregated TRAIL receptors in cholesterol-rich membrane microdomains (often called "lipid rafts") leads to the formation of complexes capable of apoptotic signalling. In contrast, receptors outside of such microdomains are mainly involved in non-apoptotic signalling [53].

2.2.4 TRAIL's Role In Vivo

Although TRAIL is mainly known for its tumour cell killing capacity it is involved in numerous other regulatory mechanisms in the human body including the defence against viral and bacterial infections as well as haematopoiesis. To exert its function as a regulator of immune responses TRAIL is expressed in different leukocytes, both from the innate and adaptive immune systems. Most important are hereby the NK and T cells, but also B cells, dendritic cells, eosinophils, neutrophils, macrophages and monocytes which all can express TRAIL after stimulation with different activating agents like interferons (IFNs) or antigens [54]. Interestingly, TRAIL seems to be not only involved in the signalling of immune cells but even in their development [55].

NK cells play an important role in the innate immune response against intracellular pathogens but are at the same time also involved in combating tumour cells. The activation status of NK cells is dependent on different activating and inhibitory receptors as well as cytokines like IFNs and interleukins (ILs). Among these, especially IFN-γ and IFN-α are known to induce TRAIL expression [56, 57]. Interestingly, it was shown that NK cells are also involved in balancing adaptive immune responses versus autoimmunity since they have been shown to limit the autoimmune response during chronic infections by TRAIL-mediated killing of T helper cells [58, 59]. Furthermore, in hepatitis B, C and lymphocytic choriomeningitis infection, NK cells not only directly eliminate virus-infected cells but also regulate T cell responses via TRAIL release [60–62]. T cells, or more precisely T helper (Th) and cytotoxic T cells are also able to express TRAIL after stimulation of the T cell receptor together with type I IFNs [63, 64]. Similar to NK cells these are also involved in the elimination of malignant and virus infected cells in the human body. Additionally, TRAIL seems to be involved in the regulation of the Th type 1 (Th1) and Th2 responses, since Th2 cells are resistant to TRAIL-mediated apoptosis but express TRAIL after T cell receptor stimulation whereas stimulated Th1 cells are sensitive for TRAIL and up-regulate FasL. Furthermore, the inhibition of TRAIL in mice which display allergic airway diseases inhibited homing of Th2 cells to the airways [65–67].

Concerning viral and bacterial infections of the human body TRAIL seems to play the role of a double-edged sword. On the one hand TRAIL is involved directly and indirectly in the elimination of infected cells, but on the other hand some viral and bacterial species manipulate TRAIL signalling to evade from the immune response and to increase replication. A participation of TRAIL in viral defence of the human body can for example be observed during influenza infection. Hereby, infected alveolar cells are eliminated by TRAIL positive cytotoxic T cells, but TRAIL is believed also to limit the immune response reducing the chance for infection-induced immunopathology [68–70]. However, it was also described that TRAIL can be released by activated alveolar macrophages leading to damage of uninfected lung tissue [71]. Also, during hyper- inflammation TRAIL might play a conflicting role, depending on the stage of the disease. At the beginning, TRAIL appears to have mainly a protective function while eliminating activated neutrophils. Later in the disease TRAIL acts as an immune suppressor, thereby, contributing to the severe development [72, 73].

Shortly after its discovery in the late nineties, TRAIL was shown to not only kill tumour cells when applied exogenously, but proved to be effective in the human body as an endogenously expressed protein leading to the suppression of tumour growth [74]. As mentioned above, cells of the immune system, especially NK cells, T cells, macrophages and neutrophils, not only kill virus infected cells but can also identify and eliminate malignant cells in vivo and in vitro by releasing TRAIL among other cytokines when activated with IFN-γ [64, 75–79].

Interestingly, TRAIL and its receptors are expressed not only on malignant cells and cells of the immune system but also in many other tissues of the human body including testis, lung, colon, kidney and endothelium [11]. Their biological functions, however, are in most cases largely undefined. In the human testis, TRAIL for example has been shown to regulate germ cell apoptosis during the first wave of spermatogenesis [80] and it was further demonstrated that high levels of TRAIL in the seminal plasma protect spermatozoa [81]. Also, the endothelium is known to express TRAIL receptors and the medial smooth cell layer of the aorta and pulmonary arteries produce the ligand TRAIL [82, 83] which was demonstrated to promote survival as well as proliferation of endothelial cells [84]. Further, TRAIL takes part in the interplay of endothelial cells with leucocytes, modelling cell adhesion by down regulation of chemokine receptors [85]. The application of TRAIL resulted in enhanced phosphorylation of oxide synthase in endothelial cells, which was shown to increase cell migration as well as cytoskeleton reorganization and might also affect blood vessel vasodilatation and angiogenesis [86, 87].

2.3 The TRAIL System in Cancer

Cancer is a major cause of death and therefore an enormous health challenge. Worldwide cancer incidents have been increased during the last decades, mostly attributable to increased average life expectancy. On the other hand, significant survival improvement could be achieved during the last 20 years by new medical diagnosis tools and better adjuvant therapies.

Cancer is treated typically by surgical resection of the tumour combined with adjuvant therapy. The classical approach is radiotherapy and chemotherapy, however, both are not cancer cell specific and in addition tumour cells can acquire resistance. To overcome these limitations, numerous novel therapeutic strategies have been developed and approved by the U.S. Food and Drug Administration during the last decade, such as targeted therapies and small molecule inhibitors [88]. In addition, much effort is put into the identification of predictive or prognostic tumour biomarkers, including characteristic genetic alterations or particular protein expression pattern. The expression of markers in different types and grades of cancers might be a rational basis to design an effective adjuvant treatment strategy and to improve the overall survival of patients [89]. For example, colorectal cancers are frequently mutated in *KRAS* and consequently patients will not respond to epidermal growth factor receptor (EGFR)-based therapies [90]. In fact, *KRAS* represents the first biomarker routinely used in clinical practice [89].

Tumours are frequently altered for p53 activity and are thus resistant to several classes of conventional chemotherapy. A promising therapeutic strategy is to trigger the extrinsic apoptotic pathway using PARAs as therapeutic agents, since cell death induced via this route is independent from p53. Consequently, the successful application of PARAs in tumour therapy requires plasma membrane expression of the respective death receptors in tumour cells and a functional downstream signalling network leading to the apoptotic machinery.

2.3.1 Predictive and Prognostic Significance of TRAIL Receptor Expression

Quite a few studies analysed patient-derived tumour tissues from different cancer types and grades, treated or untreated, for cellular TRAIL receptor expression using conventional immunohistochemistry. In addition, reports on TRAIL receptor gene expression and mutational analysis are found in the literature. These studies focused on the expression profile of pro-apoptotic proteins including TRAIL-R1, TRAIL-R2, caspase-8 and TRAIL itself as well as anti-apoptotic proteins such as TRAIL-R3, TRAIL-R4, c-Flip and Bcl-2 family members. In general, TRAIL receptors are frequently expressed in carcinomas from different origins as well as in the respective normal surrounding tissue [91–96]. Receptor expression was detected in various subcellular localizations, namely, the cytoplasm, the nucleus and membrane-bound. Interestingly, oncogenic mutations in the MAPK pathway, *KRAS* and/or *BRAF*, frequently found in colorectal tumours, were linked to high TRAIL-R1 and TRAIL-R2 expression [94].

Reports of genetic loss or mutation of TRAIL receptors have been also described, but were suggested to represent not a common event in cancer cells [97, 98].

Polymorphisms in the *TRAIL-R1* gene and a loss of function mutation of *TRAIL-R2* potentially increase the risk for development of head and neck cancer [99, 100]. A polymorphism in the *TRAIL-R4* gene appears to be associated with reduced breast cancer risk [101]. A recent study identified a single nucleotide polymorphism (SNP)-SNP interaction pair, located in the NF-kB pathway genes *TRAF2* and *TRAIL-R4*, to be correlated with improved survival in breast cancer [102]. Notably, both NF-kB and TRAIL-R4 have been rather implicated in the protection from TRAIL-induced apoptosis although constitutive activation of NF-kB signalling is associated with tumour progression.

Both negative and positive correlations of the expression pattern with the grade of malignancy and other clinical features such as overall survival have been shown for TRAIL-R1 to TRAIL-R4. But it should be mentioned that there are also reports demonstrating no correlation of either TRAIL receptor expression with grade or survival [95, 103, 104]. High TRAIL-R1 expression is correlated with tumour grade in breast cancer patients with invasive ductal carcinoma and bladder cancer [105, 106] and with an unfavourable overall survival in adjuvant treated stage III colon cancer [93]. High TRAIL-R2 expression was shown to be associated with a higher grade of malignancy in breast, bladder, hepatocellular, renal, head and neck carcinomas and with less differentiated areas of non-small cell lung cancer of different grades [92, 106–112]. Increased TRAIL-R2 expression also matched a larger tumour size in head and neck cancer tissues [113]. Accordingly, TRAIL-R2 was found to negatively correlate with overall survival in breast, renal and lung cancers. Conversely, TRAIL-R2 expression was significantly decreased in prostate cancer of higher tumour grade [114].

Reports on TRAIL receptor expression as positive prognostic markers can also be found. High TRAIL-R1 expression was correlated with well-differentiated tumours and with better prognosis in colorectal cancer patients [91, 115]. In cervical cancer, TRAIL-R1 in the nucleus might be a predictive biomarker for radiotherapy [116]. In glioblastoma multiforme, a strong membrane staining for both TRAIL-R1 and TRAIL-R2 was correlated with better survival [117]. Since TRAIL exerts its bioactivity after binding to TRAIL receptors in the plasma membrane, loss of surface expression may explain tumour resistance to TRAIL-based therapies despite uniform cellular receptor expression. In fact, a poorer prognosis for patient survival was associated with loss of membrane staining for TRAIL-R2, but also TRAIL-R1, in early-stage colorectal carcinoma, breast cancer and pancreatic carcinoma [96, 118, 119].

Quite unexpected, recent studies revealed evidence that the subcellular localization of TRAIL receptors, in particular of TRAIL-R2, is an important determinant for the signalling outcome. Nuclear TRAIL-R2 was shown to inhibit microRNA maturation thereby enhancing malignancy of tumours, however, the functional role of cytoplasmic TRAIL receptors has not been addressed so far [5]. High cytoplasmic levels of TRAIL-R1 or TRAIL-R2 correlated with an improved recurrence-free rate for bladder cancer patients [106]. Accordingly, the differential distribution of the receptors in cellular compartments could be one reason for the inconsistent correlation of receptor expression with prognosis in cancer.

Most human cell lines co-express TRAIL-R3 and TRAIL-R4, albeit at comparably low levels. Accordingly, the expression of TRAIL-R3 and TRAIL-R4 was also evaluated for prognostic impact in several studies. TRAIL-R4 expression level is increased in prostate, pancreatic, breast, hepatocellular cancers and meningioma [107, 108, 120–122]. A strong correlation of its expression with higher tumour grades as well as poor clinical outcome and decreased survival has been demonstrated. In colorectal carcinoma, high TRAIL-R3 expression, in combination with low TRAIL-R1, is linked to poor response to 5-fluorouracil and shorter progression-free survival [123]. In head and neck cancer, TRAIL-R3 and TRAIL-R4 expressions were also significantly increased but did not correlate with tumour staging or prognosis [110, 124].

Remarkably, a positive correlation was found between the expression levels of TRAIL death receptors and inhibitory receptors. TRAIL-R2 upregulation correlates with increased TRAIL-R4, as reported for meningioma, hepatocellular, pancreatic and head and neck cancers, however, without relevance for the overall patient survival [108, 122, 124]. In contrast, high TRAIL-R2 levels along with low TRAIL-R4 expression were shown to be associated with higher grade of renal cell cancer and worse survival [109]. Similarly, high levels of TRAIL-R3 are associated with low TRAIL-R1 [123]. These data appear puzzling, more knowledge about the molecular mechanisms which control expression of the individual receptors could help to understand them better.

Interestingly, the ligand itself was highlighted as a prognostic marker. Patients newly diagnosed with acute myeloid or acute lymphoblastic leukaemia have significantly lower serum concentrations of TRAIL compared to healthy volunteers [125, 126]. Upon start of the therapy an increase of TRAIL expression resulting in higher serum concentrations was predictive of better overall patient survival [126]. Higher TRAIL expression was also associated with low tumour grade and better progression-free survival in ovarian and renal cancer patients [95, 127]. Loss of TRAIL expression in oral and cervical carcinoma is an early event and is correlated with malignant progression [113, 116]. These results indicate that downregulation of TRAIL expression enables cancerous cells to evade apoptosis suggesting that TRAIL contributes to a positive therapeutic response. On the other hand, a high level of TRAIL was associated with shorter survival for patients with renal and colorectal cancers [109, 128]. It was argued that high TRAIL expression may protect cancer cells from the immune system while promoting metastasis. TRAIL was also shown to have no prognostic value [91, 93] and there was no correlation between TRAIL expression and survival [117].

In summary, numerous studies have evaluated the prognostic relevance of the expression pattern of TRAIL and TRAIL receptors in tumour entities. The results are interesting, but also very conflicting. As most data have not been confirmed in larger validation studies, their clinical value remains limited [89]. Recently, it has become evident that the subcellular localization of TRAIL receptors may regulate specific functions and thus correlates with pro-apoptotic versus pro-survival signalling. Accordingly, it will be necessary to carefully re-evaluate the pattern of TRAIL receptor staining in primary tissue to further analyse its significance on tumour growth and response to TRAIL-based therapeutics.

2.3.2 TRAIL Death Receptor Agonists

Shortly after its discovery in the late nineties, TRAIL was shown to represent a promising candidate in the battle against cancer since it selectively eliminates malignant cells while sparing normal tissue [4]. Although early reports claimed a cytotoxic effect of recombinant TRAIL in hepatocytes and cells in human brain slices, this was later shown to be caused by the protein's affinity tags resulting in the formation of supramolecular aggregates [129]. However, despite that TRAIL is well tolerated in vivo and shows cytotoxicity against tumour cells in vitro, until today there is no TRAIL-based anti-tumour drug available on the market. The main reason might be that TRAIL receptor-directed clinical studies showed only moderate effects.

Among all generated TRAIL death receptor agonists investigated so far, homotrimeric recombinant TRAIL protein (dulanermin) was one of the first. In different phase I studies dulanermin proved to be well tolerated but did not reveal any significant anti-tumour activities [129]. Likely explanations for this failure are the very short half-life of only 20 min of this molecule [4, 130] but also the fact that soluble TRAIL might only fully activate TRAIL-R1, but not TRAIL-R2 [3, 14]. To address this problem oligomerized derivatives have been produced by the addition of a leucine or isoleucine zipper domain [4, 131] or a tenascin-c (TNC) domain [132]. Approaches to prolong the half-life in vivo include coupling of TRAIL with polyethylene glycol or human serum albumin [129]. An interesting approach is the use of single-chain TRAIL (scTRAIL) which, in contrast to the classical homotrimeric TRAIL, is expressed as a single protein chain consisting of the three TRAIL "monomers" covalently connected by short peptide linkers [133]. This molecule, possessing only a single N- and C-terminus, has been further fused with the Fc portion of human IgG1 to obtain a hexameric molecule with enhanced bioactivity [134].

Beside the stability and half-life also the targeting of the molecule to cancer cells is of great interest. Fusing of the abovementioned TRAIL variants to single-chain variable fragment (scFv) domains specific for different tumour-expressed antigens such as EGFR, fibroblast activation protein, CD19, CD33, or CD20 enables targeting and enhances protein stability [129, 135]. In addition, as these constructs bind to cell surface antigens thereby increasing receptor cross linking they show enhanced bioactivities. In another approach, the TRAIL death receptor agonists were not targeted to the tumour cells but to cells of the immune systems to enhance their tumour killing capacity [136–138].

Beside the large group of TRAIL fusion proteins also antibodies specific for either TRAIL-R1 or TRAIL-R2 have been developed like mapatumumab and lexatumumab. All of them have been demonstrated to effectively kill tumour cells in vitro, but did not display compelling anti-tumour activity in clinical trials [139]. The reasons for this limited success might include insufficient receptor cross linking, i.e., the need for molecules with higher affinity/avidity, problems to reach the tumour cells at sufficient concentration and the fact that cells in a solid tumour might show a relative TRAIL resistance as indicated by data from multicellular tumour spheroids in vitro, where downregulation of TRAIL-R1 and TRAIL-R2 has been demonstrated [140, 141]. To increase the efficacy of PARAs it appears feasible to use sensitizing drugs, like bortezomib, doxorubicin, cisplatin and 5-fluorouracil, which all have been shown to enhance TRAIL-mediated apoptosis in vitro [142].

2.3.3 The Role of TRAIL-R3 and TRAIL-R4 in Resistance to TRAIL-Mediated Apoptosis

A major hurdle in developing TRAIL-based therapies is the primary or acquired resistance to TRAIL, as it has been reported that around 50% of all cancer cell lines show resistance to TRAIL treatment [4]. Clearly, TRAIL resistance can be generated at multiple levels in the apoptotic signalling network, but the first control point exists at the membrane at the level of TRAIL receptors, e.g., by overexpression of decoy receptors or downregulation of death receptors. Initial studies have proposed that high expression of decoy receptors TRAIL-R3 and/or TRAIL-R4 in normal cells would cause protection against TRAIL-induced apoptosis [18, 30]. But later on it has been clarified that the situation is not that simple since inhibition of the decoy receptors does not necessarily result in a sensitization of normal cells to TRAIL. So, their functional role and mode of action are much more complicated than what initially was proposed. Nevertheless, a broad range of studies has shown that transformed cells can evade TRAIL-induced apoptosis by overexpression of decoy receptors [143–147].

2.3.3.1 The Decoy Model for TRAIL-R3 and TRAIL-R4

Unlike other TNF receptor family members, TRAIL-R3 completely lacks a cytoplasmic domain as it is anchored in the plasma membrane by a GPI residue [27]. In contrast, TRAIL-R4 contains a cytoplasmic region representing only one-third of a typical DD and which is therefore considered to be non-functional [29]. However, the ECDs of all four membrane-bound receptors TRAIL-R1 to TRAIL-R4 show strong homologies in their structure and all consist of three CRDs. Since most of the cells simultaneously co-express both pro- and anti-apoptotic receptors on their surface, it was initially thought that TRAIL-R3 and TRAIL-R4 compete with TRAIL-R1 and TRAIL-R2 for binding of the ligand through their ECDs [148]. Consequently they were referred to as "decoy receptors". In fact, various initial in vitro studies have linked a high expression level of decoy receptors with TRAIL resistance and vice versa [145, 149]. Sanlioglu and co-workers found that the TRAIL sensitive breast cancer cell line MDA-MB-231 expresses less TRAIL-R4 on the cell surface as compared to the higher expression in the TRAIL resistant MCF7 cell line [144]. Further, enforced overexpression of TRAIL-R3 has been shown to inhibit TRAIL-mediated apoptosis induction in various cancer cells and this resistance could be abolished by cleavage of the GPI anchor to remove

TRAIL-R3 from the cell surface [150]. Although these and other studies linked the expression of the decoy receptors to TRAIL resistance, finally no significant correlation was found between TRAIL sensitivity and the expression levels of TRAIL-R3 and/or TRAIL-R4 on tumour cells [151–153].

Clearly, the principle of the proposed decoy mechanism is functional, i.e., TRAIL-R3 and TRAIL-R4 consume ligand without induction of a resulting pro-apoptotic signal, thereby reducing the ligand amount available for TRAIL-R1 and TRAIL-R2. But it is also obvious, that inhibition of TRAIL sensitivity by the decoy mechanism must be overcome when using extremely high concentrations of TRAIL which so far could not be demonstrated (Neumann, S., unpublished data). There exist some exceptional situations where one might expect the decoy mechanism to play a major role, for example in case of extremely high expression levels of these receptors and/or at very low ligand concentrations [154]. Alternatively, one might expect that the ligand binding affinity values of the decoy receptors should be significantly higher compared to those of the death receptors. The first reports determining binding affinities suggested that all four receptors bind to TRAIL with comparable affinities [27, 30]. However, later investigations demonstrated that the death receptors possess somewhat higher binding affinity values at physiological temperature as compared to the decoy receptors [155, 156], arguing further against the importance of the decoy mechanism under (patho)physiological conditions in vivo. Together, the idea that the inhibitory effects of TRAIL-R3 and TRAIL-R4 mainly depends on ligand consumption became hard to accept as a general and important mechanism.

2.3.3.2 Formation of Heteromeric Complexes Affected in Signalling

A second possibility for TRAIL-R3 and TRAIL-R4 to interfere with TRAIL-mediated apoptosis induction is the formation of heteromeric ligand/receptor complexes. As mentioned TRAIL forms homotrimers capable to bind three receptor molecules in the clefts between the individual protomers [12]. In a cell co-expressing for example equal levels of TRAIL-R1 and TRAIL-R3, four different initial complexes could be formed upon ligation: TRAIL-$(R1)_3$, TRAIL-$(R1)_2$R3, TRAIL-R1$(R3)_2$ and TRAIL-$(R3)_3$. The potential signalling capabilities of the two mixed complexes are totally unclear, but if we assume that TRAIL-R3 is incapable to signal at all, we would end up in any case with a situation of partly inhibited apoptotic signalling as compared to a cell line expressing only TRAIL-R1, but no TRAIL-R3. Additional constraints exist, however, which could regulate the efficiency of formation of the different homomeric and heteromeric complexes. First, individual receptors might be enriched in the cell membrane in different compartments, like the already mentioned cholesterol-rich microdomains. Taken as an extreme case, in our example above TRAIL-R1 and TRAIL-R3 could then be separated totally in distinct microdomains, which would not allow significant formation of heteromeric complexes upon ligand binding at all. Second, TRAIL receptors, like other members of the TNF receptor family, possess a homophilic interaction domain allowing homomultimer formation of the membrane-expressed receptors even in the absence of ligand, the PLAD. This domain is located at the membrane distal (partial) first CRD (CRD1) of the four TRAIL receptors. Moreover, in the TRAIL receptor system, but e.g., not in the TNF receptor system, this domain allows the formation of heteromeres [154, 156–158]. The PLAD has been originally detected and described in the TNF and the Fas systems [159, 160]. The stoichiometry of PLAD-mediated multimer formation is not well defined. The group of Lenardo originally described TNF receptor and Fas homotrimers, whereas later studies using TNF receptor chimeras suggested homodimers [161]. More recently, we confirmed heteromeric TRAIL receptor interactions in the absence of ligand by acceptor photobleaching fluorescence resonance energy transfer (FRET) studies and also found predominant TRAIL receptor homodimer and heterodimer formation [154]. It cannot be excluded, however, that trimer vs. dimer formation might be regulated in a cell type-specific manner or is mainly attributable to the chemical cross linker used.

Convincing evidence exists that the PLAD not only serves to mediate multimer formation of receptors in the absence of ligand, but also after ligation. Accordingly, driven by two different interaction sites which do not sterically interfere with each other, the formation of large ligand/receptor clusters is allowed. Originally proposed in the TNF system on the basis of studies with TNF receptor mutants [161], the group of Sachs later confirmed the formation of TRAIL-R2 dimers within high molecular weight ligand/receptor networks [158]. Further studies of this group with TNF-R1 and TRAIL-R2 resulted in an activation model for these receptors. According to this model unligated receptor homodimers are in an "OFF" stage when homodimerized via PLAD interaction, but are twisted to "ON" when becoming incorporated in large ligand/receptor clusters [162, 163]. In the formation of these clusters the initial step is likely the binding of one TRAIL molecule with one of its three binding sites on the "back" of the homodimerized receptor molecules (Fig. 2.3a). Mathematical modelling studies suggest that the PLAD-PLAD interaction of the receptor dimer then opens to allow binding of the second receptor to one of the two other binding sites of the TRAIL molecule as detailed in [164]. These initial complexes TRAIL-(TRAIL-R)$_2$ would then further aggregate upon diffusion in the membrane.

Affinity data obtained from plasmon resonance studies of purified soluble ECDs from TRAIL receptors indicate comparable affinity values for homomeric and heteromeric PLAD-mediated interactions and were found to be in the micromolar range [165]. These low affinity values determined, however, cannot be taken for the "effective" PLAD affinities of membrane-expressed receptor molecules, because the latter are oriented and arranged in the cell membrane, whereas one binding partner in the studies by Lee et al. freely diffused in solution, whereas the other partner was immobilized (for discussion of this point, see [154]). Notably, no measurable affinity values were found for the interaction between the ECD of TRAIL-R2 and those of the two decoy receptors. It is unlikely that some molecules in this study were simply misfolded, because proper interactions in all other eight ECD combinations could be determined. These data indicate an interesting difference between

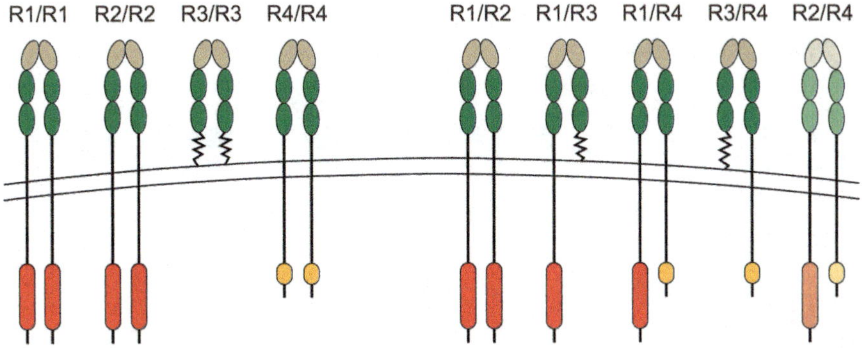

Fig. 2.2 Homotypic and heterotypic interactions between TRAIL receptor dimers. TRAIL receptors on the plasma membrane exist as pre-formed dimers in the absence of ligand, although unligated receptor trimers have also been proposed. Dimerization is mediated by the PLAD and occurs either as a homotypic (*left*) or a heterotypic (*right*) interaction between individual TRAIL receptor monomers. Note that TRAIL-R3 might be sequestered in cholesterol-rich membrane microdomains. Although heteromeric TRAIL-R3 interactions with TRAIL-R1 or TRAIL-R4 have been reported, their existence remains fairly speculative. Similarly, the heteromeric TRAIL-R2/TRAIL-R4 interaction remains inconclusive (see text for detail)

TRAIL-R1 and TRAIL-R2, the first capable to interact with all four receptors, whereas the latter can interact only with TRAIL-R1 and TRAIL-R2. However, in contrast to these data FRET and co-immunoprecipitation experiments suggested an interaction between TRAIL-R2 and TRAIL-R4 [154, 156]. Having all these facts in mind, we end up with a very complex situation: We have up to four different receptors co-expressed in a single cell, which might form up to four different homodimers and four or even five heterodimers (Fig. 2.2), which then react with the homotrimeric ligand TRAIL to finally produce large ligand/receptor clusters (Fig. 2.3).

2.3.3.3 TRAIL-R3 and TRAIL-R4 Incorporation in Ligand Receptor Clusters

Based on initial PLAD data, Clancy and colleagues introduced a new term for TRAIL-R4, "regulatory receptor" instead of "decoy receptor". They claimed that the inhibitory action of TRAIL-R4 does not entirely depend on the consumption of TRAIL, but is rather mediated by ligand independent formation of mixed complexes with TRAIL-R2 [156]. However, there are conflicting results regarding the role of TRAIL in the formation of homomeric and heteromeric complexes, as Merino and colleagues concluded that this interaction between TRAIL-R4 and TRAIL-R2 is ligand dependent while other studies suggested a ligand independent process, mediated by the PLAD [156, 157].

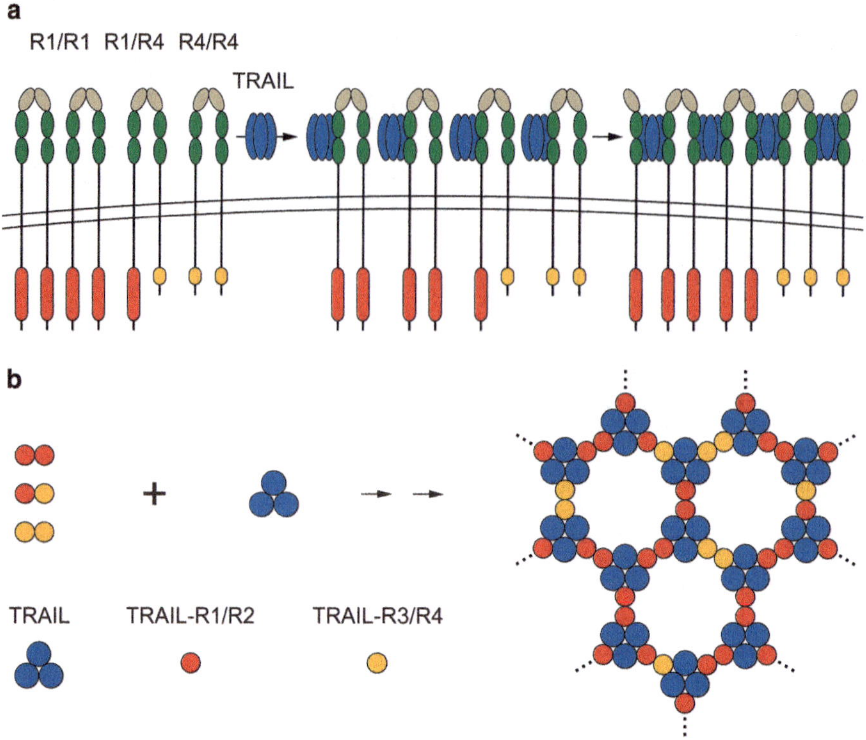

Fig. 2.3 Formation of heteromeric ligand-receptor clusters driven by PLAD-mediated receptor-receptor and ligand-receptor interaction. According to the current model, binding of TRAIL molecules (*blue*) on the "back" of pre-ligated homomeric or heteromeric receptor dimers on the cell membrane induces conformational changes of the receptors, results in opening of the PLAD-PLAD interaction and subsequent binding of a second TRAIL receptor dimer (a). Formation of large ligand-receptor clusters referred to as signalling protein oligomeric transduction structures (SPOTS) are shown in hexagonal arrangement. TRAIL-R3- and TRAIL-R4-mediated interference with death receptor signalling is based on the reduction of signalling-competent receptor complexes (b)

In a more recent work our group investigated the effects of TRAIL-R4 on TRAIL-R1 signalling in detail, aided by mathematical modelling [154]. As expected, the experimental data demonstrate that TRAIL-R4 effectively inhibited TRAIL-R1-mediated apoptosis induction, but also non-apoptotic signalling like activation of NF-κB. Moreover, these effects were not mediated by the cytoplasmic domain of TRAIL-R4 (see Sect. 2.3.3.4), i.e., signalling crosstalk, because a cytoplasmatically truncated TRAIL-R4 mutant showed comparable effects. In addition, the results from mathematical modelling clearly showed that the classical decoy mechanism must be neglectable under the experimental conditions chosen. As both, intracellular signalling by TRAIL-R4 and the decoy mechanism could be ruled out to be effective, the formation of heteromeric complexes was proposed to cause the dominant negative effects of TRAIL-R4 on TRAIL-R1 signalling (Fig. 2.3).

2.3.3.4 Activation of Pro-Survival Pathways by TRAIL-R4

TRAIL and its receptors create a highly complex signalling system not only because of the presence of multiple receptors, but also caused by the fact that individual TRAIL receptors can not only induce apoptosis but are also known to initiate survival pathways. The induction of survival pathways, like e.g., the activation of NF-κB and Akt, has been suggested as an additional mechanism contributing to the inhibitory effects of TRAIL-R4, mediated by its truncated DD suggested to be incapable to induce apoptosis. There exist conflicting results regarding the role of TRAIL-R4 in activation of the transcription factor NF-κB, as initial studies by Marsters and colleagues showed that removal of the intracellular domain of TRAIL-R4 had no effects on TRAIL-mediated apoptosis induction and NF-κB activation. Accordingly, it was proposed that the truncated DD of TRAIL-R4 is not functional and does not play any role in the inhibitory function of this receptor [29]. However, another group reported that TRAIL-R4, alike TRAIL-R1/R2 is capable to activate the NF-κB pathway via its cytoplasmic domain although the precise molecular mechanism remained unclear [30]. It was therefore proposed that NF-κB activation and subsequent transcription of various anti-apoptotic proteins could play a role in TRAIL-R4-mediated resistance against TRAIL. In our experimental systems, however, TRAIL-R1-mediated phosphorylation of inhibitor of NF-κB (IκBα), a central step in the activation of the classical NF-κB pathway, was inhibited by overexpression of both functional and cytoplasmatically deleted TRAIL-R4 [154]. Although it is generally accepted that TRAIL is not a potent inducer of NF-κB activation, this signalling pathway may be controlled in a cell specific manner similar to the activation of Akt where again conflicting results exist. TRAIL-R4 expression in HeLa cells was shown to protect from TRAIL-induced apoptosis and enhanced cell proliferation and these effects could be reversed by inhibiting Akt phosphorylation [166]. Contrary to these results we could not observe any difference in the phosphorylation of Akt in HeLa cells overexpressing TRAIL-R4 [154].

More recent data open a new facet in the field of negative TRAIL receptor interaction. In most studies which have been investigated, the interference between apoptotic and non-apoptotic TRAIL receptors took only the amounts of membrane-expressed receptor molecules into account. It is now clear, however, that TRAIL receptors including TRAIL-R3 and TRAIL-R4 also occur in intracellular compartments and may act there in a still largely undefined manner [5, 96, 119, 167]. It is, therefore, possible that the ligand TRAIL may act also as a stimulus to induce a relocalization of receptors, thereby shifting their function. Further intricate studies will be necessary to verify this hypothesis.

Taken together, three possible mechanisms have been proposed up to now that may contribute to TRAIL-resistance being mediated by TRAIL-R3/TRAIL-R4. These are the classical decoy mechanism which does occur but has been convincingly shown to play no major role under typical experimental conditions. In special (patho)physiological situations this effect could be of significance. The formation of ligand/receptor signalling clusters comprising a mixture of signal competent and incompetent receptors (TRAIL-R1/R2 and TRAIL-R3/R4, respectively) as the second proposed mechanism are believed to have a strong impact (Fig. 2.3). Molecular interactions and parameters guiding their formation are complex, however, including (co)expression levels, distribution in microdomains, PLAD-mediated interaction and finally ligand/receptor interactions. The third possible mechanism, intracellular signal induction mediated by TRAIL-R3 and TRAIL-R4, is again believed to occur in a special context only. Whereas a signalling capacity by the GPI moiety-anchored TRAIL-R3 appears speculative, the biological function of the intracellular domain of TRAIL-R4 needs to be further investigated.

2.4 Outlook

Coming to the insight that the TRAIL system is extremely complex and the role of TRAIL receptors and their crosstalk in cancer are highly undefined, it is evident that we still need much more data from experimental systems and from the clinic. Nevertheless, it appears to be a valuable therapeutic approach to induce apoptosis/necroptosis in tumour cells upon stimulation of TRAIL-R1 and/or TRAIL-R2. To successfully follow this pathway, we need strong agonists like targeted, multimerized TRAIL fusion proteins or receptor-specific agonistic antibody constructs. A multitude of such molecules has been already tested in animal models and clinical studies. In all these approaches it appears beneficial to spare the inhibitory receptors TRAIL-R3 and TRAIL-R4, which can be easily obtained using agonistic antibodies, but also by the construction of receptor-selective mutants of TRAIL.

References

1. Aggarwal BB, Gupta SC, Kim JH (2012) Historical perspectives on tumor necrosis factor and its superfamily: 25 years later, a golden journey. Blood 119(3):651–665. doi:10.1182/blood-2011-04-325225
2. Croft M, Benedict CA, Ware CF (2013) Clinical targeting of the TNF and TNFR superfamilies. Nat Rev Drug Discov 12(2):147–168. doi:10.1038/nrd3930
3. Wajant H, Moosmayer D, Wuest T, Bartke T, Gerlach E, Schonherr U, Peters N, Scheurich P, Pfizenmaier K (2001) Differential activation of TRAIL-R1 and −2 by soluble and membrane TRAIL allows selective surface antigen-directed activation of TRAIL-R2 by a soluble TRAIL derivative. Oncogene 20(30):4101–4106. doi:10.1038/sj.onc.1204558
4. Walczak H, Miller RE, Ariail K, Gliniak B, Griffith TS, Kubin M, Chin W, Jones J, Woodward A, Le T, Smith C, Smolak P, Goodwin RG, Rauch CT, Schuh JC, Lynch DH (1999) Tumoricidal activity of tumor necrosis factor-related apoptosis-inducing ligand in vivo. Nat Med 5(2):157–163. doi:10.1038/5517
5. Haselmann V, Kurz A, Bertsch U, Hubner S, Olempska-Muller M, Fritsch J, Hasler R, Pickl A, Fritsche H, Annewanter F, Engler C, Fleig B, Bernt A, Roder C, Schmidt H, Gelhaus C, Hauser C, Egberts JH, Heneweer C, Rohde AM, Boger C, Knippschild U, Rocken C, Adam D, Walczak H, Schutze S, Janssen O, Wulczyn FG, Wajant H, Kalthoff H, Trauzold A (2014) Nuclear death receptor TRAIL-R2 inhibits maturation of let-7 and promotes proliferation of pancreatic and other tumor cells. Gastroenterology 146(1):278–290. doi:10.1053/j.gastro.2013.10.009

6. Wiley SR, Schooley K, Smolak PJ, Din WS, Huang CP, Nicholl JK, Sutherland GR, Smith TD, Rauch C, Smith CA et al (1995) Identification and characterization of a new member of the TNF family that induces apoptosis. Immunity 3(6):673–682
7. Pitti RM, Marsters SA, Ruppert S, Donahue CJ, Moore A, Ashkenazi A (1996) Induction of apoptosis by Apo-2 ligand, a new member of the tumor necrosis factor cytokine family. J Biol Chem 271(22):12687–12690
8. Krieg A, Krieg T, Wenzel M, Schmitt M, Ramp U, Fang B, Gabbert HE, Gerharz CD, Mahotka C (2003) TRAIL-beta and TRAIL-gamma: two novel splice variants of the human TNF-related apoptosis-inducing ligand (TRAIL) without apoptotic potential. Br J Cancer 88(6):918–927. doi:10.1038/sj.bjc.6600772
9. Wang P, Lu Y, Li C, Li N, Yu P, Ma D (2011) Novel transcript variants of TRAIL show different activities in activation of NF-kappaB and apoptosis. Life Sci 89(23–24):839–846. doi:10.1016/j.lfs.2011.09.003
10. Krieg A, Mersch S, Wolf N, Stoecklein NH, Verde PE, am Esch JS 2nd, Heikaus S, Gabbert HE, Knoefel WT, Mahotka C (2013) Expression of TRAIL-splice variants in gastric carcinomas: identification of TRAIL-gamma as a prognostic marker. BMC Cancer 13:384. doi:10.1186/1471-2407-13-384
11. Spierings DC, de Vries EG, Vellenga E, van den Heuvel FA, Koornstra JJ, Wesseling J, Hollema H, de Jong S (2004) Tissue distribution of the death ligand TRAIL and its receptors. J Histochem Cytochem 52(6):821–831
12. Hymowitz SG, O'Connell MP, Ultsch MH, Hurst A, Totpal K, Ashkenazi A, de Vos AM, Kelley RF (2000) A unique zinc-binding site revealed by a high-resolution X-ray structure of homotrimeric Apo2L/TRAIL. Biochemistry 39(4):633–640
13. Mariani SM, Krammer PH (1998) Differential regulation of TRAIL and CD95 ligand in transformed cells of the T and B lymphocyte lineage. Eur J Immunol 28(3):973–982. doi:10.1002/(SICI)1521-4141(199803)28:03<973::AID-IMMU973>3.0.CO;2-T
14. Muhlenbeck F, Schneider P, Bodmer JL, Schwenzer R, Hauser A, Schubert G, Scheurich P, Moosmayer D, Tschopp J, Wajant H (2000) The tumor necrosis factor-related apoptosis-inducing ligand receptors TRAIL-R1 and TRAIL-R2 have distinct cross-linking requirements for initiation of apoptosis and are non-redundant in JNK activation. J Biol Chem 275(41):32208–32213. doi:10.1074/jbc.M000482200
15. Pan G, O'Rourke K, Chinnaiyan AM, Gentz R, Ebner R, Ni J, Dixit VM (1997) The receptor for the cytotoxic ligand TRAIL. Science 276(5309):111–113
16. Sheridan JP, Marsters SA, Pitti RM, Gurney A, Skubatch M, Baldwin D, Ramakrishnan L, Gray CL, Baker K, Wood WI, Goddard AD, Godowski P, Ashkenazi A (1997) Control of TRAIL-induced apoptosis by a family of signaling and decoy receptors. Science 277(5327): 818–821
17. Screaton GR, Mongkolsapaya J, Xu XN, Cowper AE, McMichael AJ, Bell JI (1997) TRICK2, a new alternatively spliced receptor that transduces the cytotoxic signal from TRAIL. Curr Biol 7(9):693–696
18. Pan G, Ni J, Wei YF, Yu G, Gentz R, Dixit VM (1997) An antagonist decoy receptor and a death domain-containing receptor for TRAIL. Science 277(5327):815–818
19. MacFarlane M, Ahmad M, Srinivasula SM, Fernandes-Alnemri T, Cohen GM, Alnemri ES (1997) Identification and molecular cloning of two novel receptors for the cytotoxic ligand TRAIL. J Biol Chem 272(41):25417–25420
20. Schneider P, Bodmer JL, Thome M, Hofmann K, Holler N, Tschopp J (1997) Characterization of two receptors for TRAIL. FEBS Lett 416(3):329–334
21. Chaudhary PM, Eby M, Jasmin A, Bookwalter A, Murray J, Hood L (1997) Death receptor 5, a new member of the TNFR family, and DR4 induce FADD-dependent apoptosis and activate the NF-kappaB pathway. Immunity 7(6):821–830
22. Wu GS, Burns TF, McDonald ER 3rd, Jiang W, Meng R, Krantz ID, Kao G, Gan DD, Zhou JY, Muschel R, Hamilton SR, Spinner NB, Markowitz S, Wu G, el-Deiry WS (1997) KILLER/DR5 is a DNA damage-inducible p53-regulated death receptor gene. Nat Genet 17(2):141–143. doi:10.1038/ng1097-141

23. Picarda G, Surget S, Guiho R, Teletchea S, Berreur M, Tirode F, Pellat-Deceunynck C, Heymann D, Trichet V, Redini F (2012) A functional, new short isoform of death receptor 4 in Ewing's sarcoma cell lines may be involved in TRAIL sensitivity/resistance mechanisms. Mol Cancer Res 10(3):336–346. doi:10.1158/1541-7786.MCR-11-0390
24. van Roosmalen IA, Quax WJ, Kruyt FA (2014) Two death-inducing human TRAIL receptors to target in cancer: similar or distinct regulation and function? Biochem Pharmacol 91(4):447–456. doi:10.1016/j.bcp.2014.08.010
25. Bertsch U, Roder C, Kalthoff H, Trauzold A (2014) Compartmentalization of TNF-related apoptosis-inducing ligand (TRAIL) death receptor functions: emerging role of nuclear TRAIL-R2. Cell Death Dis 5:e1390. doi:10.1038/cddis.2014.351
26. von Karstedt S, Conti A, Nobis M, Montinaro A, Hartwig T, Lemke J, Legler K, Annewanter F, Campbell AD, Taraborrelli L, Grosse-Wilde A, Coy JF, El-Bahrawy MA, Bergmann F, Koschny R, Werner J, Ganten TM, Schweiger T, Hoetzenecker K, Kenessey I, Hegedus B, Bergmann M, Hauser C, Egberts JH, Becker T, Rocken C, Kalthoff H, Trauzold A, Anderson KI, Sansom OJ, Walczak H (2015) Cancer cell-autonomous TRAIL-R signaling promotes KRAS-driven cancer progression, invasion, and metastasis. Cancer Cell 27(4):561–573. doi:10.1016/j.ccell.2015.02.014
27. Degli-Esposti MA, Smolak PJ, Walczak H, Waugh J, Huang CP, DuBose RF, Goodwin RG, Smith CA (1997) Cloning and characterization of TRAIL-R3, a novel member of the emerging TRAIL receptor family. J Exp Med 186(7):1165–1170
28. Mongkolsapaya J, Cowper AE, Xu XN, Morris G, McMichael AJ, Bell JI, Screaton GR (1998) Lymphocyte inhibitor of TRAIL (TNF-related apoptosis-inducing ligand): a new receptor protecting lymphocytes from the death ligand TRAIL. J Immunol 160(1):3–6
29. Marsters SA, Sheridan JP, Pitti RM, Huang A, Skubatch M, Baldwin D, Yuan J, Gurney A, Goddard AD, Godowski P, Ashkenazi A (1997) A novel receptor for Apo2L/TRAIL contains a truncated death domain. Curr Biol 7(12):1003–1006
30. Degli-Esposti MA, Dougall WC, Smolak PJ, Waugh JY, Smith CA, Goodwin RG (1997) The novel receptor TRAIL-R4 induces NF-kappaB and protects against TRAIL-mediated apoptosis, yet retains an incomplete death domain. Immunity 7(6):813–820
31. Pan G, Ni J, Yu G, Wei YF, Dixit VM (1998) TRUNDD, a new member of the TRAIL receptor family that antagonizes TRAIL signalling. FEBS Lett 424(1–2):41–45
32. Kimberley FC, Screaton GR (2004) Following a TRAIL: update on a ligand and its five receptors. Cell Res 14(5):359–372. doi:10.1038/sj.cr.7290236
33. Krieg A, Schulte am Esch J 2nd, Ramp U, Hosch SB, Knoefel WT, Gabbert HE, Mahotka C (2006) TRAIL-R4-beta: a new splice variant of TRAIL-receptor 4 lacking the cysteine rich domain 1. Biochem Biophys Res Commun 349(1):115–121. doi:10.1016/j.bbrc.2006.08.031
34. Boyle WJ, Simonet WS, Lacey DL (2003) Osteoclast differentiation and activation. Nature 423(6937):337–342. doi:10.1038/nature01658
35. Emery JG, McDonnell P, Burke MB, Deen KC, Lyn S, Silverman C, Dul E, Appelbaum ER, Eichman C, DiPrinzio R, Dodds RA, James IE, Rosenberg M, Lee JC, Young PR (1998) Osteoprotegerin is a receptor for the cytotoxic ligand TRAIL. J Biol Chem 273(23):14363–14367
36. Candido R (2014) The osteoprotegerin/tumor necrosis factor related apoptosis-inducing ligand axis in the kidney. Curr Opin Nephrol Hypertens 23(1):69–74. doi:10.1097/01.mnh.0000437611.42417.7a
37. Pitti RM, Marsters SA, Lawrence DA, Roy M, Kischkel FC, Dowd P, Huang A, Donahue CJ, Sherwood SW, Baldwin DT, Godowski PJ, Wood WI, Gurney AL, Hillan KJ, Cohen RL, Goddard AD, Botstein D, Ashkenazi A (1998) Genomic amplification of a decoy receptor for Fas ligand in lung and colon cancer. Nature 396(6712):699–703. doi:10.1038/25387
38. Arakawa Y, Tachibana O, Hasegawa M, Miyamori T, Yamashita J, Hayashi Y (2005) Frequent gene amplification and overexpression of decoy receptor 3 in glioblastoma. Acta Neuropathol 109(3):294–298. doi:10.1007/s00401-004-0956-6

39. Yu KY, Kwon B, Ni J, Zhai Y, Ebner R, Kwon BS (1999) A newly identified member of tumor necrosis factor receptor superfamily (TR6) suppresses LIGHT-mediated apoptosis. J Biol Chem 274(20):13733–13736
40. Migone TS, Zhang J, Luo X, Zhuang L, Chen C, Hu B, Hong JS, Perry JW, Chen SF, Zhou JX, Cho YH, Ullrich S, Kanakaraj P, Carrell J, Boyd E, Olsen HS, Hu G, Pukac L, Liu D, Ni J, Kim S, Gentz R, Feng P, Moore PA, Ruben SM, Wei P (2002) TL1A is a TNF-like ligand for DR3 and TR6/DcR3 and functions as a T cell costimulator. Immunity 16(3):479–492
41. Wang W, Zhang M, Sun W, Yang S, Su Y, Zhang H, Liu C, Li X, Lin L, Kim S, Okunieff P, Zhang Z, Zhang L (2013) Reduction of decoy receptor 3 enhances TRAIL-mediated apoptosis in pancreatic cancer. PLoS One 8(10):e74272. doi:10.1371/journal.pone.0074272
42. Zhou J, Song S, He S, Wang Z, Zhang B, Li D, Zhu D (2013) Silencing of decoy receptor 3 (DcR3) expression by siRNA in pancreatic carcinoma cells induces Fas ligand-mediated apoptosis in vitro and in vivo. Int J Mol Med 32(3):653–660. doi:10.3892/ijmm.2013.1437
43. Kerr JF, Wyllie AH, Currie AR (1972) Apoptosis: a basic biological phenomenon with wide-ranging implications in tissue kinetics. Br J Cancer 26(4):239–257
44. Davidovich P, Kearney CJ, Martin SJ (2014) Inflammatory outcomes of apoptosis, necrosis and necroptosis. Biol Chem 395(10):1163–1171. doi:10.1515/hsz-2014-0164
45. Renehan AG, Booth C, Potten CS (2001) What is apoptosis, and why is it important? BMJ 322(7301):1536–1538
46. Elmore S (2007) Apoptosis: a review of programmed cell death. Toxicol Pathol 35(4):495–516. doi:10.1080/01926230701320337
47. Ouyang L, Shi Z, Zhao S, Wang FT, Zhou TT, Liu B, Bao JK (2012) Programmed cell death pathways in cancer: a review of apoptosis, autophagy and programmed necrosis. Cell Prolif 45(6):487–498. doi:10.1111/j.1365-2184.2012.00845.x
48. Chen D, Yu J, Zhang L (2016) Necroptosis: an alternative cell death program defending against cancer. Biochim Biophys Acta 1865(2):228–236. doi:10.1016/j.bbcan.2016.03.003
49. Azijli K, Weyhenmeyer B, Peters GJ, de Jong S, Kruyt FA (2013) Non-canonical kinase signaling by the death ligand TRAIL in cancer cells: discord in the death receptor family. Cell Death Differ 20(7):858–868. doi:10.1038/cdd.2013.28
50. Varfolomeev E, Maecker H, Sharp D, Lawrence D, Renz M, Vucic D, Ashkenazi A (2005) Molecular determinants of kinase pathway activation by Apo2 ligand/tumor necrosis factor-related apoptosis-inducing ligand. J Biol Chem 280(49):40599–40608. doi:10.1074/jbc.M509560200
51. Grunert M, Gottschalk K, Kapahnke J, Gundisch S, Kieser A, Jeremias I (2012) The adaptor protein FADD and the initiator caspase-8 mediate activation of NF-kappaB by TRAIL. Cell Death Dis 3:e414. doi:10.1038/cddis.2012.154
52. Zhang L, Blackwell K, Workman LM, Chen S, Pope MR, Janz S, Habelhah H (2015) RIP1 cleavage in the kinase domain regulates TRAIL-induced NF-kappaB activation and lymphoma survival. Mol Cell Biol 35(19):3324–3338. doi:10.1128/MCB.00692-15
53. Song JH, Tse MC, Bellail A, Phuphanich S, Khuri F, Kneteman NM, Hao C (2007) Lipid rafts and nonrafts mediate tumor necrosis factor related apoptosis-inducing ligand induced apoptotic and nonapoptotic signals in non small cell lung carcinoma cells. Cancer Res 67(14):6946–6955. doi:10.1158/0008-5472.CAN-06-3896
54. Collison A, Foster PS, Mattes J (2009) Emerging role of tumour necrosis factor-related apoptosis-inducing ligand (TRAIL) as a key regulator of inflammatory responses. Clin Exp Pharmacol Physiol 36(11):1049–1053. doi:10.1111/j.1440-1681.2009.05258.x
55. Mizrahi K, Askenasy N (2014) Physiological functions of TNF family receptor/ligand interactions in hematopoiesis and transplantation. Blood 124(2):176–183. doi:10.1182/blood-2014-03-559641
56. Sato K, Hida S, Takayanagi H, Yokochi T, Kayagaki N, Takeda K, Yagita H, Okumura K, Tanaka N, Taniguchi T, Ogasawara K (2001) Antiviral response by natural killer cells through TRAIL gene induction by IFN-alpha/beta. Eur J Immunol 31(11):3138–3146. doi:10.1002/1521-4141(200111)31:11<3138::AID-IMMU3138>3.0.CO;2-B

57. Stegmann KA, Bjorkstrom NK, Veber H, Ciesek S, Riese P, Wiegand J, Hadem J, Suneetha PV, Jaroszewicz J, Wang C, Schlaphoff V, Fytili P, Cornberg M, Manns MP, Geffers R, Pietschmann T, Guzman CA, Ljunggren HG, Wedemeyer H (2010) Interferon-alpha-induced TRAIL on natural killer cells is associated with control of hepatitis C virus infection. Gastroenterology 138(5):1885–1897. doi:10.1053/j.gastro.2010.01.051
58. Schuster IS, Wikstrom ME, Brizard G, Coudert JD, Estcourt MJ, Manzur M, O'Reilly LA, Smyth MJ, Trapani JA, Hill GR, Andoniou CE, Degli-Esposti MA (2014) TRAIL+ NK cells control CD4+ T cell responses during chronic viral infection to limit autoimmunity. Immunity 41(4):646–656. doi:10.1016/j.immuni.2014.09.013
59. Cook KD, Kline HC, Whitmire JK (2015) NK cells inhibit humoral immunity by reducing the abundance of CD4+ T follicular helper cells during a chronic virus infection. J Leukoc Biol 98(2):153–162. doi:10.1189/jlb.4HI1214-594R
60. Waggoner SN, Cornberg M, Selin LK, Welsh RM (2011) Natural killer cells act as rheostats modulating antiviral T cells. Nature 481(7381):394–398. doi:10.1038/nature10624
61. Lang PA, Lang KS, Xu HC, Grusdat M, Parish IA, Recher M, Elford AR, Dhanji S, Shaabani N, Tran CW, Dissanayake D, Rahbar R, Ghazarian M, Brustle A, Fine J, Chen P, Weaver CT, Klose C, Diefenbach A, Haussinger D, Carlyle JR, Kaech SM, Mak TW, Ohashi PS (2012) Natural killer cell activation enhances immune pathology and promotes chronic infection by limiting CD8+ T-cell immunity. Proc Natl Acad Sci U S A 109(4):1210–1215. doi:10.1073/pnas.1118834109
62. Peppa D, Gill US, Reynolds G, Easom NJ, Pallett LJ, Schurich A, Micco L, Nebbia G, Singh HD, Adams DH, Kennedy PT, Maini MK (2013) Up-regulation of a death receptor renders antiviral T cells susceptible to NK cell-mediated deletion. J Exp Med 210(1):99–114. doi:10.1084/jem.20121172
63. Jeremias I, Herr I, Boehler T, Debatin KM (1998) TRAIL/Apo-2-ligand-induced apoptosis in human T cells. Eur J Immunol 28(1):143–152. doi:10.1002/(SICI)1521-4141(199801)28:01<143::AID-IMMU143>3.0.CO;2-3
64. Kayagaki N, Yamaguchi N, Nakayama M, Eto H, Okumura K, Yagita H (1999) Type I interferons (IFNs) regulate tumor necrosis factor-related apoptosis-inducing ligand (TRAIL) expression on human T cells: a novel mechanism for the antitumor effects of type I IFNs. J Exp Med 189(9):1451–1460
65. Zhang XR, Zhang LY, Devadas S, Li L, Keegan AD, Shi YF (2003) Reciprocal expression of TRAIL and CD95L in Th1 and Th2 cells: role of apoptosis in T helper subset differentiation. Cell Death Differ 10(2):203–210. doi:10.1038/sj.cdd.4401138
66. Roberts AI, Devadas S, Zhang X, Zhang L, Keegan A, Greeneltch K, Solomon J, Wei L, Das J, Sun E, Liu C, Yuan Z, Zhou JN, Shi Y (2003) The role of activation-induced cell death in the differentiation of T-helper-cell subsets. Immunol Res 28(3):285–293. doi:10.1385/IR:28:3:285
67. Weckmann M, Collison A, Simpson JL, Kopp MV, Wark PA, Smyth MJ, Yagita H, Matthaei KI, Hansbro N, Whitehead B, Gibson PG, Foster PS, Mattes J (2007) Critical link between TRAIL and CCL20 for the activation of TH2 cells and the expression of allergic airway disease. Nat Med 13(11):1308–1315. doi:10.1038/nm1660
68. Mirandola P, Ponti C, Gobbi G, Sponzilli I, Vaccarezza M, Cocco L, Zauli G, Secchiero P, Manzoli FA, Vitale M (2004) Activated human NK and CD8+ T cells express both TNF-related apoptosis-inducing ligand (TRAIL) and TRAIL receptors but are resistant to TRAIL-mediated cytotoxicity. Blood 104(8):2418–2424. doi:10.1182/blood-2004-04-1294
69. Brincks EL, Gurung P, Langlois RA, Hemann EA, Legge KL, Griffith TS (2011) The magnitude of the T cell response to a clinically significant dose of influenza virus is regulated by TRAIL. J Immunol 187(9):4581–4588. doi:10.4049/jimmunol.1002241
70. Brincks EL, Katewa A, Kucaba TA, Griffith TS, Legge KL (2008) CD8 T cells utilize TRAIL to control influenza virus infection. J Immunol 181(7):4918–4925
71. Herold S, Steinmueller M, von Wulffen W, Cakarova L, Pinto R, Pleschka S, Mack M, Kuziel WA, Corazza N, Brunner T, Seeger W, Lohmeyer J (2008) Lung epithelial apoptosis

in influenza virus pneumonia: the role of macrophage-expressed TNF-related apoptosis-inducing ligand. J Exp Med 205(13):3065–3077. doi:10.1084/jem.20080201
72. Gurung P, Rai D, Condotta SA, Babcock JC, Badovinac VP, Griffith TS (2011) Immune unresponsiveness to secondary heterologous bacterial infection after sepsis induction is TRAIL dependent. J Immunol 187(5):2148–2154. doi:10.4049/jimmunol.1101180
73. Beyer K, Poetschke C, Partecke LI, von Bernstorff W, Maier S, Broeker BM, Heidecke CD (2014) TRAIL induces neutrophil apoptosis and dampens sepsis-induced organ injury in murine colon ascendens stent peritonitis. PLoS One 9(6):e97451. doi:10.1371/journal.pone.0097451
74. Falschlehner C, Schaefer U, Walczak H (2009) Following TRAIL's path in the immune system. Immunology 127(2):145–154. doi:10.1111/j.1365-2567.2009.03058.x
75. Fanger NA, Maliszewski CR, Schooley K, Griffith TS (1999) Human dendritic cells mediate cellular apoptosis via tumor necrosis factor-related apoptosis-inducing ligand (TRAIL). J Exp Med 190(8):1155–1164
76. Griffith TS, Wiley SR, Kubin MZ, Sedger LM, Maliszewski CR, Fanger NA (1999) Monocyte-mediated tumoricidal activity via the tumor necrosis factor-related cytokine, TRAIL. J Exp Med 189(8):1343–1354
77. Takeda K, Hayakawa Y, Smyth MJ, Kayagaki N, Yamaguchi N, Kakuta S, Iwakura Y, Yagita H, Okumura K (2001) Involvement of tumor necrosis factor-related apoptosis-inducing ligand in surveillance of tumor metastasis by liver natural killer cells. Nat Med 7(1):94–100. doi:10.1038/83416
78. Lelaidier M, Diaz-Rodriguez Y, Cordeau M, Cordeiro P, Haddad E, Herblot S, Duval M (2015) TRAIL-mediated killing of acute lymphoblastic leukemia by plasmacytoid dendritic cell-activated natural killer cells. Oncotarget 6(30):29440–29455. doi:10.18632/oncotarget.4984
79. Tecchio C, Scapini P, Pizzolo G, Cassatella MA (2013) On the cytokines produced by human neutrophils in tumors. Semin Cancer Biol 23(3):159–170. doi:10.1016/j.semcancer.2013.02.004
80. Lin YC, Richburg JH (2014) Characterization of the role of tumor necrosis factor apoptosis inducing ligand (TRAIL) in spermatogenesis through the evaluation of trail gene-deficient mice. PLoS One 9(4):e93926. doi:10.1371/journal.pone.0093926
81. Zauli G, Celeghini C, Monasta L, Martinelli M, Luppi S, Gonelli A, Grill V, Ricci G, Secchiero P (2014) Soluble TRAIL is present at high concentrations in seminal plasma and promotes spermatozoa survival. Reproduction 148(2):191–198. doi:10.1530/REP-14-0144
82. Zhang XD, Nguyen T, Thomas WD, Sanders JE, Hersey P (2000) Mechanisms of resistance of normal cells to TRAIL induced apoptosis vary between different cell types. FEBS Lett 482(3):193–199
83. Gochuico BR, Zhang J, Ma BY, Marshak-Rothstein A, Fine A (2000) TRAIL expression in vascular smooth muscle. Am J Physiol Lung Cell Mol Physiol 278(5):L1045–L1050
84. Secchiero P, Gonelli A, Carnevale E, Milani D, Pandolfi A, Zella D, Zauli G (2003) TRAIL promotes the survival and proliferation of primary human vascular endothelial cells by activating the Akt and ERK pathways. Circulation 107(17):2250–2256. doi:10.1161/01.CIR.0000062702.60708.C4
85. Secchiero P, Corallini F, di Iasio MG, Gonelli A, Barbarotto E, Zauli G (2005) TRAIL counteracts the proadhesive activity of inflammatory cytokines in endothelial cells by down-modulating CCL8 and CXCL10 chemokine expression and release. Blood 105(9):3413–3419. doi:10.1182/blood-2004-10-4111
86. Zauli G, Pandolfi A, Gonelli A, Di Pietro R, Guarnieri S, Ciabattoni G, Rana R, Vitale M, Secchiero P (2003) Tumor necrosis factor-related apoptosis-inducing ligand (TRAIL) sequentially upregulates nitric oxide and prostanoid production in primary human endothelial cells. Circ Res 92(7):732–740. doi:10.1161/01.RES.0000067928.83455.9C
87. Di Pietro R, Mariggio MA, Guarnieri S, Sancilio S, Giardinelli A, Di Silvestre S, Consoli A, Zauli G, Pandolfi A (2006) Tumor necrosis factor-related apoptosis-inducing ligand

(TRAIL) regulates endothelial nitric oxide synthase (eNOS) activity and its localization within the human vein endothelial cells (HUVEC) in culture. J Cell Biochem 97(4):782–794. doi:10.1002/jcb.20686

88. Baudino TA (2015) Targeted cancer therapy: the next generation of cancer treatment. Curr Drug Discov Technol 12(1):3–20
89. Johnston PG (2014) Identification of clinically relevant molecular subtypes in colorectal cancer: the dawning of a new era. Oncologist 19(5):568–573. doi:10.1634/theoncologist.2014-038
90. Siena S, Sartore-Bianchi A, Di Nicolantonio F, Balfour J, Bardelli A (2009) Biomarkers predicting clinical outcome of epidermal growth factor receptor-targeted therapy in metastatic colorectal cancer. J Natl Cancer Inst 101(19):1308–1324. doi:10.1093/jnci/djp280
91. Strater J, Hinz U, Walczak H, Mechtersheimer G, Koretz K, Herfarth C, Moller P, Lehnert T (2002) Expression of TRAIL and TRAIL receptors in colon carcinoma: TRAIL-R1 is an independent prognostic parameter. Clin Cancer Res 8(12):3734–3740
92. McCarthy MM, Sznol M, DiVito KA, Camp RL, Rimm DL, Kluger HM (2005) Evaluating the expression and prognostic value of TRAIL-R1 and TRAIL-R2 in breast cancer. Clin Cancer Res 11(14):5188–5194. doi:10.1158/1078-0432.CCR-05-0158
93. van Geelen CM, Westra JL, de Vries EG, Boersma-van Ek W, Zwart N, Hollema H, Boezen HM, Mulder NH, Plukker JT, de Jong S, Kleibeuker JH, Koornstra JJ (2006) Prognostic significance of tumor necrosis factor-related apoptosis-inducing ligand and its receptors in adjuvantly treated stage III colon cancer patients. J Clin Oncol Off J Am Soc Clin Oncol 24(31):4998–5004. doi:10.1200/JCO.2006.06.8809
94. Oikonomou E, Kosmidou V, Katseli A, Kothonidis K, Mourtzoukou D, Kontogeorgos G, Andera L, Zografos G, Pintzas A (2009) TRAIL receptor upregulation and the implication of KRAS/BRAF mutations in human colon cancer tumors. Int J Cancer 125(9):2127–2135. doi:10.1002/ijc.24613
95. Duiker EW, van der Zee AG, de Graeff P, Boersma-van Ek W, Hollema H, de Bock GH, de Jong S, de Vries EG (2010) The extrinsic apoptosis pathway and its prognostic impact in ovarian cancer. Gynecol Oncol 116(3):549–555. doi:10.1016/j.ygyno.2009.09.014
96. Gallmeier E, Bader DC, Kriegl L, Berezowska S, Seeliger H, Goke B, Kirchner T, Bruns C, De Toni EN (2013) Loss of TRAIL-receptors is a recurrent feature in pancreatic cancer and determines the prognosis of patients with no nodal metastasis after surgery. PLoS One 8(2):e56760. doi:10.1371/journal.pone.0056760
97. Shin MS, Kim HS, Lee SH, Park WS, Kim SY, Park JY, Lee JH, Lee SK, Lee SN, Jung SS, Han JY, Kim H, Lee JY, Yoo NJ (2001) Mutations of tumor necrosis factor-related apoptosis-inducing ligand receptor 1 (TRAIL-R1) and receptor 2 (TRAIL-R2) genes in metastatic breast cancers. Cancer Res 61(13):4942–4946
98. Jeng YM, Hsu HC (2002) Mutation of the DR5/TRAIL receptor 2 gene is infrequent in hepatocellular carcinoma. Cancer Lett 181(2):205–208
99. Teng MS, Brandwein-Gensler MS, Teixeira MS, Martignetti JA, Duffey DC (2005) A study of TRAIL receptors in squamous cell carcinoma of the head and neck. Arch Otolaryngol Head Neck Surg 131(5):407–412. doi:10.1001/archotol.131.5.407
100. Pai SI, Wu GS, Ozoren N, Wu L, Jen J, Sidransky D, El-Deiry WS (1998) Rare loss-of-function mutation of a death receptor gene in head and neck cancer. Cancer Res 58(16):3513–3518
101. Martinez-Ferrandis JI, Rodriguez-Lopez R, Milne RL, Gonzalez E, Cebolla E, Chirivella I, Zamora P, Arias JI, Palacios S, Cervantes A, Diez O, Benitez J, Armengod ME (2007) Polymorphisms in TRAIL receptor genes and risk of breast cancer in Spanish women. Cancer Biomark 3(2):89–93
102. Jamshidi M, Fagerholm R, Khan S, Aittomaki K, Czene K, Darabi H, Li J, Andrulis IL, Chang-Claude J, Devilee P, Fasching PA, Michailidou K, Bolla MK, Dennis J, Wang Q, Guo Q, Rhenius V, Cornelissen S, Rudolph A, Knight JA, Loehberg CR, Burwinkel B, Marme F, Hopper JL, Southey MC, Bojesen SE, Flyger H, Brenner H, Holleczek B, Margolin S, Mannermaa A, Kosma VM, kConFab I, Van Dyck L, Nevelsteen I, Couch FJ, Olson JE, Giles GG, McLean C, Haiman CA, Henderson BE, Winqvist R, Pylkas K, Tollenaar RA, Garcia-Closas M, Figueroa J, Hooning MJ, Martens JW, Cox A, Cross SS, Simard J, Dunning AM,

Easton DF, Pharoah PD, Hall P, Blomqvist C, Schmidt MK, Nevanlinna H (2015) SNP-SNP interaction analysis of NF-kappaB signaling pathway on breast cancer survival. Oncotarget 6(35):37979–37994. doi:10.18632/oncotarget.4991

103. Min YJ, Lee JH, Choi SJ, Chi HS, Lee JS, Kim WK, Lee KH (2004) Prognostic significance of Fas (CD95) and TRAIL receptors (DR4/DR5) expression in acute myelogenous leukemia. Leuk Res 28(4):359–365. doi:10.1016/j.leukres.2003.08.015
104. Koornstra JJ, Kleibeuker JH, van Geelen CM, Rijcken FE, Hollema H, de Vries EG, de Jong S (2003) Expression of TRAIL (TNF-related apoptosis-inducing ligand) and its receptors in normal colonic mucosa, adenomas, and carcinomas. J Pathol 200(3):327–335. doi:10.1002/path.1364
105. Sanlioglu AD, Korcum AF, Pestereli E, Erdogan G, Karaveli S, Savas B, Griffith TS, Sanlioglu S (2007) TRAIL death receptor-4 expression positively correlates with the tumor grade in breast cancer patients with invasive ductal carcinoma. Int J Radiat Oncol Biol Phys 69(3):716–723. doi:10.1016/j.ijrobp.2007.03.057
106. Li Y, Jin X, Li J, Jin X, Yu J, Sun X, Chu Y, Xu C, Li X, Wang X, Kakehi Y, Wu X (2012) Expression of TRAIL, DR4, and DR5 in bladder cancer: correlation with response to adjuvant therapy and implications of prognosis. Urology 79(4):968.e967–968.e915. doi:10.1016/j.urology.2011.11.011
107. Ganten TM, Sykora J, Koschny R, Batke E, Aulmann S, Mansmann U, Stremmel W, Sinn HP, Walczak H (2009) Prognostic significance of tumour necrosis factor-related apoptosis-inducing ligand (TRAIL) receptor expression in patients with breast cancer. J Mol Med 87(10):995–1007. doi:10.1007/s00109-009-0510-z
108. Koschny R, Brost S, Hinz U, Sykora J, Batke EM, Singer S, Breuhahn K, Stremmel W, Walczak H, Schemmer P, Schirmacher P, Ganten TM (2013) Cytosolic and nuclear caspase-8 have opposite impact on survival after liver resection for hepatocellular carcinoma. BMC Cancer 13:532. doi:10.1186/1471-2407-13-532
109. Macher-Goeppinger S, Aulmann S, Tagscherer KE, Wagener N, Haferkamp A, Penzel R, Brauckhoff A, Hohenfellner M, Sykora J, Walczak H, Teh BT, Autschbach F, Herpel E, Schirmacher P, Roth W (2009) Prognostic value of tumor necrosis factor-related apoptosis-inducing ligand (TRAIL) and TRAIL receptors in renal cell cancer. Clin Cancer Res 15(2):650–659. doi:10.1158/1078-0432.CCR-08-0284
110. Yoldas B, Ozer C, Ozen O, Canpolat T, Dogan I, Griffith TS, Sanlioglu S, Ozluoglu LN (2011) Clinical significance of TRAIL and TRAIL receptors in patients with head and neck cancer. Head Neck 33(9):1278–1284. doi:10.1002/hed.21598
111. Spierings DC, de Vries EG, Timens W, Groen HJ, Boezen HM, de Jong S (2003) Expression of TRAIL and TRAIL death receptors in stage III non-small cell lung cancer tumors. Clin Cancer Res 9(9):3397–3405
112. Cooper WA, Kohonen-Corish MR, Zhuang L, McCaughan B, Kennedy C, Screaton G, Sutherland RL, Lee CS (2008) Role and prognostic significance of tumor necrosis factor-related apoptosis-inducing ligand death receptor DR5 in nonsmall-cell lung cancer and precursor lesions. Cancer 113(1):135–142. doi:10.1002/cncr.23528
113. Vigneswaran N, Baucum DC, Wu J, Lou Y, Bouquot J, Muller S, Zacharias W (2007) Repression of tumor necrosis factor-related apoptosis-inducing ligand (TRAIL) but not its receptors during oral cancer progression. BMC Cancer 7:108. doi:10.1186/1471-2407-7-108
114. Hernandez-Cueto A, Hernandez-Cueto D, Antonio-Andres G, Mendoza-Marin M, Jimenez-Gutierrez C, Sandoval-Mejia AL, Mora-Campos R, Gonzalez-Bonilla C, Vega MI, Bonavida B, Huerta-Yepez S (2014) Death receptor 5 expression is inversely correlated with prostate cancer progression. Mol Med Rep 10(5):2279–2286. doi:10.3892/mmr.2014.2504
115. Bavi P, Prabhakaran SE, Abubaker J, Qadri Z, George T, Al-Sanea N, Abduljabbar A, Ashari LH, Alhomoud S, Al-Dayel F, Hussain AR, Uddin S, Al-Kuraya KS (2010) Prognostic significance of TRAIL death receptors in middle eastern colorectal carcinomas and their correlation to oncogenic KRAS alterations. Mol Cancer 9:203. doi:10.1186/1476-4598-9-203
116. Yao Q, Du J, Lin J, Luo Y, Wang Y, Liu Y, Zhang B, Ren C, Liu C (2016) Prognostic significance of TRAIL signalling molecules in cervical squamous cell carcinoma. J Clin Pathol 69(2):122–127. doi:10.1136/jclinpath-2014-202811

117. Kuijlen JM, Mooij JJ, Platteel I, Hoving EW, van der Graaf WT, Span MM, Hollema H, den Dunnen WF (2006) TRAIL-receptor expression is an independent prognostic factor for survival in patients with a primary glioblastoma multiforme. J Neurooncol 78(2):161–171. doi:10.1007/s11060-005-9081-1
118. Kriegl L, Jung A, Horst D, Rizzani A, Jackstadt R, Hermeking H, Gallmeier E, Gerbes AL, Kirchner T, Goke B, De Toni EN (2012) Microsatellite instability, KRAS mutations and cellular distribution of TRAIL-receptors in early stage colorectal cancer. PLoS One 7(12):e51654. doi:10.1371/journal.pone.0051654
119. Chen JJ, Shen HC, Rivera Rosado LA, Zhang Y, Di X, Zhang B (2012) Mislocalization of death receptors correlates with cellular resistance to their cognate ligands in human breast cancer cells. Oncotarget 3(8):833–842. doi:10.18632/oncotarget.542
120. Koksal IT, Sanlioglu AD, Karacay B, Griffith TS, Sanlioglu S (2008) Tumor necrosis factor-related apoptosis inducing ligand-R4 decoy receptor expression is correlated with high Gleason scores, prostate-specific antigen recurrence, and decreased survival in patients with prostate carcinoma. Urol Oncol 26(2):158–165. doi:10.1016/j.urolonc.2007.01.022
121. Sanlioglu AD, Dirice E, Elpek O, Korcum AF, Ozdogan M, Suleymanlar I, Balci MK, Griffith TS, Sanlioglu S (2009) High TRAIL death receptor 4 and decoy receptor 2 expression correlates with significant cell death in pancreatic ductal adenocarcinoma patients. Pancreas 38(2):154–160. doi:10.1097/MPA.0b013e31818db9e3
122. Koschny R, Krupp W, Xu LX, Mueller WC, Bauer M, Sinn P, Keller M, Koschny T, Walczak H, Bruckner T, Ganten TM, Holland H (2015) WHO grade related expression of TRAIL-receptors and apoptosis regulators in meningioma. Pathol Res Pract 211(2):109–116. doi:10.1016/j.prp.2014.11.002
123. Granci V, Bibeau F, Kramar A, Boissiere-Michot F, Thezenas S, Thirion A, Gongora C, Martineau P, Del Rio M, Ychou M (2008) Prognostic significance of TRAIL-R1 and TRAIL-R3 expression in metastatic colorectal carcinomas. Eur J Cancer 44(15):2312–2318. doi:10.1016/j.ejca.2008.06.042
124. Erkul E, Kucukodaci Z, Pinar D, Gungor A, Alparslan Babayigit M, Kurt O, Cincik H (2016) TRAIL and TRAIL receptors in patients with laryngeal cancer. Head Neck 38(Suppl 1):E535–E541. doi:10.1002/hed.24035
125. Bolkun L, Lemancewicz D, Jablonska E, Szumowska A, Bolkun-Skornicka U, Moniuszko M, Dzieciol J, Kloczko J (2015) Prognostic significance of ligands belonging to tumour necrosis factor superfamily in acute lymphoblastic leukaemia. Leuk Res 39(3):290–295. doi:10.1016/j.leukres.2014.12.012
126. Bolkun L, Lemancewicz D, Jablonska E, Szumowska A, Bolkun-Skornicka U, Ratajczak-Wrona W, Dzieciol J, Kloczko J (2015) The impact of TNF superfamily molecules on overall survival in acute myeloid leukaemia: correlation with biological and clinical features. Ann Hematol 94(1):35–43. doi:10.1007/s00277-014-2178-x
127. Toiyama D, Takaha N, Shinnoh M, Ueda T, Kimura Y, Nakamura T, Hongo F, Mikami K, Kamoi K, Kawauchi A, Miki T (2013) Significance of serum tumor necrosis factor-related apoptosis-inducing ligand as a prognostic biomarker for renal cell carcinoma. Mol Clin Oncol 1(1):69–74. doi:10.3892/mco.2012.35
128. McLornan DP, Barrett HL, Cummins R, McDermott U, McDowell C, Conlon SJ, Coyle VM, Van Schaeybroeck S, Wilson R, Kay EW, Longley DB, Johnston PG (2010) Prognostic significance of TRAIL signaling molecules in stage II and III colorectal cancer. Clin Cancer Res 16(13):3442–3451. doi:10.1158/1078-0432.CCR-10-0052
129. de Miguel D, Lemke J, Anel A, Walczak H, Martinez-Lostao L (2016) Onto better TRAILs for cancer treatment. Cell Death Differ 23(5):733–747. doi:10.1038/cdd.2015.174
130. Kelley SK, Harris LA, Xie D, Deforge L, Totpal K, Bussiere J, Fox JA (2001) Preclinical studies to predict the disposition of Apo2L/tumor necrosis factor-related apoptosis-inducing ligand in humans: characterization of in vivo efficacy, pharmacokinetics, and safety. J Pharmacol Exp Ther 299(1):31–38
131. Ganten TM, Koschny R, Sykora J, Schulze-Bergkamen H, Buchler P, Haas TL, Schader MB, Untergasser A, Stremmel W, Walczak H (2006) Preclinical differentiation between appar-

ently safe and potentially hepatotoxic applications of TRAIL either alone or in combination with chemotherapeutic drugs. Clin Cancer Res 12(8):2640–2646. doi:10.1158/1078-0432.CCR-05-2635
132. Berg D, Lehne M, Muller N, Siegmund D, Munkel S, Sebald W, Pfizenmaier K, Wajant H (2007) Enforced covalent trimerization increases the activity of the TNF ligand family members TRAIL and CD95L. Cell Death Differ 14(12):2021–2034. doi:10.1038/sj.cdd.4402213
133. Schneider B, Munkel S, Krippner-Heidenreich A, Grunwald I, Wels WS, Wajant H, Pfizenmaier K, Gerspach J (2010) Potent antitumoral activity of TRAIL through generation of tumor-targeted single-chain fusion proteins. Cell Death Dis 1:e68. doi:10.1038/cddis.2010.45
134. Gieffers C, Kluge M, Merz C, Sykora J, Thiemann M, Schaal R, Fischer C, Branschadel M, Abhari BA, Hohenberger P, Fulda S, Fricke H, Hill O (2013) APG350 induces superior clustering of TRAIL receptors and shows therapeutic antitumor efficacy independent of cross-linking via Fcgamma receptors. Mol Cancer Ther 12(12):2735–2747. doi:10.1158/1535-7163.MCT-13-0323
135. Siegemund M, Pollak N, Seifert O, Wahl K, Hanak K, Vogel A, Nussler AK, Gottsch D, Munkel S, Bantel H, Kontermann RE, Pfizenmaier K (2012) Superior antitumoral activity of dimerized targeted single-chain TRAIL fusion proteins under retention of tumor selectivity. Cell Death Dis 3:e295. doi:10.1038/cddis.2012.29
136. de Bruyn M, Wei Y, Wiersma VR, Samplonius DF, Klip HG, van der Zee AG, Yang B, Helfrich W, Bremer E (2011) Cell surface delivery of TRAIL strongly augments the tumoricidal activity of T cells. Clin Cancer Res 17(17):5626–5637. doi:10.1158/1078-0432.CCR-11-0303
137. El-Mesery M, Trebing J, Schafer V, Weisenberger D, Siegmund D, Wajant H (2013) CD40-directed scFv-TRAIL fusion proteins induce CD40-restricted tumor cell death and activate dendritic cells. Cell Death Dis 4:e916. doi:10.1038/cddis.2013.402
138. Wiersma VR, de Bruyn M, Shi C, Gooden MJ, Wouters MC, Samplonius DF, Hendriks D, Nijman HW, Wei Y, Zhou J, Helfrich W, Bremer E (2015) C-type lectin-like molecule-1 (CLL1)-targeted TRAIL augments the tumoricidal activity of granulocytes and potentiates therapeutic antibody-dependent cell-mediated cytotoxicity. MAbs 7(2):321–330. doi:10.1080/19420862.2015.1007811
139. Lemke J, von Karstedt S, Zinngrebe J, Walczak H (2014) Getting TRAIL back on track for cancer therapy. Cell Death Differ 21(9):1350–1364. doi:10.1038/cdd.2014.81
140. Yang TM, Barbone D, Fennell DA, Broaddus VC (2009) Bcl-2 family proteins contribute to apoptotic resistance in lung cancer multicellular spheroids. Am J Respir Cell Mol Biol 41(1):14–23. doi:10.1165/rcmb.2008-0320OC
141. Chandrasekaran S, Marshall JR, Messing JA, Hsu JW, King MR (2014) TRAIL-mediated apoptosis in breast cancer cells cultured as 3D spheroids. PLoS One 9(10):e111487. doi:10.1371/journal.pone.0111487
142. Newsom-Davis T, Prieske S, Walczak H (2009) Is TRAIL the holy grail of cancer therapy? Apoptosis 14(4):607–623. doi:10.1007/s10495-009-0321-2
143. Bernard D, Quatannens B, Vandenbunder B, Abbadie C (2001) Rel/NF-kappaB transcription factors protect against tumor necrosis factor (TNF)-related apoptosis-inducing ligand (TRAIL)-induced apoptosis by up-regulating the TRAIL decoy receptor DcR1. J Biol Chem 276(29):27322–27328. doi:10.1074/jbc.M011183200
144. Sanlioglu AD, Dirice E, Aydin C, Erin N, Koksoy S, Sanlioglu S (2005) Surface TRAIL decoy receptor-4 expression is correlated with TRAIL resistance in MCF7 breast cancer cells. BMC Cancer 5:54. doi:10.1186/1471-2407-5-54
145. Riccioni R, Pasquini L, Mariani G, Saulle E, Rossini A, Diverio D, Pelosi E, Vitale A, Chierichini A, Cedrone M, Foa R, Lo Coco F, Peschle C, Testa U (2005) TRAIL decoy receptors mediate resistance of acute myeloid leukemia cells to TRAIL. Haematologica 90(5):612–624
146. Sanlioglu AD, Karacay B, Koksal IT, Griffith TS, Sanlioglu S (2007) DcR2 (TRAIL-R4) siRNA and adenovirus delivery of TRAIL (Ad5hTRAIL) break down in vitro tumorigenic

potential of prostate carcinoma cells. Cancer Gene Ther 14(12):976–984. doi:10.1038/sj.cgt.7701087
147. Chamuleau ME, Ossenkoppele GJ, van Rhenen A, van Dreunen L, Jirka SM, Zevenbergen A, Schuurhuis GJ, van de Loosdrecht AA (2011) High TRAIL-R3 expression on leukemic blasts is associated with poor outcome and induces apoptosis-resistance which can be overcome by targeting TRAIL-R2. Leuk Res 35(6):741–749. doi:10.1016/j.leukres.2010.12.032
148. Ashkenazi A, Dixit VM (1999) Apoptosis control by death and decoy receptors. Curr Opin Cell Biol 11(2):255–260
149. Morizot A, Merino D, Lalaoui N, Jacquemin G, Granci V, Iessi E, Lanneau D, Bouyer F, Solary E, Chauffert B, Saas P, Garrido C, Micheau O (2011) Chemotherapy overcomes TRAIL-R4-mediated TRAIL resistance at the DISC level. Cell Death Differ 18(4):700–711. doi:10.1038/cdd.2010.144
150. Wada S, Manabe N, Nakayama M, Inou N, Matsui T, Miyamoto H (2002) TRAIL-decoy receptor 1 plays inhibitory role in apoptosis of granulosa cells from pig ovarian follicles. J Vet Med Sci 64(5):435–439
151. Griffith TS, Rauch CT, Smolak PJ, Waugh JY, Boiani N, Lynch DH, Smith CA, Goodwin RG, Kubin MZ (1999) Functional analysis of TRAIL receptors using monoclonal antibodies. J Immunol 162(5):2597–2605
152. Zhang XD, Franco A, Myers K, Gray C, Nguyen T, Hersey P (1999) Relation of TNF-related apoptosis-inducing ligand (TRAIL) receptor and FLICE-inhibitory protein expression to TRAIL-induced apoptosis of melanoma. Cancer Res 59(11):2747–2753
153. Wuchter C, Krappmann D, Cai Z, Ruppert V, Scheidereit C, Dorken B, Ludwig WD, Karawajew L (2001) In vitro susceptibility to TRAIL-induced apoptosis of acute leukemia cells in the context of TRAIL receptor gene expression and constitutive NF-kappa B activity. Leukemia 15(6):921–928
154. Neumann S, Hasenauer J, Pollak N, Scheurich P (2014) Dominant negative effects of tumor necrosis factor (TNF)-related apoptosis-inducing ligand (TRAIL) receptor 4 on TRAIL receptor 1 signaling by formation of heteromeric complexes. J Biol Chem 289(23):16576–16587. doi:10.1074/jbc.M114.559468
155. Truneh A, Sharma S, Silverman C, Khandekar S, Reddy MP, Deen KC, McLaughlin MM, Srinivasula SM, Livi GP, Marshall LA, Alnemri ES, Williams WV, Doyle ML (2000) Temperature-sensitive differential affinity of TRAIL for its receptors. DR5 is the highest affinity receptor. J Biol Chem 275(30):23319–23325. doi:10.1074/jbc.M910438199
156. Clancy L, Mruk K, Archer K, Woelfel M, Mongkolsapaya J, Screaton G, Lenardo MJ, Chan FK (2005) Preligand assembly domain-mediated ligand-independent association between TRAIL receptor 4 (TR4) and TR2 regulates TRAIL-induced apoptosis. Proc Natl Acad Sci U S A 102(50):18099–18104. doi:10.1073/pnas.0507329102
157. Merino D, Lalaoui N, Morizot A, Schneider P, Solary E, Micheau O (2006) Differential inhibition of TRAIL-mediated DR5-DISC formation by decoy receptors 1 and 2. Mol Cell Biol 26(19):7046–7055. doi:10.1128/MCB.00520-06
158. Valley CC, Lewis AK, Mudaliar DJ, Perlmutter JD, Braun AR, Karim CB, Thomas DD, Brody JR, Sachs JN (2012) Tumor necrosis factor-related apoptosis-inducing ligand (TRAIL) induces death receptor 5 networks that are highly organized. J Biol Chem 287(25):21265–21278. doi:10.1074/jbc.M111.306480
159. Chan FK (2000) The pre-ligand binding assembly domain: a potential target of inhibition of tumour necrosis factor receptor function. Ann Rheum Dis 59(Suppl 1):i50–i53
160. Siegel RM, Frederiksen JK, Zacharias DA, Chan FK, Johnson M, Lynch D, Tsien RY, Lenardo MJ (2000) Fas preassociation required for apoptosis signaling and dominant inhibition by pathogenic mutations. Science 288(5475):2354–2357
161. Branschadel M, Aird A, Zappe A, Tietz C, Krippner-Heidenreich A, Scheurich P (2010) Dual function of cysteine rich domain (CRD) 1 of TNF receptor type 1: conformational stabilization of CRD2 and control of receptor responsiveness. Cell Signal 22(3):404–414. doi:10.1016/j.cellsig.2009.10.011

162. Lewis AK, Valley CC, Sachs JN (2012) TNFR1 signaling is associated with backbone conformational changes of receptor dimers consistent with overactivation in the R92Q TRAPS mutant. Biochemistry 51(33):6545–6555. doi:10.1021/bi3006626
163. Lewis AK, James ZM, McCaffrey JE, Braun AR, Karim CB, Thomas DD, Sachs JN (2014) Open and closed conformations of the isolated transmembrane domain of death receptor 5 support a new model of activation. Biophys J 106(6):L21–L24. doi:10.1016/j.bpj.2014.01.044
164. Winkel C, Neumann S, Surulescu C, Scheurich P (2012) A minimal mathematical model for the initial molecular interactions of death receptor signalling. Math Biosci Eng 9(3):663–683. doi:10.3934/mbe.2012.9.663
165. Lee HW, Lee SH, Lee HW, Ryu YW, Kwon MH, Kim YS (2005) Homomeric and heteromeric interactions of the extracellular domains of death receptors and death decoy receptors. Biochem Biophys Res Commun 330(4):1205–1212. doi:10.1016/j.bbrc.2005.03.101
166. Lalaoui N, Morle A, Merino D, Jacquemin G, Iessi E, Morizot A, Shirley S, Robert B, Solary E, Garrido C, Micheau O (2011) TRAIL-R4 promotes tumor growth and resistance to apoptosis in cervical carcinoma HeLa cells through AKT. PLoS One 6(5):e19679. doi:10.1371/journal.pone.0019679
167. Zhang XD, Franco AV, Nguyen T, Gray CP, Hersey P (2000) Differential localization and regulation of death and decoy receptors for TNF-related apoptosis-inducing ligand (TRAIL) in human melanoma cells. J Immunol 164(8):3961–3970

Chapter 3
IAPs and Resistance to Death Receptors in Cancer

Laurence Dubrez and Simone Fulda

Abstract Since their identification in mammal cells, IAPs emerged have as potent regulators of death receptor signalling pathways, determining the cell fate in response to receptor stimulation. Among IAPs, cIAP1 and cIAP2 are active components of receptor-associated signalling complexes able to promote the activation of ubiquitin-dependent survival signalling pathways. For its part, XIAP is an important regulator of caspase activity, determining the apoptotic signalling pathway engaged after death receptor stimulation. The use of IAP antagonists is a promising strategy in order to overcome the resistance of tumor cells to death receptor stimulation.

Keywords IAPs • Smac mimetics • NF-κB • Apoptosis • Necroptosis • RIPK1

3.1 Introduction

Inhibitors of apoptosis (IAPs) constitute a family of proteins highly conserved throughout evolution. They were discovered in 1993 in baculoviruses because of their capacity to prevent apoptosis of infected insect cells, allowing for viral propagation [1]. Then, based on functional or structural homologies, IAPs were identified in flies, yeasts, worms, fish, and mammals. Eight human members of the IAP family have been described and include neuronal apoptosis inhibitory protein (NAIP, also known as BIRC1) [2], cellular

L. Dubrez (✉)
Université de Bourgogne Franche-Comté, LNC UMR1231, 21000 Dijon, France

Institut National de la Santé et de la Recherche Médicale (Inserm), LNC UMR1231, Dijon, France
e-mail: ldubrez@u-bourgogne.fr

S. Fulda (✉)
Institute for Experimental Cancer Research in Pediatrics, Goethe-University Frankfurt, Komturstrasse 3a, 60528 Frankfurt, Germany

German Cancer Consortium (DKTK), Heidelberg, Germany

German Cancer Research Center (DKFZ), Heidelberg, Germany
e-mail: fulda@em.uni-frankfurt.de

O. Micheau (ed.), *TRAIL, Fas Ligand, TNF and TLR3 in Cancer*, Resistance to Targeted Anti-Cancer Therapeutics, DOI 10.1007/978-3-319-56805-8_3

IAP1 (cIAP1, also known as BIRC2, HIAP2, or MIHB) [3–5], cIAP2 (also known as BIRC3, HIAP1, or MIHC) [3–5], X-chromosome-linked IAP (XIAP, also known as BIRC4, hILP, or MIHA) [4–6], survivin (also known as BIRC5 or TIAP) [7], Apollon (also known as BIRC6 or Bruce) [8, 9], melanoma IAP (ML-IAP, also known as BIRC7, livin, or KIAP) [10–12], and IAP-like protein 2 (ILP2, BIRC8) [13]. Although all of them retain the ability to regulate cell death [4, 5, 14, 15], only XIAP appears to be the most efficient in inhibiting apoptotic signalling pathways by directly blocking caspases-3, -7, and -9 activities (for review, see [16]). The main function of most IAP proteins is not related to their anti-apoptotic activity, but to the regulation of ubiquitin-dependent signalling events. cIAPs, XIAP, ML-IAP, and ILP2 harbor a Really Interesting New Gene (RING) domain in the C-terminal position that confers to them an E3-ligase activity in the ubiquitination reaction. They have the capacity to bind several cell signalling intermediates and catalyze the conjugation of ubiquitin chains that modulates the stability and activity of protein partners and/or the assembly of multiprotein signalling platforms. Thus, IAPs are involved in inflammation, cell differentiation, cell cycle regulation, and cell migration (for review, see [17–19]). Since their discovery in 1995 as tumor necrosis factor receptor (TNFR)-associated factor (TRAF) partners [3, 20], cIAPs have been linked to death receptor (DR) signalling pathways. Because of their capacity to regulate both cell death and nonapoptotic signalling pathways, IAPs have emerged as a central determinant of the response of cells to DR stimulation and modulation of IAPs is a very promising strategy to sensitize tumor cells to DR-induced cell death [21].

3.2 Structure and Molecular Functions

The IAP family is defined by the presence of at least one conserved domain named BIR (baculoviral IAP repeat) (Fig. 3.1) (for review, see [22]). BIR domains contain approximately 80 amino-acid residues forming three short-stranded antiparallel β-sheets and 4–5 α-helices, stabilized by the presence of Zn^{2+} atom that coordinates three Cys and one His residues [23]. The BIRs are critical for the interaction of IAPs with multiple protein partners. Two distinct modes of interaction of the BIRs with protein partners have been described. The first one involves a deep hydrophobic groove found in the BIR2 and BIR3 domains of cIAPs and XIAP and in the only BIR domain of ML-IAP (also referred to as type II BIRs). This pocket specifically anchors a conserved short linear motif called IAP-binding motif (IBM) [24–26]. The main characteristic of IBMs is the presence of an N-terminal alanine or, for a few of them, a serine residue that have to be exposed to get inserted into the BIR pocket [27]. A number of mammal IBM-bearing proteins have been identified [27, 28], the best characterized of them are the apoptotic caspases-3, -7 and -9 [26, 29, 30] and the IAP antagonists second mitochondrial activator of caspases (Smac, also named Diablo (Direct IAP binding protein with low pI)) [24, 25, 31, 32] and the high temperature requirement protein A2 (HtrA2) [33–37] that compete with caspases for IAP binding. The IBM is normally hidden in native proteins and requires N-terminal exposure for recognition and binding by IAPs. Caspase IBMs, found in the extreme N-terminus of active subunits, become exposed upon apoptotic proteolytic processing while the IBM

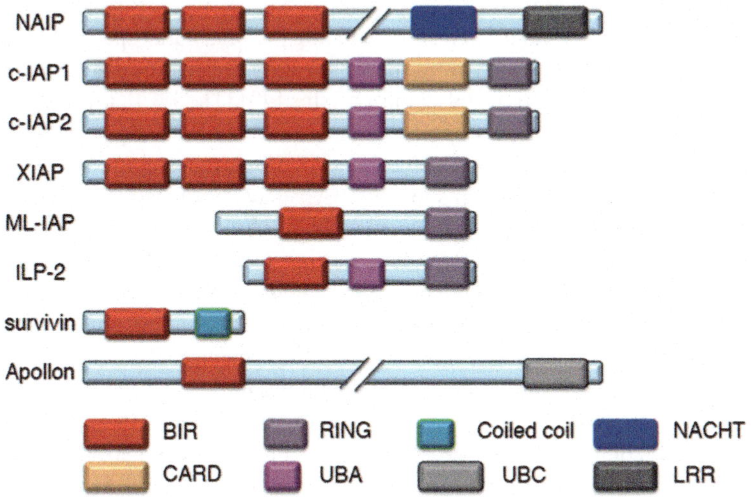

Fig. 3.1 Structure of human IAP proteins. All IAP proteins contain at least one baculoviral IAP repeat (BIR) domain. Additional domains are NACHT (domain present in NAIP, MHC class II transactivator (CIITA), 20-hydroxyeicosatetraenoic acid synthase (HET-E) and transition protein 1 (TP1)), leucine-rich repeat (LRR), ubiquitin-associated (UBA), caspase recruitment domain (CARD), ubiquitin-conjugating (UBC), and RING

of Smac and HtrA2 is unmasked by removing the N-terminal mitochondrial localization signal peptide. IBM-carrying proteins display a differential affinity for specific BIRs, depending on the primary sequence of IBM peptide and the dimerization status of the client IBM-proteins [38]. For example, the second BIR of XIAP preferentially binds caspase-3 and -7, while the third BIR specifically binds caspase-9. IAP antagonists have a higher affinity for the BIR3 than for the BIR2 domain. Unconventional IBMs have also been described that extend the spectrum of potential IAP interacting partners [39]. The second interacting mode is IBM-independent and involves the BIR1 devoid of the IBM-binding pocket (also referred to as type I BIR) of cIAPs and XIAP. The BIR1-dependent interaction is devoted to cell signalling intermediates. For instance, the BIR1 domain of cIAP1 and cIAP2 allows their interaction with TRAF2 [40, 41] and the XIAP BIR1 is required for the binding to TAB1 (Transforming growth factor-β activated kinase 1 (TAK1) Binding Protein 1) [42], an upstream adaptor of TAK1.

Another very important functional domain is the RING domain carried by cIAP1, cIAP2, XIAP, ML-IAP and ILP2 (Fig. 3.1). RING is a well-characterized Zinc finger domain that confers an E3-ligase activity in the ubiquitination process. Ubiquitination consists in a multistep enzymatic cascade involving an ubiquitin-activating (E1), an ubiquitin-conjugating (E2) and an E3-ubiquitin ligase, and results in a covalent attachment of the small protein modifier ubiquitin to a lysine residue of a substrate protein. The Ubiquitin contains seven lysine residues and a free N-terminus that can serve as an acceptor site for another ubiquitin, forming a variety of combinations of ubiquitin chains with distinct topologies. At least eight varieties of ubiquitin chains have been described (named M1, K6, K11, K27, K29, K33, K48, and K63) in function of the linking residue, each corresponding to a signal that specifically affects the protein fate modifying the stability, the localization, the recruitment in the signalling platform and/or the activity of client proteins [43]. The E3 ligases confer substrate specificity. They recruit target proteins and ubiquitin-charged E2 and they promote the formation of an isopeptide bond between the ubiquitin's C-terminal glycine and a lysine of the protein substrate. IAPs have been shown to promote the conjugation of a single ubiquitin molecule (mono-ubiquitination), K11-, K48- or K63-linked polyubiquitin chains to protein partners recruited via the BIR domains.

The E3-ubiquitin ligase activity of IAPs depends on their capacity to dimerize via the RING domain [44–47]. In resting conditions, cIAPs are maintained in inactive, monomer conformation because of an intramolecular interaction between the BIR3 and the RING domains. The substrate binding to the BIRs modifies the protein conformation and promotes RING dimerization that is essential for the recruitment of the E2-conjugating enzyme and for the ubiquitin conjugation to the target substrate lysine [45, 48]. The IAP E3-ligase activity is controlled by the UBA (Ubiquitin-associated) domain that facilitates the recruitment of the ubiquitin-charged E2-conjugating enzyme [49] and the CARD (Caspase Recruitment Domain) that stabilizes cIAPs in inactive, monomer conformation [49, 50].

3.3 Regulation of DR Signalling Pathways by IAPs

3.3.1 Regulation of RIPK-Dependent Signalling Complex

TNF can bind two related surface membrane receptors: the ubiquitous TNFR1 contains a cytoplasmic death domain (DD) that characterizes DR (for review, see [51]), and the TNFR2 devoid of DD, whose expression is restricted mostly to lymphocytes and endothelial cells. Stimulation of TNFR1 primarily induces the activation of canonical nuclear factor kappaB (NF-κB), JNK (c-jun amino-terminal kinase) and p38 signalling pathways that culminate in cytokine, survival, and differentiation factor gene expression. When the NF-κB signalling is blocked or in the absence of survival factors, TNFR1 engagement triggers apoptotic or necrotic cell death (for review, see [52]). In 1995, Rothe et al. isolated two novel components of the TNFR2 signalling complex using a GST-hTNFR2 fusion protein affinity column, which they named cIAP1 and cIAP2 because of the structural homologies with the baculoviral IAPs [3]. cIAPs do not directly interact with TNFR2 but are recruited to the membrane receptor complex through interaction with TRAFs. In the same time, Uren et al. [4] used an in silico strategy to identify mammalian homologs of viral IAPs which they named MIHA, MIHB, and MIHC (corresponding to XIAP, cIAP1, and cIAP2) and confirmed that, in contrast to XIAP, cIAPs are able to bind TRAF1 and TRAF2. TRAF2, known as a signalling adaptor, directly interacts with the DD-containing adaptor TNFR-associated death domain (TRADD) that specifically binds the DD of TNFR1 [53] (Fig. 3.2). The recruitment of cIAP1 along with TRAF2

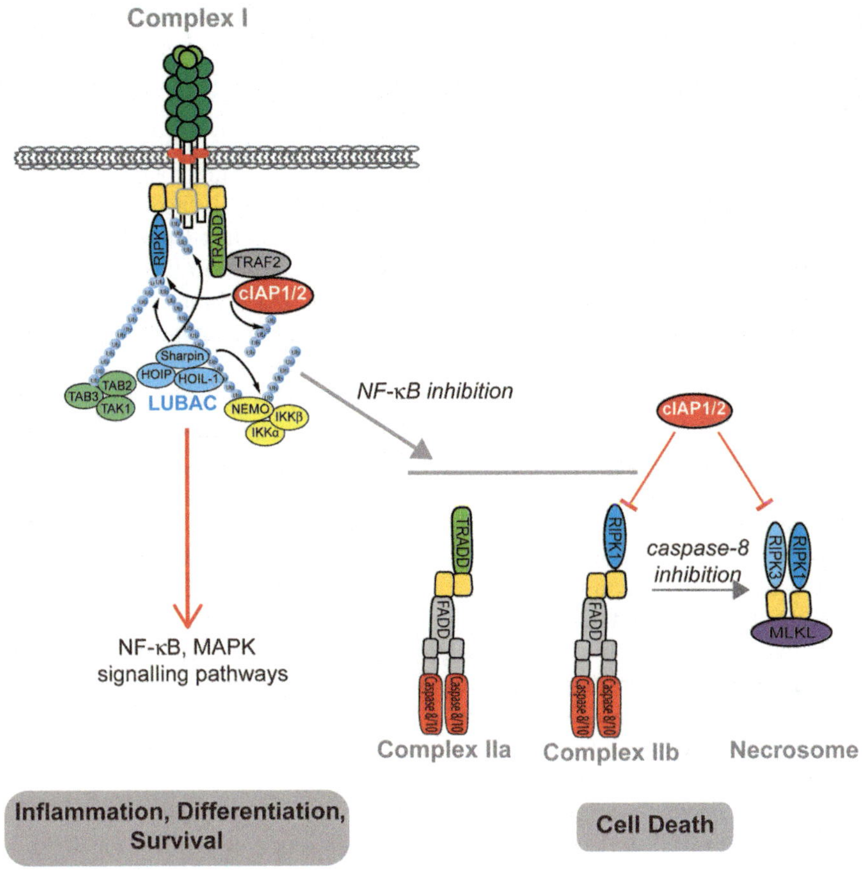

Fig. 3.2 TNFR1 signalling pathway. TNFRI engagement leads to the recruitment to its cytoplasmic DD of the kinase RIPK1 and the adaptor TRADD that in turn binds TRAF2 and cIAP1/2 (Complex I). cIAPs mediate the conjugation of different types of ubiquitin chains on cIAPs themselves and on RIPK1. Then, the LUBAC composed of Sharpin, HOIP, and HOIL1 is recruited thanks to the presence of ubiquitin binding domains on HOIL/Sharpin and adds linear ubiquitin chains to complex I components. These different ubiquitin chains are recognized by the ubiquitin binding domains of TABs and IKK, allowing the assembly of a signalling platform containing LUBAC (linear ubiquitin chain assembly complex), NEMO/IKKs (NF-κB essential modulator/IκB kinases), and TABs/TAK1 complexes and leading to NF-kB and MAPK (Mitogen-activated protein kinase) signalling pathway activation. In case of blockage of NF-kB signalling pathway, TRADD and RIPK1 are released from the complex I and recruit FADD (Fas-Associated protein with Death Domain) and caspase-8, forming secondary cytoplasmic complexes named complex II that lead to caspase-8 activation and apoptosis. Inhibition of caspase-8 can lead to the assembly of necrosome formed of RIPK1/RIPK3 and MLKL (Mixed Lineage Kinase Domain Like Pseudokinase) that promotes necroptotic cell death

into the TNFR1 signalling complex in response to TNF stimulation has been demonstrated [54], as well as a function of cIAPs as an inhibitor of TNFR1-mediated caspase-8 activation [55]. However, the mechanisms involved in the regulation of DR-signalling pathways by cIAPs have been deciphered only a decade later thanks to the availability of IAP antagonists [56–59] and the demonstration that the Receptor-interacting protein kinase 1 (RIPK1) is an ubiquitin target of cIAP1 [59, 60]. The importance of IAPs in TNFR1 and RIPK regulation has thereafter been strengthened by the combined deletion of IAPs in mice showing that embryonic lethality of cIAP1/cIAP2 and cIAP1/XIAP double knock-out mice was rescued by deletion of TNFR1 or RIPK1 [61].

The mechanism of assembly of the membrane TNFR1-signalling complex I has been extensively investigated (for review, see [51, 52]) (Fig. 3.2). TNF engagement triggers the TNFR1 oligomerization and the recruitment of the cytosolic adaptor TRADD and the kinase RIPK1 via homotypic DD interaction. In turn, TRADD binds TRAF2 that serves as an adaptor for the recruitment of cIAP1 and cIAP2. In the complex, cIAPs promote the conjugation of K63-, K11-, and K48-linked ubiquitin chains on cIAPs themselves and on RIPK1 [59, 60, 62]. These ubiquitin chains allow the recruitment of an Ub-E3 complex named Linear Ubiquitin chain Assembly Complex (LUBAC) that adds exclusively linear-ubiquitin chains to complex I components [57, 63–66]. The ubiquitin chains generated by cIAPs and LUBAC cooperate to form a platform for the recruitment of both NEMO/IKKs and TAK/TABs kinase complexes, resulting in NF-κB and mitogen-activated protein kinase (MAPK) activation [63, 67, 68] (Fig. 3.2).

When NF-κB signalling is blocked, cell death-induced secondary cytoplasmic complexes (known as complexes II) are generated from the TNFR1 complex I [69]. Complex II consists in homotypic DD association of either TRADD (complex IIa) or RIPK1 (Complex IIb), and the adaptor FAS-Associated via Death Domain (FADD), the latter recruiting and activating caspase-8 and/or -10. RIPK1 ubiquitination prevents the formation of RIPK1-containing complex II (Fig. 3.2). Thus, downregulation of cIAPs by using IAP antagonists [56–58, 70], or deficiency in cIAP1 [61] or LUBAC components [71–73] in mice promote the formation of the RIPK1 kinase activity-dependent caspase-8-activating complex and, therefore, sensitizes cells to TNF-induced apoptosis. In the presence of RIPK3, the RIPK1-dependent complex II can also result in necroptosis (for review, see [52, 74]).

In contrast to TNF, CD95L and TNF-related apoptosis-inducing ligand (TRAIL) first elicit pro-apoptotic response through the formation of a membrane receptor-associated death-inducing signal complex (DISC). CD95L and TRAIL stimulation can also trigger pro-inflammatory, proliferative, and pro-migratory signals (for review, see [75]) as a result of the release of FADD from the DISC and the recruitment of TRADD, TRAF2, cIAPs, RIPK1 to form the cytoplasmic complex II, leading to the activation of NF-κB and MAPK [76, 77] (Fig. 3.3). The regulatory mechanisms of differential responses to CD95 or TRAIL stimulation are not yet fully understood: however, as in the TNFR1 complex I, cIAPs appear to regulate RIPK1-dependent signalling events [76, 78].

3.3.2 Regulation of DR-Induced Apoptosis by IAPs

The recruitment of caspase-8 into the DISC upon CD95L or TRAIL stimulation leads to the activating oligomerization of caspase-8 to specifically activate, via proteolytic processing, effector caspases-3 and -7 and the BH3-only protein from the Bcl-2

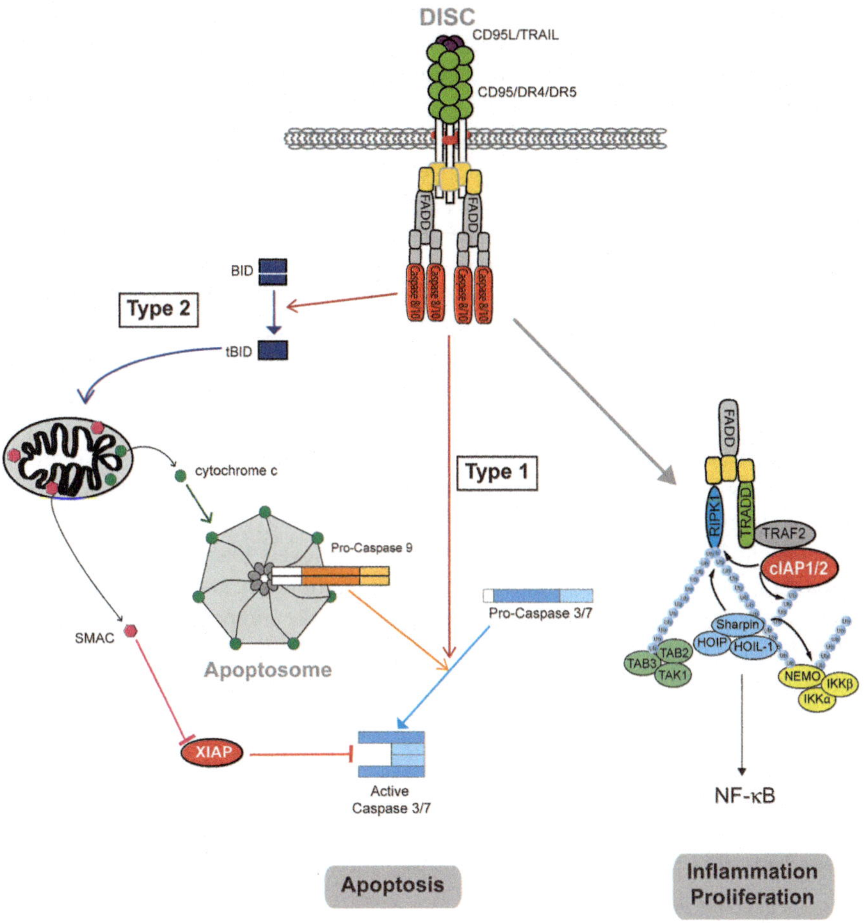

Fig. 3.3 Regulation of type I and type 2 CD-95-mediated apoptosis signalling pathways by IAPs. CD95 or TRAIL stimulation leads to the recruitment of the adaptor TRADD that in turn binds and allows the activating oligomerization of caspase-8. In type 1 cells, caspase-8 activates via proteolytic cleavage effector caspase-3 and -7, leading to apoptosis. In type 2, effector caspases are neutralized by binding to XIAP. Caspase-8 induces the cleavage of the BH3-protein BID. The truncated form of BID activates the release, from the mitochondria intermembrane space to the cytosol, of (1) Smac that sequesters XIAP and releases effector caspase-3 and -7; and (2) cytochrome c that engages the formation of apoptosome allowing caspase-9 oligomerization and activation that in turn activates effector caspases. In some conditions, a secondary cytoplasmic complex can be formed from the DISC that contains FADD, RIPKI, TRADD, TRAF2 and cIAP1/2. As in complex I TNFR1, cIAPs promote the ubiquitination of RIPK1 and allow NF-κB activation

protein family Bid (Fig. 3.3). In turn, effector caspases cleave a broad spectrum of vital intracellular proteins that culminate in cell dismantlement and apoptosis (also called type 1 apoptosis). On its part, truncated BID (tBID) generates an amplification loop of apoptosis (named type 2 apoptosis) in which it activates the release of apoptogenic factors that include cytochrome c and Smac from the mitochondrial intermembrane space to the cytosol. Cytosolic cytochrome c initiates the assembly of the caspase-9 activating complex named apoptosome that results in the activation of the effector caspases-3 and -7 (Fig. 3.3) while Smac neutralizes XIAP.

Cells can be discriminated into type 1 (e.g., thymocytes and resting T-cells) and type 2 (e.g., hepatocytes and pancreatic β-cells) depending on the prevailing activated apoptotic signalling pathway. The magnitude and kinetics of DISC formation and caspase-8 activation, the available activated caspase-8 and the expression levels of specific inhibitors such as Bcl-x_L and Bcl-2 that block the mitochondrial step of apoptosis can partly explain this discrepancy. More recently, a key role in determining type 1 versus type 2 CD95-mediated apoptotic signalling pathways has been attributed to XIAP [79]. Most IAPs have the ability to directly bind caspases-3, -7, and -9 [25, 30, 38, 80]; however, only XIAP can directly inhibit their enzymatic activity [81–84]. Other IAPs including cIAPs and ML-IAP can indirectly regulate caspase activity by sequestering the IAP antagonist Smac and HtrA2, thereby preventing them from inhibiting XIAP anti-caspase activity. In type 2 cells, CD95 engagement leads to an increase in XIAP protein levels that neutralizes effector caspases-3 and -7. Caspase-8-mediated tBID generation activates the mitochondrial pathway of apoptosis leading to the release of Smac that competes with caspases for XIAP binding thereby releasing caspases-3 and -7 and allowing apoptosis to occur. Thus, depletion of XIAP or Smac mimetics can convert type 2 cells into type 1 cells, which ultimately results in a sensitization of cells to CD95- and TRAIL-induced cell death [79, 85–87].

3.4 Sensitization to Death Receptor-Induced Cell Death by Smac Mimetics

3.4.1 Smac Mimetics in Combination with Tumor Necrosis Factor (TNF)

The capacity of Smac to block the anti-apoptotic activity of XIAP has been exploited to design IAP antagonists named Smac mimetics. Unexpectedly, cell treatment with Smac mimetics alone appeared to induce cell death in cancer cells via proteasomal degradation of cIAP proteins, followed by NF-κB activation and upregulation of TNFα which in turn triggers cell death in an autocrine or paracrine manner [56, 58, 70, 88]. There is a strong rationale to combine Smac mimetics with TNFα. Indeed, addition of TNFα has been shown to increase the antitumor activity of Smac mimetics in various cancer models [56, 58, 70, 88]. A screening of the cytotoxic responsiveness of a diverse panel of 51 cancer cell lines showed synergistic effects between the Smac mimetic

AEG40730 and TNFα depending on the expression levels of the cellular FLICE (FADD-like IL-1β-converting enzyme)-inhibitory protein (cFLIP), and downregulation of cFLIP has been described to enhance cell death induced by AEG40730/TNFα cotreatment [89]. Testing of the Smac mimetic birinapant against a panel of childhood cancer cells lines revealed that birinapant acted in concert with TNFα to induce cell death in acute lymphoblastic leukemia (ALL) as well as in some solid cancer cell lines [90]. In addition, birinapant in combination with TNFα has been reported to exhibit a strong anti-melanoma effect in vitro and in vivo, including melanoma cells with acquired resistance to BRAF (V-raf murine sarcoma viral oncogene homolog B1) inhibitors [91].

In addition to Smac mimetic-mediated sensitization for apoptosis in combination with death receptor ligands, cells depleted of cIAP proteins by treatment with Smac mimetics or by genetic knockdown have shown to be sensitized for TNFα-induced necroptosis [92]. Synergistic induction of necroptosis by Smac mimetic/TNFα cotreatment has been shown to require RIPK3 as a key determinant for cellular necroptosis [93]. In apoptosis-resistant ALL cells deficient in key apoptosis regulatory proteins such as FADD or caspase-8, Smac mimetics even bypassed apoptosis resistance by priming cells for TNFα-induced necroptosis [78], indicating that Smac mimetics may overcome at least some types of apoptosis resistance by engaging necroptosis as an alternative form of cell death.

3.4.2 Smac Mimetics in Combination with CD95

Furthermore, several studies showed that Smac mimetics can prime cancer cell death induced by CD95 ligation. In childhood acute leukemia, Smac mimetics at subtoxic concentrations, but not a structurally related control compound, acted synergistically with agonistic anti-CD95 antibodies or MegaFasL, a hexameric form of CD95 ligand, to induce apoptosis [94]. Importantly, a similar sensitization for CD95-induced cell death was found in primary leukemic samples that were freshly derived from ALL patients, underscoring the clinical significance of this targeted therapy [94]. In contrast, Smac mimetics failed to increase the susceptibility of apoptosis-resistant ALL cells with deficiency in FADD or caspase-8 to CD95-mediated apoptosis [95]. The combination of Smac mimetics with Fas ligand has been described to synergistically stimulate cancer cell death independently of TNFα by amplifying the apoptotic signal via caspase-8-mediated activation of Bid and subsequent activation of the caspase-9-dependent mitochondrial apoptotic pathway [96]. Also, the loss of cIAP proteins has been shown to result in a potent sensitization to CD95 ligand (CD95L)-mediated cell death in a RIPK1-dependent manner independently of TNFα signalling in squamous cell carcinoma cells [78].

3.4.3 Smac Mimetics in Combination with TNF-Related Apoptosis-Inducing Ligand (TRAIL)

Among the death receptor ligands, TRAIL is considered as the most promising candidate for Smac-mimetic-based combination treatments, because it preferentially targets tumor versus nonmalignant cells. An initial proof-of-concept study has demonstrated that a cell-permeable Smac peptide mimicking the N-terminal four amino acids of Smac can potentiate the antitumor activity of TRAIL against glioblastoma in vitro and in vivo, leading to tumor eradication in an orthotopic mouse glioblastoma model [78, 97]. Subsequent studies confirmed the cooperative antitumor activity of Smac mimetics together with soluble TRAIL ligand or agonistic TRAIL receptor antibodies against glioblastoma cells [98, 99].

In ALL, Smac mimetics at low concentrations have been shown to synergize together with TRAIL to trigger apoptosis and to inhibit clonogenic survival of acute leukemia cells, whereas they did not affect the viability of normal peripheral blood lymphocytes, suggesting some tumor selectivity [87]. This Smac mimetic-mediated sensitization to TRAIL has also been found in a panel of primary leukemic samples as well as in vivo in a patient-derived ALL mouse model, underlining the clinical relevance [87]. This Smac mimetic/TRAIL combination was even able to overcome Bcl-2-mediated resistance to TRAIL by enhancing Bcl-2 cleavage and Bak conformational change [87]. Similarly, a series of Smac mimetics has been shown to potentiate the antileukemic activity of TRAIL [100]. Also in multiple myeloma, the Smac mimetic LBW242 together with TRAIL proved to be a potent combination to engage apoptosis [101]. In primary chronic lymphocytic leukemia (CLL) samples, Smac mimetics have been shown to synergistically trigger apoptosis in combination with TRAIL even in resistant forms and poor prognostic subgroups of CLL, including samples from patients with 17p deletion, TP53 mutation, unmutated V(H) genes or chemotherapy-refractory disease [94]. Similarly, an XIAP inhibitor has been described to act in concert with TRAIL in CLL cases with poor prognosis [102].

In pancreatic cancer, which harbors high expression levels of XIAP, Smac mimetics have been described to synergize with TRAIL to induce apoptosis and to inhibit long-term clonogenic survival. Also, Smac mimetics have been shown to cooperate with TRAIL to trigger apoptosis and suppress pancreatic carcinoma growth in vivo in two preclinical models, which was associated with increased caspase-3 activation and apoptosis induction, as shown by parallel immunohistochemistry of tumor tissue under therapy [85]. Besides soluble TRAIL ligand, the agonistic antibody Mapatumumab that is directed against TRAIL-receptor 2 (TRAIL-R2/DR5) has been shown to cooperate with Smac mimetics to engage caspase-dependent apoptosis in pancreatic cancer cell lines as well as in primary cultured pancreatic carcinoma cells derived from tumor samples [103]. By comparison, additional cross-linking was required for maximal antitumor activity of the TRAIL-receptor 1 (TRAIL-R1/DR4) agonistic antibody lexatumumab together with Smac mimetics against pancreatic cancer cells [103]. Interestingly, targeting of XIAP by Smac mimetics proved to be capable of eliminating the requirement of mitochondrial signalling to

TRAIL-triggered apoptosis by converting 'type 2', which depends on mitochondrial signalling, to 'type 1' cells, where death receptor-stimulated apoptosis occurs independently of mitochondrial events (Fig. 3.3). This has initially been shown in pancreatic carcinoma and ALL, where Bcl-2 failed to protect against TRAIL-induced apoptosis in the presence of Smac mimetics [85, 87] and in Bax/Bak double-deficient colon carcinoma cells [86].

Smac mimetics or IAP inhibitors have been shown to act in concert with TRAIL or TRAIL-R2 antibody in preclinical in vitro models of colon carcinoma [85, 96, 104]. Autocrine/paracrine TNFα signalling, known to be critical for single agent activity of Smac mimetics in various models, has been reported to be dispensable for the cooperative induction of cell death by Smac mimetics and the agonistic TRAIL-R2 antibody drozitumab against colon carcinoma cells [96]. In cholangiocarcinoma, the Smac mimetic JP1584 did not sensitize cells to TRAIL-induced apoptosis, but reduced TRAIL-stimulated metastatic behavior both in vitro and in vivo [105].

The potency of a combination approach with Smac mimetics together with TRAIL in preclinical models of breast cancer has been documented in several studies. For example, the Smac mimetic SM-164 acted in concert with TRAIL to trigger apoptosis not only in TRAIL-sensitive but also in TRAIL-resistant breast cancer cell lines [104]. This combination also induced tumor regression in an in vivo model of breast cancer [104]. Besides TRAIL the agonistic TRAIL-R2 antibody Drozitumab has been shown to cooperate with the Smac mimetic BV6 to elicit apoptosis in breast carcinoma cells and to cause tumor growth suppression in an in vivo mouse model [96]. A synergistic interaction resulting in increased cytotoxicity has similarly been reported for the Smac mimetic AT-406 and the TRAIL-R2 antibody TRA-8 [106]. In combinational treatments with TRAIL the Smac mimetic compound 3 interacted with TRAIL to induce apoptosis via caspase-3 activation in breast carcinoma cells [107].

In ovarian cancer, different Smac mimetics have been shown to strongly synergize with TRAIL or the agonistic TRAIL-R2 antibody lexatumumab in inducing apoptosis [108, 109]. A significant inhibition of ovarian cancer growth in vivo by Smac mimetic together with TRAIL has been reported by Gatti et al. [110].

A synergistic activity of Smac mimetics together with TRAIL agonists has also been reported in pediatric cancers such as neuroblastoma and rhabdomyosarcoma or in neck squamous cell carcinoma, nasopharyngeal carcinoma, bladder carcinoma or melanoma cells [111–116].

While the function of IAPs in the TNFR signalling pathway has been extensively studied, more investigations will be required to improve our understanding of the regulation of Fas and TRAIL-dependent signalling pathways, mainly non apoptotic signalling pathways, by IAPs. Considering the importance of IAPs in DR signalling pathways and the promising results of preclinical analysis, many hopes and expectations are resting on the therapeutic approach combining DR agonists and IAP antagonists for cancer treatment. For example, a phase I clinical trial combining the DR5 antagonist conatumumab (AMG 655) and birinapant is ongoing in patients with relapsed ovarian cancer (ClinicalTrials.gov Identifier: NCT01940172). Future clinical trials will reveal the utility of such an approach.

Acknowledgments The research teams has partially been supported by grants from the "Comités de Côte d'Or et de Saône-et-Loire of the Ligue Contre le Cancer" (to L.D.), the "Association pour la Recherche sur le Cancer" (to L.D.), the French National Research Agency ("Investissements d'Avenir" program; ANR-11-LABX-0021) (to L.D.), the European Union (to L.D.) the "Conseil Régional de Bourgogne" (to L.D.), BMBF (to S.F.), IUAP VII (to S.F.), and Wilhelm Sander-Stiftung (to S.F.).

References

1. Crook NE, Clem RJ, Miller LK (1993) An apoptosis-inhibiting baculovirus gene with a zinc finger-like motif. J Virol 67(4):2168–2174
2. Roy N, Mahadevan MS, McLean M, Shutler G, Yaraghi Z, Farahani R, Baird S, Besner-Johnston A, Lefebvre C, Kang X et al (1995) The gene for neuronal apoptosis inhibitory protein is partially deleted in individuals with spinal muscular atrophy. Cell 80(1):167–178
3. Rothe M, Pan MG, Henzel WJ, Ayres TM, Goeddel DV (1995) The TNFR2-TRAF signaling complex contains two novel proteins related to baculoviral inhibitor of apoptosis proteins. Cell 83(7):1243–1252
4. Uren AG, Pakusch M, Hawkins CJ, Puls KL, Vaux DL (1996) Cloning and expression of apoptosis inhibitory protein homologs that function to inhibit apoptosis and/or bind tumor necrosis factor receptor-associated factors. Proc Natl Acad Sci U S A 93(10):4974–4978
5. Liston P, Roy N, Tamai K, Lefebvre C, Baird S, Cherton-Horvat G, Farahani R, McLean M, Ikeda JE, MacKenzie A, Korneluk RG (1996) Suppression of apoptosis in mammalian cells by NAIP and a related family of IAP genes. Nature 379(6563):349–353. doi:10.1038/379349a0
6. Duckett CS, Nava VE, Gedrich RW, Clem RJ, Van Dongen JL, Gilfillan MC, Shiels H, Hardwick JM, Thompson CB (1996) A conserved family of cellular genes related to the baculovirus iap gene and encoding apoptosis inhibitors. EMBO J 15(11):2685–2694
7. Ambrosini G, Adida C, Altieri DC (1997) A novel anti-apoptosis gene, survivin, expressed in cancer and lymphoma. Nat Med 3(8):917–921
8. Hauser HP, Bardroff M, Pyrowolakis G, Jentsch S (1998) A giant ubiquitin-conjugating enzyme related to IAP apoptosis inhibitors. J Cell Biol 141(6):1415–1422
9. Chen Z, Naito M, Hori S, Mashima T, Yamori T, Tsuruo T (1999) A human IAP-family gene, apollon, expressed in human brain cancer cells. Biochem Biophys Res Commun 264(3):847–854. doi:10.1006/bbrc.1999.1585
10. Vucic D, Stennicke HR, Pisabarro MT, Salvesen GS, Dixit VM (2000) ML-IAP, a novel inhibitor of apoptosis that is preferentially expressed in human melanomas. Curr Biol 10(21):1359–1366
11. Lin JH, Deng G, Huang Q, Morser J (2000) KIAP, a novel member of the inhibitor of apoptosis protein family. Biochem Biophys Res Commun 279(3):820–831. doi:10.1006/bbrc.2000.4027
12. Kasof GM, Gomes BC (2001) Livin, a novel inhibitor of apoptosis protein family member. J Biol Chem 276(5):3238–3246. doi:10.1074/jbc.M003670200
13. Richter BW, Mir SS, Eiben LJ, Lewis J, Reffey SB, Frattini A, Tian L, Frank S, Youle RJ, Nelson DL, Notarangelo LD, Vezzoni P, Fearnhead HO, Duckett CS (2001) Molecular cloning of ILP-2, a novel member of the inhibitor of apoptosis protein family. Mol Cell Biol 21(13):4292–4301. doi:10.1128/MCB.21.13.4292-4301.2001
14. Vucic D, Kaiser WJ, Miller LK (1998) Inhibitor of apoptosis proteins physically interact with and block apoptosis induced by Drosophila proteins HID and GRIM. Mol Cell Biol 18(6):3300–3309
15. Lagace M, Xuan JY, Young SS, McRoberts C, Maier J, Rajcan-Separovic E, Korneluk RG (2001) Genomic organization of the X-linked inhibitor of apoptosis and identification of a novel testis-specific transcript. Genomics 77(3):181–188. doi:10.1006/geno.2001.6635

16. Eckelman BP, Salvesen GS, Scott FL (2006) Human inhibitor of apoptosis proteins: why XIAP is the black sheep of the family. EMBO Rep 7(10):988–994
17. Dubrez L, Rajalingam K (2015) IAPs and cell migration. Semin Cell Dev Biol 39:124–131. doi:10.1016/j.semcdb.2015.02.015
18. Kocab AJ, Duckett CS (2016) Inhibitor of apoptosis proteins as intracellular signaling intermediates. FEBS J 283(2):221–231. doi:10.1111/febs.13554
19. Estornes Y, Bertrand MJ (2015) IAPs, regulators of innate immunity and inflammation. Semin Cell Dev Biol 39:106–114. doi:10.1016/j.semcdb.2014.03.035
20. Shu HB, Takeuchi M, Goeddel DV (1996) The tumor necrosis factor receptor 2 signal transducers TRAF2 and c-IAP1 are components of the tumor necrosis factor receptor 1 signaling complex. Proc Natl Acad Sci U S A 93(24):13973–13978
21. Fulda S (2015) Smac mimetics as IAP antagonists. Semin Cell Dev Biol 39:132–138. doi:10.1016/j.semcdb.2014.12.005
22. Budhidarmo R, Day CL (2015) IAPs: modular regulators of cell signalling. Semin Cell Dev Biol 39:80–90. doi:10.1016/j.semcdb.2014.12.002
23. Hinds MG, Norton RS, Vaux DL, Day CL (1999) Solution structure of a baculoviral inhibitor of apoptosis (IAP) repeat. Nat Struct Biol 6(7):648–651. doi:10.1038/10701
24. Wu G, Chai J, Suber TL, Wu JW, Du C, Wang X, Shi Y (2000) Structural basis of IAP recognition by Smac/DIABLO. Nature 408(6815):1008–1012. doi:10.1038/35050012
25. Liu Z, Sun C, Olejniczak ET, Meadows RP, Betz SF, Oost T, Herrmann J, Wu JC, Fesik SW (2000) Structural basis for binding of Smac/DIABLO to the XIAP BIR3 domain. Nature 408(6815):1004–1008. doi:10.1038/35050006
26. Kulathila R, Vash B, Sage D, Cornell-Kennon S, Wright K, Koehn J, Stams T, Clark K, Price A (2009) The structure of the BIR3 domain of cIAP1 in complex with the N-terminal peptides of SMAC and caspase-9. Acta Crystallogr D Biol Crystallogr 65(Pt 1):58–66. doi:10.1107/S0907444908039243
27. Verhagen AM, Kratina TK, Hawkins CJ, Silke J, Ekert PG, Vaux DL (2007) Identification of mammalian mitochondrial proteins that interact with IAPs via N-terminal IAP binding motifs. Cell Death Differ 14(2):348–357. doi:10.1038/sj.cdd.4402001
28. Zhuang M, Guan S, Wang H, Burlingame AL, Wells JA (2013) Substrates of IAP ubiquitin ligases identified with a designed orthogonal E3 ligase, the NEDDylator. Mol Cell 49(2):273–282. doi:10.1016/j.molcel.2012.10.022
29. Huang Y, Park YC, Rich RL, Segal D, Myszka DG, Wu H (2001) Structural basis of caspase inhibition by XIAP: differential roles of the linker versus the BIR domain. Cell 104(5):781–790
30. Srinivasula SM, Hegde R, Saleh A, Datta P, Shiozaki E, Chai J, Lee RA, Robbins PD, Fernandes-Alnemri T, Shi Y, Alnemri ES (2001) A conserved XIAP-interaction motif in caspase-9 and Smac/DIABLO regulates caspase activity and apoptosis. Nature 410(6824):112–116. doi:10.1038/35065125
31. Verhagen AM, Ekert PG, Pakusch M, Silke J, Connolly LM, Reid GE, Moritz RL, Simpson RJ, Vaux DL (2000) Identification of DIABLO, a mammalian protein that promotes apoptosis by binding to and antagonizing IAP proteins. Cell 102(1):43–53
32. Du C, Fang M, Li Y, Li L, Wang X (2000) Smac, a mitochondrial protein that promotes cytochrome c-dependent caspase activation by eliminating IAP inhibition. Cell 102(1):33–42
33. Martins LM, Iaccarino I, Tenev T, Gschmeissner S, Totty NF, Lemoine NR, Savopoulos J, Gray CW, Creasy CL, Dingwall C, Downward J (2002) The serine protease Omi/HtrA2 regulates apoptosis by binding XIAP through a reaper-like motif. J Biol Chem 277(1):439–444
34. van Loo G, van Gurp M, Depuydt B, Srinivasula SM, Rodriguez I, Alnemri ES, Gevaert K, Vandekerckhove J, Declercq W, Vandenabeele P (2002) The serine protease Omi/HtrA2 is released from mitochondria during apoptosis. Omi interacts with caspase-inhibitor XIAP and induces enhanced caspase activity. Cell Death Differ 9(1):20–26. doi:10.1038/sj.cdd.4400970

35. Suzuki Y, Imai Y, Nakayama H, Takahashi K, Takio K, Takahashi R (2001) A serine protease, HtrA2, is released from the mitochondria and interacts with XIAP, inducing cell death. Mol Cell 8(3):613–621
36. Hegde R, Srinivasula SM, Zhang Z, Wassell R, Mukattash R, Cilenti L, DuBois G, Lazebnik Y, Zervos AS, Fernandes-Alnemri T, Alnemri ES (2002) Identification of Omi/HtrA2 as a mitochondrial apoptotic serine protease that disrupts inhibitor of apoptosis protein-caspase interaction. J Biol Chem 277(1):432–438
37. Verhagen AM, Silke J, Ekert PG, Pakusch M, Kaufmann H, Connolly LM, Day CL, Tikoo A, Burke R, Wrobel C, Moritz RL, Simpson RJ, Vaux DL (2002) HtrA2 promotes cell death through its serine protease activity and its ability to antagonize inhibitor of apoptosis proteins. J Biol Chem 277(1):445–454. doi:10.1074/jbc.M109891200
38. Eckelman BP, Drag M, Snipas SJ, Salvesen GS (2008) The mechanism of peptide-binding specificity of IAP BIR domains. Cell Death Differ 15(5):920–928. doi:10.1038/cdd.2008.6
39. Kurakin A, Bredesen DE (2007) An unconventional IAP-binding motif revealed by target-assisted iterative screening (TAIS) of the BIR3-cIAP1 domain. J Mol Recognit 20(1):39–50
40. Samuel T, Welsh K, Lober T, Togo SH, Zapata JM, Reed JC (2006) Distinct BIR domains of cIAP1 mediate binding to and ubiquitination of tumor necrosis factor receptor-associated factor 2 and second mitochondrial activator of caspases. J Biol Chem 281(2):1080–1090. doi:10.1074/jbc.M509381200
41. Varfolomeev E, Wayson SM, Dixit VM, Fairbrother WJ, Vucic D (2006) The inhibitor of apoptosis protein fusion c-IAP2.MALT1 stimulates NF-kappaB activation independently of TRAF1 AND TRAF2. J Biol Chem 281(39):29022–29029. doi:10.1074/jbc.M605116200
42. Lu M, Lin SC, Huang Y, Kang YJ, Rich R, Lo YC, Myszka D, Han J, Wu H (2007) XIAP induces NF-kappaB activation via the BIR1/TAB1 interaction and BIR1 dimerization. Mol Cell 26(5):689–702. doi:10.1016/j.molcel.2007.05.006
43. Heride C, Urbe S, Clague MJ (2014) Ubiquitin code assembly and disassembly. Curr Biol 24(6):R215–R220. doi:10.1016/j.cub.2014.02.002
44. Silke J, Kratina T, Chu D, Ekert PG, Day CL, Pakusch M, Huang DC, Vaux DL (2005) Determination of cell survival by RING-mediated regulation of inhibitor of apoptosis (IAP) protein abundance. Proc Natl Acad Sci U S A 102(45):16182–16187
45. Feltham R, Bettjeman B, Budhidarmo R, Mace PD, Shirley S, Condon SM, Chunduru SK, McKinlay MA, Vaux DL, Silke J, Day CL (2011) Smac mimetics activate the E3 ligase activity of cIAP1 protein by promoting RING domain dimerization. J Biol Chem 286(19):17015–17028. doi:10.1074/jbc.M111.222919
46. Dou H, Buetow L, Sibbet GJ, Cameron K, Huang DT (2012) BIRC7-E2 ubiquitin conjugate structure reveals the mechanism of ubiquitin transfer by a RING dimer. Nat Struct Mol Biol 19(9):876–883. doi:10.1038/nsmb.2379
47. Mace PD, Linke K, Feltham R, Schumacher FR, Smith CA, Vaux DL, Silke J, Day CL (2008) Structures of the cIAP2 RING domain reveal conformational changes associated with ubiquitin-conjugating enzyme (E2) recruitment. J Biol Chem 283(46):31633–31640. doi:10.1074/jbc.M804753200
48. Dueber EC, Schoeffler AJ, Lingel A, Elliott JM, Fedorova AV, Giannetti AM, Zobel K, Maurer B, Varfolomeev E, Wu P, Wallweber HJ, Hymowitz SG, Deshayes K, Vucic D, Fairbrother WJ (2011) Antagonists induce a conformational change in cIAP1 that promotes autoubiquitination. Science 334(6054):376–380. doi:10.1126/science.1207862
49. Budhidarmo R, Day CL (2014) The ubiquitin-associated domain of cellular inhibitor of apoptosis proteins facilitates ubiquitylation. J Biol Chem 289(37):25721–25736. doi:10.1074/jbc.M113.545475
50. Lopez J, John SW, Tenev T, Rautureau GJ, Hinds MG, Francalanci F, Wilson R, Broemer M, Santoro MM, Day CL, Meier P (2011) CARD-mediated autoinhibition of cIAP1's E3 ligase activity suppresses cell proliferation and migration. Mol Cell 42(5):569–583. doi:10.1016/j.molcel.2011.04.008

51. Walczak H (2013) Death receptor-ligand systems in cancer, cell death, and inflammation. Cold Spring Harb Perspect Biol 5(5):a008698. doi:10.1101/cshperspect.a008698
52. Dondelinger Y, Darding M, Bertrand MJ, Walczak H (2016) Poly-ubiquitination in TNFR1-mediated necroptosis. Cell Mol Life Sci 73(11–12):2165–2176. doi:10.1007/s00018-016-2191-4
53. Hsu H, Xiong J, Goeddel DV (1995) The TNF receptor 1-associated protein TRADD signals cell death and NF-kappa B activation. Cell 81(4):495–504. doi:10.1016/0092-8674(95)90070-5. 0092-8674(95)90070-5 [pii]
54. Hsu H, Shu HB, Pan MG, Goeddel DV (1996) TRADD-TRAF2 and TRADD-FADD interactions define two distinct TNF receptor 1 signal transduction pathways. Cell 84(2):299–308. doi:10.1016/S0092-8674(00)80984-8. S0092-8674(00)80984-8 [pii]
55. Wang CY, Mayo MW, Korneluk RG, Goeddel DV, Baldwin AS Jr (1998) NF-kappaB antiapoptosis: induction of TRAF1 and TRAF2 and c-IAP1 and c-IAP2 to suppress caspase-8 activation. Science 281(5383):1680–1683
56. Petersen SL, Wang L, Yalcin-Chin A, Li L, Peyton M, Minna J, Harran P, Wang X (2007) Autocrine TNFalpha signaling renders human cancer cells susceptible to Smac-mimetic-induced apoptosis. Cancer Cell 12(5):445–456
57. Gaither A, Porter D, Yao Y, Borawski J, Yang G, Donovan J, Sage D, Slisz J, Tran M, Straub C, Ramsey T, Iourgenko V, Huang A, Chen Y, Schlegel R, Labow M, Fawell S, Sellers WR, Zawel L (2007) A Smac mimetic rescue screen reveals roles for inhibitor of apoptosis proteins in tumor necrosis factor-alpha signaling. Cancer Res 67(24):11493–11498
58. Vince JE, Wong WW, Khan N, Feltham R, Chau D, Ahmed AU, Benetatos CA, Chunduru SK, Condon SM, McKinlay M, Brink R, Leverkus M, Tergaonkar V, Schneider P, Callus BA, Koentgen F, Vaux DL, Silke J (2007) IAP antagonists target cIAP1 to induce TNFalpha-dependent apoptosis. Cell 131(4):682–693
59. Bertrand MJ, Milutinovic S, Dickson KM, Ho WC, Boudreault A, Durkin J, Gillard JW, Jaquith JB, Morris SJ, Barker PA (2008) cIAP1 and cIAP2 facilitate cancer cell survival by functioning as E3 ligases that promote RIP1 ubiquitination. Mol Cell 30(6):689–700
60. Varfolomeev E, Goncharov T, Fedorova AV, Dynek JN, Zobel K, Deshayes K, Fairbrother WJ, Vucic D (2008) c-IAP1 and c-IAP2 are critical mediators of tumor necrosis factor alpha (TNFalpha)-induced NF-kappaB activation. J Biol Chem 283(36):24295–24299. doi:10.1074/jbc.C800128200
61. Moulin M, Anderton H, Voss AK, Thomas T, Wong WW, Bankovacki A, Feltham R, Chau D, Cook WD, Silke J, Vaux DL (2012) IAPs limit activation of RIP kinases by TNF receptor 1 during development. EMBO J 31(7):1679–1691. doi:10.1038/emboj.2012.18
62. Mahoney DJ, Cheung HH, Mrad RL, Plenchette S, Simard C, Enwere E, Arora V, Mak TW, Lacasse EC, Waring J, Korneluk RG (2008) Both cIAP1 and cIAP2 regulate TNFalpha-mediated NF-kappaB activation. Proc Natl Acad Sci U S A 105(33):11778–11783. doi:10.1073/pnas.0711122105. 0711122105 [pii]
63. Haas TL, Emmerich CH, Gerlach B, Schmukle AC, Cordier SM, Rieser E, Feltham R, Vince J, Warnken U, Wenger T, Koschny R, Komander D, Silke J, Walczak H (2009) Recruitment of the linear ubiquitin chain assembly complex stabilizes the TNF-R1 signaling complex and is required for TNF-mediated gene induction. Mol Cell 36(5):831–844. doi:10.1016/j.molcel.2009.10.013. S1097-2765(09)00778-3 [pii]
64. Ikeda F, Deribe YL, Skanland SS, Stieglitz B, Grabbe C, Franz-Wachtel M, van Wijk SJ, Goswami P, Nagy V, Terzic J, Tokunaga F, Androulidaki A, Nakagawa T, Pasparakis M, Iwai K, Sundberg JP, Schaefer L, Rittinger K, Macek B, Dikic I (2011) SHARPIN forms a linear ubiquitin ligase complex regulating NF-kappaB activity and apoptosis. Nature 471(7340):637–641. doi:10.1038/nature09814
65. Tokunaga F, Nakagawa T, Nakahara M, Saeki Y, Taniguchi M, Sakata S, Tanaka K, Nakano H, Iwai K (2011) SHARPIN is a component of the NF-kappaB-activating linear ubiquitin chain assembly complex. Nature 471(7340):633–636. doi:10.1038/nature09815
66. Tokunaga F, Sakata S, Saeki Y, Satomi Y, Kirisako T, Kamei K, Nakagawa T, Kato M, Murata S, Yamaoka S, Yamamoto M, Akira S, Takao T, Tanaka K, Iwai K (2009) Involvement of

linear polyubiquitylation of NEMO in NF-kappaB activation. Nat Cell Biol 11(2):123–132. doi:10.1038/ncb1821. ncb1821 [pii]
67. Dynek JN, Goncharov T, Dueber EC, Fedorova AV, Izrael-Tomasevic A, Phu L, Helgason E, Fairbrother WJ, Deshayes K, Kirkpatrick DS, Vucic D (2010) c-IAP1 and UbcH5 promote K11-linked polyubiquitination of RIP1 in TNF signalling. EMBO J 29(24):4198–4209. doi:10.1038/emboj.2010.300
68. Gerlach B, Cordier SM, Schmukle AC, Emmerich CH, Rieser E, Haas TL, Webb AI, Rickard JA, Anderton H, Wong WW, Nachbur U, Gangoda L, Warnken U, Purcell AW, Silke J, Walczak H (2011) Linear ubiquitination prevents inflammation and regulates immune signalling. Nature 471(7340):591–596. doi:10.1038/nature09816
69. Micheau O, Tschopp J (2003) Induction of TNF receptor I-mediated apoptosis via two sequential signaling complexes. Cell 114(2):181–190. doi:S009286740300521X [pii]
70. Varfolomeev E, Blankenship JW, Wayson SM, Fedorova AV, Kayagaki N, Garg P, Zobel K, Dynek JN, Elliott LO, Wallweber HJ, Flygare JA, Fairbrother WJ, Deshayes K, Dixit VM, Vucic D (2007) IAP antagonists induce autoubiquitination of c-IAPs, NF-kappaB activation, and TNFalpha-dependent apoptosis. Cell 131(4):669–681. doi:10.1016/j.cell.2007.10.030
71. Peltzer N, Rieser E, Taraborrelli L, Draber P, Darding M, Pernaute B, Shimizu Y, Sarr A, Draberova H, Montinaro A, Martinez-Barbera JP, Silke J, Rodriguez TA, Walczak H (2014) HOIP deficiency causes embryonic lethality by aberrant TNFR1-mediated endothelial cell death. Cell Rep 9(1):153–165. doi:10.1016/j.celrep.2014.08.066
72. Rickard JA, Anderton H, Etemadi N, Nachbur U, Darding M, Peltzer N, Lalaoui N, Lawlor KE, Vanyai H, Hall C, Bankovacki A, Gangoda L, Wong WW, Corbin J, Huang C, Mocarski ES, Murphy JM, Alexander WS, Voss AK, Vaux DL, Kaiser WJ, Walczak H, Silke J (2014) TNFR1-dependent cell death drives inflammation in Sharpin-deficient mice. eLife 3:e03464. doi:10.7554/eLife.03464
73. Berger SB, Kasparcova V, Hoffman S, Swift B, Dare L, Schaeffer M, Capriotti C, Cook M, Finger J, Hughes-Earle A, Harris PA, Kaiser WJ, Mocarski ES, Bertin J, Gough PJ (2014) Cutting edge: RIP1 kinase activity is dispensable for normal development but is a key regulator of inflammation in SHARPIN-deficient mice. J Immunol 192(12):5476–5480. doi:10.4049/jimmunol.1400499
74. Liu X, Shi F, Li Y, Yu X, Peng S, Li W, Luo X, Cao Y (2016) Post-translational modifications as key regulators of TNF-induced necroptosis. Cell Death Dis 7(7):e2293. doi:10.1038/cddis.2016.197
75. Fouque A, Debure L, Legembre P (2014) The CD95/CD95L signaling pathway: a role in carcinogenesis. Biochim Biophys Acta 1846(1):130–141. doi:10.1016/j.bbcan.2014.04.007
76. Cullen SP, Henry CM, Kearney CJ, Logue SE, Feoktistova M, Tynan GA, Lavelle EC, Leverkus M, Martin SJ (2013) Fas/CD95-induced chemokines can serve as "find-me" signals for apoptotic cells. Mol Cell 49(6):1034–1048. doi:10.1016/j.molcel.2013.01.025
77. Varfolomeev E, Maecker H, Sharp D, Lawrence D, Renz M, Vucic D, Ashkenazi A (2005) Molecular determinants of kinase pathway activation by Apo2 ligand/tumor necrosis factor-related apoptosis-inducing ligand. J Biol Chem 280(49):40599–40608. doi:10.1074/jbc.M509560200. M509560200 [pii]
78. Geserick P, Hupe M, Moulin M, Wong WW, Feoktistova M, Kellert B, Gollnick H, Silke J, Leverkus M (2009) Cellular IAPs inhibit a cryptic CD95-induced cell death by limiting RIP1 kinase recruitment. J Cell Biol 187(7):1037–1054. doi:10.1083/jcb.200904158. jcb.200904158 [pii]
79. Jost PJ, Grabow S, Gray D, McKenzie MD, Nachbur U, Huang DC, Bouillet P, Thomas HE, Borner C, Silke J, Strasser A, Kaufmann T (2009) XIAP discriminates between type I and type II FAS-induced apoptosis. Nature 460(7258):1035–1039. doi:10.1038/nature08229
80. Tenev T, Zachariou A, Wilson R, Ditzel M, Meier P (2005) IAPs are functionally non-equivalent and regulate effector caspases through distinct mechanisms. Nat Cell Biol 7(1):70–77. doi:10.1038/ncb1204

81. Scott FL, Denault JB, Riedl SJ, Shin H, Renatus M, Salvesen GS (2005) XIAP inhibits caspase-3 and -7 using two binding sites: evolutionarily conserved mechanism of IAPs. EMBO J 24(3):645–655. doi:10.1038/sj.emboj.7600544
82. Shiozaki EN, Chai J, Rigotti DJ, Riedl SJ, Li P, Srinivasula SM, Alnemri ES, Fairman R, Shi Y (2003) Mechanism of XIAP-mediated inhibition of caspase-9. Mol Cell 11(2):519–527
83. Riedl SJ, Renatus M, Schwarzenbacher R, Zhou Q, Sun C, Fesik SW, Liddington RC, Salvesen GS (2001) Structural basis for the inhibition of caspase-3 by XIAP. Cell 104(5):791–800
84. Broemer M, Tenev T, Rigbolt KT, Hempel S, Blagoev B, Silke J, Ditzel M, Meier P (2010) Systematic in vivo RNAi analysis identifies IAPs as NEDD8-E3 ligases. Mol Cell 40(5):810–822. doi:10.1016/j.molcel.2010.11.011
85. Vogler M, Walczak H, Stadel D, Haas TL, Genze F, Jovanovic M, Bhanot U, Hasel C, Moller P, Gschwend JE, Simmet T, Debatin KM, Fulda S (2009) Small molecule XIAP inhibitors enhance TRAIL-induced apoptosis and antitumor activity in preclinical models of pancreatic carcinoma. Cancer Res 69(6):2425–2434. doi:10.1158/0008-5472.CAN-08-2436
86. Gillissen B, Richter A, Overkamp T, Essmann F, Hemmati PG, Preissner R, Belka C, Daniel PT (2013) Targeted therapy of the XIAP/proteasome pathway overcomes TRAIL-resistance in carcinoma by switching apoptosis signaling to a Bax/Bak-independent 'type I' mode. Cell Death Dis 4:e643. doi:10.1038/cddis.2013.67
87. Fakler M, Loeder S, Vogler M, Schneider K, Jeremias I, Debatin KM, Fulda S (2009) Small molecule XIAP inhibitors cooperate with TRAIL to induce apoptosis in childhood acute leukemia cells and overcome Bcl-2-mediated resistance. Blood 113(8):1710–1722. doi:10.1182/blood-2007-09-114314
88. Wang L, Du F, Wang X (2008) TNF-alpha induces two distinct caspase-8 activation pathways. Cell 133(4):693–703. doi:10.1016/j.cell.2008.03.036
89. Cheung HH, Mahoney DJ, Lacasse EC, Korneluk RG (2009) Down-regulation of c-FLIP enhances death of cancer cells by smac mimetic compound. Cancer Res 69(19):7729–7738. doi:10.1158/0008-5472.CAN-09-1794
90. Smith MA, Carol H, Evans K, Richmond J, Kang M, Reynolds CP, Chunduru S, Graham MA, Geier B, Kurmasheva R, Houghton PJ, Lock RB (2012) Birinapant (TL32711), a small molecule smac mimetic, induces regressions in childhood acute lymphoblastic leukemia (ALL) xenografts that express TNF alpha and synergizes with TNF alpha in vitro—a report from the Pediatric Preclinical Testing Program (PPTP). Blood 120(21):3565
91. Krepler C, Chunduru SK, Halloran MB, He X, Xiao M, Vultur A, Villanueva J, Mitsuuchi Y, Neiman EM, Benetatos C, Nathanson KL, Amaravadi RK, Pehamberger H, McKinlay M, Herlyn M (2013) The novel SMAC mimetic birinapant exhibits potent activity against human melanoma cells. Clin Cancer Res 19(7):1784–1794. doi:10.1158/1078-0432.CCR-12-2518
92. Vanlangenakker N, Vanden Berghe T, Bogaert P, Laukens B, Zobel K, Deshayes K, Vucic D, Fulda S, Vandenabeele P, Bertrand MJ (2011) cIAP1 and TAK1 protect cells from TNF-induced necrosis by preventing RIP1/RIP3-dependent reactive oxygen species production. Cell Death Differ 18(4):656–665. doi:10.1038/cdd.2010.138
93. He S, Wang L, Miao L, Wang T, Du F, Zhao L, Wang X (2009) Receptor interacting protein kinase-3 determines cellular necrotic response to TNF-alpha. Cell 137(6):1100–1111. doi:10.1016/j.cell.2009.05.021
94. Loeder S, Drensek A, Jeremias I, Debatin KM, Fulda S (2010) Small molecule XIAP inhibitors sensitize childhood acute leukemia cells for CD95-induced apoptosis. Int J Cancer 126(9):2216–2228. doi:10.1002/ijc.24816
95. Laukens B, Jennewein C, Schenk B, Vanlangenakker N, Schier A, Cristofanon S, Zobel K, Deshayes K, Vucic D, Jeremias I, Bertrand MJ, Vandenabeele P, Fulda S (2011) Smac mimetic bypasses apoptosis resistance in FADD- or caspase-8-deficient cells by priming for tumor necrosis factor alpha-induced necroptosis. Neoplasia 13(10):971–979
96. Varfolomeev E, Alicke B, Elliott JM, Zobel K, West K, Wong H, Scheer JM, Ashkenazi A, Gould SE, Fairbrother WJ, Vucic D (2009) X chromosome-linked inhibitor of apoptosis regu-

lates cell death induction by proapoptotic receptor agonists. J Biol Chem 284(50):34553–34560. doi:10.1074/jbc.M109.040139
97. Fulda S, Wick W, Weller M, Debatin KM (2002) Smac agonists sensitize for Apo2L/TRAIL- or anticancer drug-induced apoptosis and induce regression of malignant glioma in vivo. Nat Med 8(8):808–815
98. Wang G, Wang X, Yu H, Wei S, Williams N, Holmes DL, Halfmann R, Naidoo J, Wang L, Li L, Chen S, Harran P, Lei X (2013) Small-molecule activation of the TRAIL receptor DR5 in human cancer cells. Nat Chem Biol 9(2):84–89. doi:10.1038/nchembio.1153
99. Li L, Thomas RM, Suzuki H, De Brabander JK, Wang X, Harran PG (2004) A small molecule Smac mimic potentiates TRAIL- and TNFalpha-mediated cell death. Science 305(5689):1471–1474
100. Servida F, Lecis D, Scavullo C, Drago C, Seneci P, Carlo-Stella C, Manzoni L, Polli E, Lambertenghi Deliliers G, Delia D, Onida F (2011) Novel second mitochondria-derived activator of caspases (Smac) mimetic compounds sensitize human leukemic cell lines to conventional chemotherapeutic drug-induced and death receptor-mediated apoptosis. Investig New Drugs 29(6):1264–1275. doi:10.1007/s10637-010-9475-6
101. Chauhan D, Neri P, Velankar M, Podar K, Hideshima T, Fulciniti M, Tassone P, Raje N, Mitsiades C, Mitsiades N, Richardson P, Zawel L, Tran M, Munshi N, Anderson KC (2007) Targeting mitochondrial factor Smac/DIABLO as therapy for multiple myeloma (MM). Blood 109(3):1220–1227. doi:10.1182/blood-2006-04-015149
102. Frenzel LP, Patz M, Pallasch CP, Brinker R, Claasen J, Schulz A, Hallek M, Kashkar H, Wendtner CM (2011) Novel X-linked inhibitor of apoptosis inhibiting compound as sensitizer for TRAIL-mediated apoptosis in chronic lymphocytic leukaemia with poor prognosis. Br J Haematol 152(2):191–200. doi:10.1111/j.1365-2141.2010.08426.x
103. Stadel D, Mohr A, Ref C, MacFarlane M, Zhou S, Humphreys R, Bachem M, Cohen G, Moller P, Zwacka RM, Debatin KM, Fulda S (2010) TRAIL-induced apoptosis is preferentially mediated via TRAIL receptor 1 in pancreatic carcinoma cells and profoundly enhanced by XIAP inhibitors. Clin Cancer Res 16(23):5734–5749. doi:10.1158/1078-0432.CCR-10-0985. 1078-0432.CCR-10-0985 [pii]
104. Lu J, McEachern D, Sun H, Bai L, Peng Y, Qiu S, Miller R, Liao J, Yi H, Liu M, Bellail A, Hao C, Sun SY, Ting AT, Wang S (2011) Therapeutic potential and molecular mechanism of a novel, potent, nonpeptide, Smac mimetic SM-164 in combination with TRAIL for cancer treatment. Mol Cancer Ther 10(5):902–914. doi:10.1158/1535-7163.MCT-10-0864
105. Fingas CD, Blechacz BR, Smoot RL, Guicciardi ME, Mott J, Bronk SF, Werneburg NW, Sirica AE, Gores GJ (2010) A smac mimetic reduces TNF related apoptosis inducing ligand (TRAIL)-induced invasion and metastasis of cholangiocarcinoma cells. Hepatology 52(2):550–561. doi:10.1002/hep.23729
106. Amm HM, Zhou T, Steg AD, Kuo H, Li Y, Buchsbaum DJ (2011) Mechanisms of drug sensitization to TRA-8, an agonistic death receptor 5 antibody, involve modulation of the intrinsic apoptotic pathway in human breast cancer cells. Mol Cancer Res 9(4):403–417. doi:10.1158/1541-7786.MCR-10-0133
107. Bockbrader KM, Tan M, Sun Y (2005) A small molecule Smac-mimic compound induces apoptosis and sensitizes TRAIL- and etoposide-induced apoptosis in breast cancer cells. Oncogene 24(49):7381–7388. doi:10.1038/sj.onc.1208888
108. Petrucci E, Pasquini L, Petronelli A, Saulle E, Mariani G, Riccioni R, Biffoni M, Ferretti G, Benedetti-Panici P, Cognetti F, Scambia G, Humphreys R, Peschle C, Testa U (2007) A small molecule Smac mimic potentiates TRAIL-mediated cell death of ovarian cancer cells. Gynecol Oncol 105(2):481–492. doi:10.1016/j.ygyno.2007.01.011
109. Petrucci E, Pasquini L, Bernabei M, Saulle E, Biffoni M, Accarpio F, Sibio S, Di Giorgio A, Di Donato V, Casorelli A, Benedetti-Panici P, Testa U (2012) A small molecule SMAC mimic LBW242 potentiates TRAIL- and anticancer drug-mediated cell death of ovarian cancer cells. PLoS One 7(4):e35073. doi:10.1371/journal.pone.0035073

110. Gatti L, De Cesare M, Ciusani E, Corna E, Arrighetti N, Cominetti D, Belvisi L, Potenza D, Moroni E, Vasile F, Lecis D, Delia D, Castiglioni V, Scanziani E, Seneci P, Zaffaroni N, Perego P (2014) Antitumor activity of a novel homodimeric SMAC mimetic in ovarian carcinoma. Mol Pharm 11(1):283–293. doi:10.1021/mp4004578
111. Lecis D, Drago C, Manzoni L, Seneci P, Scolastico C, Mastrangelo E, Bolognesi M, Anichini A, Kashkar H, Walczak H, Delia D (2010) Novel SMAC-mimetics synergistically stimulate melanoma cell death in combination with TRAIL and Bortezomib. Br J Cancer 102(12):1707–1716. doi:10.1038/sj.bjc.6605687
112. Ren X, Xu Z, Myers JN, Wu X (2007) Bypass NFkappaB-mediated survival pathways by TRAIL and Smac. Cancer Biol Ther 6(7):1031–1035
113. Metwalli AR, Khanbolooki S, Jinesh G, Sundi D, Shah JB, Shrader M, Choi W, Lashinger LM, Chunduru S, McConkey DJ, McKinlay M, Kamat AM (2010) Smac mimetic reverses resistance to TRAIL and chemotherapy in human urothelial cancer cells. Cancer Biol Ther 10(9):885–892. doi:10.4161/cbt.10.9.13237
114. Wu MS, Wang GF, Zhao ZQ, Liang Y, Wang HB, Wu MY, Min P, Chen LZ, Feng QS, Bei JX, Zeng YX, Yang D (2013) Smac mimetics in combination with TRAIL selectively target cancer stem cells in nasopharyngeal carcinoma. Mol Cancer Ther 12(9):1728–1737. doi:10.1158/1535-7163.MCT-13-0017
115. Abhari BA, Cristofanon S, Kappler R, von Schweinitz D, Humphreys R, Fulda S (2013) RIP1 is required for IAP inhibitor-mediated sensitization for TRAIL-induced apoptosis via a RIP1/FADD/caspase-8 cell death complex. Oncogene 32(27):3263–3273. doi:10.1038/onc.2012.337
116. Basit F, Humphreys R, Fulda S (2012) RIP1 protein-dependent assembly of a cytosolic cell death complex is required for inhibitor of apoptosis (IAP) inhibitor-mediated sensitization to lexatumumab-induced apoptosis. J Biol Chem 287(46):38767–38777. doi:10.1074/jbc.M112.398966

Chapter 4
Bcl-2 Proteins and TRAIL Resistance in Melanoma

Jürgen Eberle

Abstract Melanoma of the skin is still characterized by high mortality, despite the recent developments of improved targeted therapies. TNF-related apoptosis-inducing ligand (TRAIL) represents a promising and additional antitumor strategy, which may also apply to metastatic melanoma. A major problem, however, results from inducible TRAIL resistance, which limits its clinical application. Addressing this issue, previous work clearly demonstrated that combinations with survival pathway inhibitors can efficiently sensitize tumor cells for TRAIL-induced apoptosis. For melanoma, the dysregulation of antiapoptotic and proapoptotic Bcl-2 proteins was identified as particularly critical. Thus, inducible TRAIL resistance in melanoma may be explained by three major steps, namely, high levels of antiapoptotic Bcl-2 proteins, high levels of inhibitor of apoptosis proteins (cIAPs) and suppressed Bax activity. These three barriers can be overcome by combinations of TRAIL and pathway inhibitors, to allow an opening for the caspase cascade and efficient induction of apoptosis, suggestive for combination therapy.

Keywords Melanoma • Bcl-2 • Apoptosis • cIAPs • Resistance • Skin

4.1 Apoptosis Deficiency: A Major Issue in Melanoma Therapy Resistance

In contrast to other solid tumors that showed decreased or stabilized incidence in the last decades, melanoma incidence still continued to rise [1]. Its high mortality results from early metastasis associated with pronounced therapy resistance. Thus, neither chemotherapy regimens nor biotherapy (IL-2 and IFN-α) or vaccination protocols could significantly improve the fatal situation of metastasized melanoma patients in the past [2]. Fortunately, this has changed in the last years due to the development of

J. Eberle (✉)
Department of Dermatology and Allergy, Skin Cancer Center Charité, Charité-Universitätsmedizin Berlin, Chariteplatz 1, 10117 Berlin, Germany
e-mail: juergen.eberle@charite.de

O. Micheau (ed.), *TRAIL, Fas Ligand, TNF and TLR3 in Cancer*, Resistance to Targeted Anti-Cancer Therapeutics, DOI 10.1007/978-3-319-56805-8_4

(1) selective BRAF inhibitors as well as (2) targeted immune modulators such as anti-CTLA4 and anti-PD1, resulting in significantly improved survival rates [3, 4]. Nevertheless, after initial tumor reduction and clinical improvement, tumor relapse and therapy resistance frequently follow within only a few months [5], thus challenging for combination therapies that may further improve the clinical outcome.

Although different cellular mechanisms do contribute to therapy resistance of cancer, apoptosis deficiency appears as the major cause. This may be explained by the need to finally eliminate cancer cells through proapoptotic programs, a common end path of most anticancer therapies. For example, chemotherapeutic drugs cause cellular or DNA damage, which induces cell-intrinsic, proapoptotic pathways [6], and also BRAF inhibition has been related to an induction of apoptosis and a sensitization for proapoptotic effectors [7–9]. Finally, immune stimulation results in cytotoxic T-lymphocytes, which express death ligands to trigger extrinsic proapoptotic pathways in target cancer cells [10]. This is suggestive for therapeutic strategies that aim at a more efficient apoptosis induction and/or apoptosis sensitization.

4.2 Control ofApoptosis

Two major proapoptotic pathways (extrinsic/intrinsic) have been reported, which are particularly mediated via death receptors and mitochondria, respectively (Fig. 4.1). Extrinsic pathways are initiated by binding of death ligands as TNF-α, CD95L/FasL or TRAIL (TNF-related apoptosis-inducing ligand) to their respective death receptors, leading to the formation of a death-inducing signalling complex and activation of initiator caspase-8 [11]. On the other hand, intrinsic pathways are initiated by different kinds of cellular dysregulation and DNA damage, which results in proapoptotic mitochondrial activation. Key events here are depolarization of the mitochondrial membrane potential ($\Delta\psi m$) and the release of proapoptotic mitochondrial factors as cytochrome c and Smac (second mitochondria-derived activator of caspases).

Cytochrome c activates initiator caspase-9 through the formation of the apoptosome, a multiprotein complex enclosing Apaf-1. On the other hand, Smac functions as antagonist of cIAPs (cellular inhibitor of apoptosis proteins), for example of XIAP, which prevents effector caspase activation [12]. Thus, cytochrome c and Smac commonly contribute to caspase activation (Fig. 4.1). A cross-link between extrinsic and intrinsic pathways results from the activation of Bid through processing by caspase-8 [13]. Initiator caspases activated in both pathways drive the processing and activation of effector caspases, such as caspase-3, which cleaves a large number of the so-called death substrates to set apoptosis into work [14].

The mitochondrial apoptosis pathways are critically controlled by the large family of Bcl-2 proteins, which enclose antiapoptotic proteins (Bcl-2, Mcl-1, Bcl-x_L, Bcl-w, and A1), proapoptotic multidomain (Bax and Bak) and proapoptotic BH3-only proteins (e.g., Bid, Bim, Bad, Puma and Noxa) [15]. Apoptosis deficiency may result both from the activation of antiapoptotic factors and from the inactivation of proapoptotic factors. Bcl-2 proteins are particularly involved and are tightly regulated by survival pathways (Fig. 4.1). In normal tissue, homeostasis is maintained by a well-balanced equilibrium of cell proliferation and cell death. In this way, programmed cell death (apoptosis) is an active cellular process, whose physiological endpoint is phagocytosis by macrophages or neighboring cells [16]. Due to this key function, apoptosis pathways are tightly regulated. Various cellular options for counter-regulation, necessary for the survival of normal cells, also allow tumor cells to escape from apoptosis control.

4.3 Aberrant Regulation of Apoptosis: A Hallmark in Cancer

As apoptosis serves as an important safeguard mechanism for the elimination of potentially harmful cells, defective proapoptotic signalling represents a critical hallmark in cancer allowing cancer cells to survive [17]. Thus, apoptosis deficiency

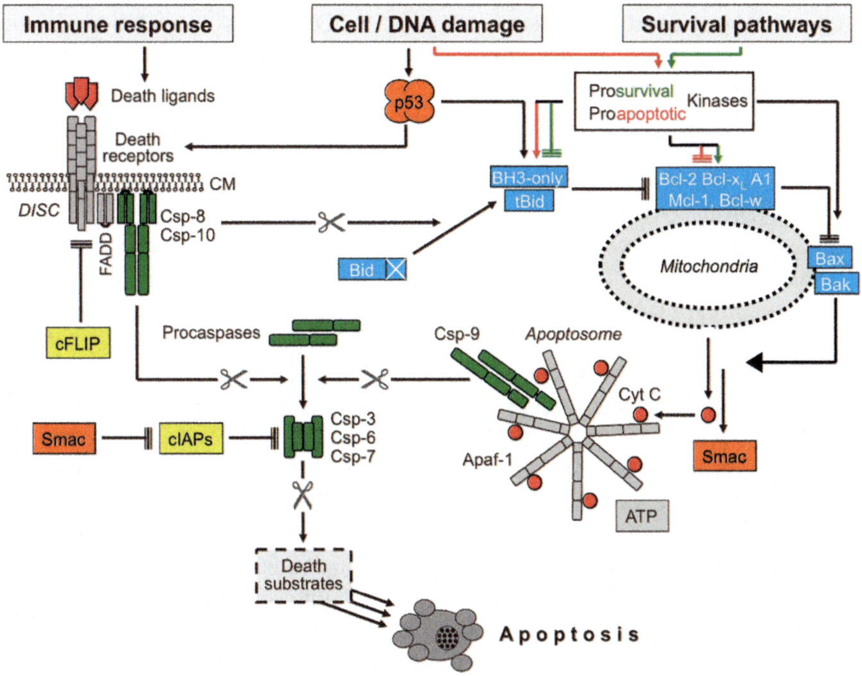

Fig. 4.1 Proapoptotic signalling pathways. Csp-3, -6, -7, -8, -9, -10, caspases; c-FLIP, cellular FLICE-inhibitory protein; *Cyt c* cytochrome c, *Smac* second mitochondria-derived activator of caspase, *cIAPs* cellular inhibitor of apoptosis proteins, *scissors* indicate protease activity, *tBid,* truncated Bid; *FADD,* Fas-associated death domain, *DISC,* death-inducing signalling complex. Please find further explanations in the text

initially supports tumor growth and at the end also provides the basis for therapy resistance. As for melanoma, its pronounced clinical chemoresistance is highly suggestive for deficient apoptosis programs [7].

Survival pathways as the RAS/RAF/MEK/ERK and the PI3K/AKT/mTOR pathways are constitutively active in many tumors, resulting in uncontrolled cell proliferation and resistance to apoptosis [18, 19]. For melanoma, activating mutations in N-RAS (10–25%) and BRAF (40–60%) appear of particular importance [20], which has resulted in the development of selective BRAF inhibitors as vemurafenib and dabrafenib [21, 22]. The downstream kinase MEK represents an additional promising target, and combinations of inhibitors for the two kinases as well as combinations of BRAF and PI3K/mTOR inhibitors are presently evaluated [23, 24].

4.4 Efficiency of TRAIL in Melanoma Cells but also Permanent and Inducible Resistance

Activation of death receptors in cancer cells by the respective ligands represents an attractive strategy to trigger apoptosis independently of p53 and may thus overcome drug resistance related to p53 inactivation [25]. CD95 ligand and TNF-α may be excluded from systemic treatment due to severe side effects such as liver toxicity and increased inflammation [26, 27].

In clear contrast, TRAIL induces apoptosis in a variety of cancer cells, while normal cells are largely spared [26, 28]. Thus, TRAIL was well tolerated in clinical studies [29–31]. In melanoma, TRAIL may induce apoptosis via both agonistic receptors, DR4/TRAIL-R1 and DR5/TRAIL-R2. Despite constitutive expression of DR5, melanoma cells with sole DR5 expression may also reveal intrinsic TRAIL resistance. On the other hand, all melanoma cell lines with additional DR4 expression reveal initial TRAIL sensitivity [32]. Resistant melanoma cells were characterized by elevated levels of XIAP and survivin [33]. Reduced expression of TRAIL receptors is seen in resistant cells of small cell lung carcinoma [34], whereas loss of caspase-10 and Bid as well as constitutive expression of the caspase-8/-10 inhibitor c-FLIP were seen in resistant cutaneous lymphoma cells [35].

Besides intrinsic resistance in some tumor cells, initially sensitive cells may also develop an inducible resistance upon TRAIL treatment, as reported for breast, colon and ovarian cancer cells [36, 37]. Inducible resistance may explain the only limited efficacy of TRAIL or TRAIL receptor agonistic antibodies so far in clinical trials performed for solid cancers and non-small cell lung cancer [29–31]. Also, in DR4-positive melanoma cells, inducible TRAIL resistance was found, which correlated to downregulation of TRAIL receptors and initiator caspases as well as proapoptotic Bcl-2 proteins as Bax, Bid and Bim [38, 39]. In relation to the role of mitochondrial pathways, knockdown of Bax prevented the release of Smac from the mitochondria and, thus, prevented an enhancement of TRAIL-induced apoptosis by pathway inhibitors [40–42].

4.5 Multiple Strategies to Sensitize Melanoma Cells for TRAIL

Many strategies were evaluated to overcome inducible TRAIL resistance. Surprisingly, melanoma cells could be sensitized for TRAIL by clearly distinct strategies as chemotherapeutics, irradiation, HDAC inhibitors, signalling inhibitors, metabolic inhibitors and ER stress inducers (for review see [43]). These strategies also included a number of targeted survival pathway inhibitors, as for BRAF and MEK [40, 44], PI3K/Akt [42], ABL [45], ATM [46], PKC [47], and IKK-β [40]. The multitude of largely unrelated strategies demanded the unravelling of common principles. In melanoma cells, this appeared to be the inhibition of cell proliferation, as proven by growing cells at high density and under serum starvation. Thus, the common principle of above-listed, different strategies for TRAIL sensitization appeared to be cell cycle inhibition [48].

4.6 Importance of Mitochondrial Pathways

In melanoma, activation of mitochondrial pathways is essential for full induction of apoptosis by death ligands [7], and mitochondrial activation was found for many strategies that resulted in TRAIL sensitization, as by kinase inhibitors. Indicators were loss of the mitochondrial membrane potential and release of proapoptotic mitochondrial factors (cytochrome c and Smac). However, mitochondrial activation alone appeared as not sufficient for apoptosis induction, and the inhibitors themselves often only insufficiently induced apoptosis in melanoma cells, as antiapoptotic Bcl-2 proteins were still active (Fig. 4.2).

Processing of caspase-8 and of Bid are characteristic steps in melanoma cells in response to TRAIL and were frequently seen even in resistant melanoma cells. Bid may further antagonize Bcl-2, which however also appeared as not sufficient for apoptosis induction in resistant cells. Although not sufficient, Bid was essential for apoptosis induction by combinations of TRAIL and pathway inhibitors, as shown by Bid knockdown [40, 41].

Another critical role in TRAIL resistance of melanoma cells is suspected for XIAP (Fig. 4.2). This may be concluded from the frequently seen incomplete processing of caspase-3 upon TRAIL treatment, despite caspase-8 was activated [40, 41, 49]. Several strategies for TRAIL sensitization coincided with a downregulation of XIAP as reported for UVB, IFN-β, HDAC inhibitors, chemotherapeutics, ADI-PEG, and kinase inhibitors. These drugs in combination with TRAIL then also enabled complete processing of caspase-3. In this relation, overexpression of XIAP protected melanoma cells from TRAIL-induced apoptosis [40, 41, 50], whereas its siRNA-mediated knockdown could sensitize melanoma cells for TRAIL [51].

As XIAP is antagonized by Smac, release of Smac should represent a critical step in TRAIL sensitivity. The important role of the Smac/XIAP rheostat was demonstrated

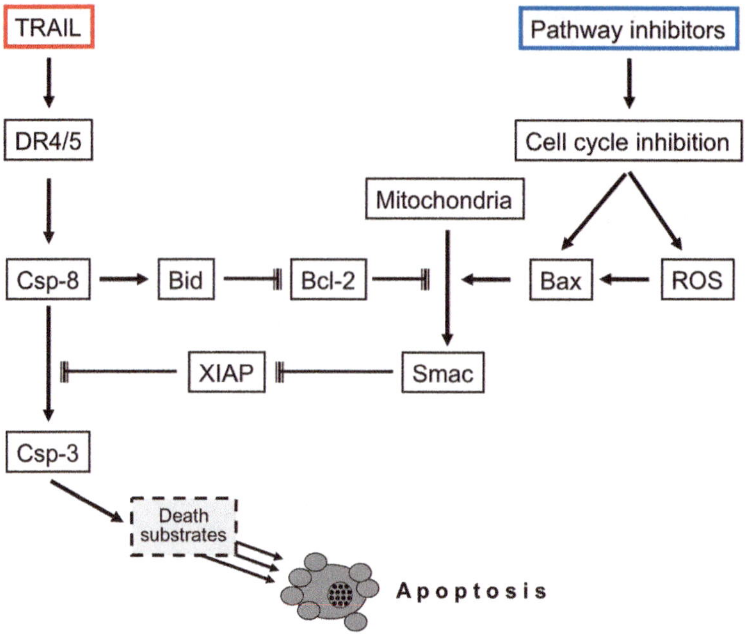

Fig. 4.2 Relevant pathways for TRAIL sensitization in melanoma. *DR4/5*, death receptors 4 and 5; *Csp-3*, *-8*, caspases; *Smac*, second mitochondria-derived activator of caspase; *XIAP*, X-linked inhibitor of apoptosis protein; *ROS*, reactive oxygen species. Please find further explanations in the text

in pancreatic and bladder cancers by using small molecule inhibitors for XIAP or Smac mimetics, which both enhanced TRAIL sensitivity [52, 53]. In melanoma cells, the essential role of Smac for enhancement of TRAIL-induced apoptosis was proven by knockdown strategies [43].

4.7 The Critical Contribution of Bcl-2 Proteins

According to generally accepted models, the mitochondrial gate is controlled by a rheostat of proapoptotic and antiapoptotic Bcl-2 proteins, and also TRAIL-induced apoptosis is blocked by Bcl-2 overexpression [40–42, 50, 54]. In aggreement, downregulation of antiapoptotic Bcl-2 proteins (Bcl-2, Mcl-1, and Bcl-x_L) is seen in melanoma cells upon treatment with different sensitizing strategies as chemotherapeutics, HDAC, metabolism and kinase inhibitors [43].

On the other hand, proapoptotic BH3-only proteins are frequently upregulated in the course of TRAIL sensitization. Particularly important roles are attributed to Bim and Puma, as both may interact with all antiapoptotic Bcl-2 family members [55]. Of note, these proteins were upregulated in the course of TRAIL sensitization by HDAC, BRAF, and cell cycle inhibition [8, 40, 48, 56]. The relation of Bim and

MAP kinases is based on ERK-mediated phosphorylation of Bim, which triggers its proteasomal degradation [57]. Considering the large number of other BH3-only proteins that have not been sufficiently investigated in most studies, one may expect even more impact from these important triggers in apoptosis in future studies.

4.8 Bax: A Master Regulator of TRAIL Sensitivity in Melanoma Cells

Sensitization of melanoma cells for TRAIL-induced apoptosis appeared as particularly dependent on Bax. Thus, mitochondrial Bax translocation was observed by different combinations of TRAIL and pathway inhibitors as imatinib, TRAM-34, HDAC inhibitors, U0126, wortmannin, and BMS-345541. In addition, Bax conformational changes, characteristic for its activation (Bax-NT), were seen after treatment with inhibitors for HDACs, PI3K/AKT, BRAF, and IKK. Of note, Bax activation is usually seen as an initial, early event (within 1–2 h), thus not reflecting induced apoptosis but clearly suggesting a mechanism that allows mitochondrial activation in melanoma cells and sensitization for TRAIL-induced apoptosis [43].

In agreement with its critical role, siRNA-mediated Bax knockdown abrogated apoptosis induction in melanoma cells by combinations of TRAIL and the different inhibitors [40, 42]. For the regulation of Bax, an inactivating phosphorylation at Ser-184 as well as an activating phosphorylation at Thr-167 had been reported [58, 59]. By using Bax phosphorylation-specific antibodies and flow cytometry, we could prove that Bax activation by IKK, PI3K, and AKT inhibitors was correlated with suppressed Ser-184 phosphorylation and enhanced Thr-167 phosphorylation. Both changes appeared as immediate effects (within 1–2 h) and were independent of induced apoptosis [40, 42].

The inhibitory phosphorylation at Ser-184 has been previously related to AKT activity [59], whereas the activating phosphorylation at Thr-167 was related to JNK, p38, and ERK pathways [58, 60]. For melanoma cells, we proved that Thr-167 phosphorylation in the course of PI3K inhibition was dependent on the production of intracellular reactive oxygen species (ROS). Thus, antioxidants prevented Thr-167 phosphorylation and partially rescued melanoma cells from wortmannin/TRAIL-induced apoptosis [42]. The significance of ROS for apoptosis regulation in melanoma cells has been previously reported [61, 62], and ROS was also involved in sensitization for TRAIL by cell cycle inhibition [48].

4.9 Conclusions

TRAIL appears as a promising antitumor strategy, which may also accomplish targeted therapies for melanoma. Many investigations therefore aimed at the sensitization of melanoma cells for TRAIL-induced apoptosis. These data provide a suitable basis for the identification of common principles that mediate TRAIL resistance in melanoma cells. Four critical steps were identified, namely, death receptor downregulation, high Bcl-2 expression, Bax inactivation, and high levels of XIAP.

In response to TRAIL, caspase-8 is activated and Bid is cleaved. However, caspase-3 activation is prevented by XIAP, and the antagonizing effect of Bid on Bcl-2 is not sufficient for opening the mitochondrial gate, as Bax is still inactive. This changes under conditions of combination treatments. Now Bax is activated by pathway inhibitors in addition of Bcl-2 inactivation through Bid. This finally opens the mitochondrial gate for Smac release, which then can angagonize XIAP. Now, caspase-3 can also be completely processed and activated to efficiently induce apoptosis (Fig. 4.2). This understanding throws new light on the mechanisms of targeted therapeutic strategies in melanoma cells that may activate Bax and sensitize for TRAIL. This should finally lead to the development of new combination strategies.

References

1. Siegel R, Ma J, Zou Z, Jemal A (2014) Cancer statistics, 2014. CA Cancer J Clin 64(1):9–29. doi:10.3322/caac.21208
2. Garbe C, Peris K, Hauschild A, Saiag P, Middleton M, Bastholt L, Grob JJ, Malvehy J, Newton-Bishop J, Stratigos AJ, Pehamberger H, Eggermont AM, European Dermatology F, European Association of D-O, European Organisation for R, Treatment of C (2016) Diagnosis and treatment of melanoma. European consensus-based interdisciplinary guideline - update 2016. Eur J Cancer 63:201–217. doi:10.1016/j.ejca.2016.05.005
3. Menzies AM, Long GV (2014) Systemic treatment for BRAF-mutant melanoma: where do we go next? Lancet Oncol 15(9):e371–e381. doi:10.1016/S1470-2045(14)70072-5
4. Hughes T, Klairmont M, Sharfman WH, Kaufman HL (2015) Interleukin-2, Ipilimumab, and anti-PD-1: clinical management and the evolving role of immunotherapy for the treatment of patients with metastatic melanoma. Cancer Biol Ther. doi:10.1080/15384047.2015.1095401
5. Chen G, Davies MA (2014) Targeted therapy resistance mechanisms and therapeutic implications in melanoma. Hematol Oncol Clin North Am 28(3):523–536. doi:10.1016/j.hoc.2014.03.001
6. Johnstone RW, Ruefli AA, Lowe SW (2002) Apoptosis: a link between cancer genetics and chemotherapy. Cell 108(2):153–164
7. Eberle J, Kurbanov BM, Hossini AM, Trefzer U, Fecker LF (2007) Overcoming apoptosis deficiency of melanoma-hope for new therapeutic approaches. Drug Resist Updat 10(6):218–234. doi:10.1016/j.drup.2007.09.001
8. Beck D, Niessner H, Smalley KS, Flaherty K, Paraiso KH, Busch C, Sinnberg T, Vasseur S, Iovanna JL, Driessen S, Stork B, Wesselborg S, Schaller M, Biedermann T, Bauer J, Lasithiotakis K, Weide B, Eberle J, Schittek B, Schadendorf D, Garbe C, Kulms D, Meier F (2013) Vemurafenib potently induces endoplasmic reticulum stress-mediated apoptosis in BRAFV600E melanoma cells. Sci Signal 6(260):ra7. doi:10.1126/scisignal.2003057
9. Berger A, Quast SA, Plotz M, Kuhn NF, Trefzer U, Eberle J (2014) RAF inhibition overcomes resistance to TRAIL-induced apoptosis in melanoma cells. J Invest Dermatol 134(2):430–440. doi:10.1038/jid.2013.347
10. Martinez-Lostao L, Anel A, Pardo J (2015) How do cytotoxic lymphocytes kill cancer cells? Clin Cancer Res 21(22):5047–5056. doi:10.1158/1078-0432.CCR-15-0685
11. Krammer PH, Arnold R, Lavrik IN (2007) Life and death in peripheral T cells. Nat Rev Immunol 7(7):532–542. doi:10.1038/nri2115

12. Fulda S, Vucic D (2012) Targeting IAP proteins for therapeutic intervention in cancer. Nat Rev Drug Discov 11(2):109–124. doi:10.1038/nrd3627
13. Li H, Zhu H, Xu CJ, Yuan J (1998) Cleavage of BID by caspase 8 mediates the mitochondrial damage in the Fas pathway of apoptosis. Cell 94(4):491–501
14. Fischer U, Janicke RU, Schulze-Osthoff K (2003) Many cuts to ruin: a comprehensive update of caspase substrates. Cell Death Differ 10(1):76–100. doi:10.1038/sj.cdd.4401160
15. Chipuk JE, Moldoveanu T, Llambi F, Parsons MJ, Green DR (2010) The BCL-2 family reunion. Mol Cell 37(3):299–310. doi:10.1016/j.molcel.2010.01.025
16. Kerr JF, Wyllie AH, Currie AR (1972) Apoptosis: a basic biological phenomenon with wide-ranging implications in tissue kinetics. Br J Cancer 26(4):239–257
17. Hanahan D, Weinberg RA (2011) Hallmarks of cancer: the next generation. Cell 144(5):646–674. doi:10.1016/j.cell.2011.02.013
18. Inamdar GS, Madhunapantula SV, Robertson GP (2010) Targeting the MAPK pathway in melanoma: why some approaches succeed and other fail. Biochem Pharmacol 80(5):624–637. doi:10.1016/j.bcp.2010.04.029
19. Wallin JJ, Edgar KA, Guan J, Berry M, Prior WW, Lee L, Lesnick JD, Lewis C, Nonomiya J, Pang J, Salphati L, Olivero AG, Sutherlin DP, O'Brien C, Spoerke JM, Patel S, Lensun L, Kassees R, Ross L, Lackner MR, Sampath D, Belvin M, Friedman LS (2011) GDC-0980 is a novel class I PI3K/mTOR kinase inhibitor with robust activity in cancer models driven by the PI3K pathway. Mol Cancer Ther 10(12):2426–2436. doi:10.1158/1535-7163.MCT-11-0446
20. Davies H, Bignell GR, Cox C, Stephens P, Edkins S, Clegg S, Teague J, Woffendin H, Garnett MJ, Bottomley W, Davis N, Dicks E, Ewing R, Floyd Y, Gray K, Hall S, Hawes R, Hughes J, Kosmidou V, Menzies A, Mould C, Parker A, Stevens C, Watt S, Hooper S, Wilson R, Jayatilake H, Gusterson BA, Cooper C, Shipley J, Hargrave D, Pritchard-Jones K, Maitland N, Chenevix-Trench G, Riggins GJ, Bigner DD, Palmieri G, Cossu A, Flanagan A, Nicholson A, Ho JW, Leung SY, Yuen ST, Weber BL, Seigler HF, Darrow TL, Paterson H, Marais R, Marshall CJ, Wooster R, Stratton MR, Futreal PA (2002) Mutations of the BRAF gene in human cancer. Nature 417(6892):949–954. doi:10.1038/nature00766
21. Hauschild A, Grob JJ, Demidov LV, Jouary T, Gutzmer R, Millward M, Rutkowski P, Blank CU, Miller WH Jr, Kaempgen E, Martin-Algarra S, Karaszewska B, Mauch C, Chiarion-Sileni V, Martin AM, Swann S, Haney P, Mirakhur B, Guckert ME, Goodman V, Chapman PB (2012) Dabrafenib in BRAF-mutated metastatic melanoma: a multicentre, open-label, phase 3 randomised controlled trial. Lancet 380(9839):358–365. doi:10.1016/S0140-6736(12)60868-X
22. Sosman JA, Kim KB, Schuchter L, Gonzalez R, Pavlick AC, Weber JS, McArthur GA, Hutson TE, Moschos SJ, Flaherty KT, Hersey P, Kefford R, Lawrence D, Puzanov I, Lewis KD, Amaravadi RK, Chmielowski B, Lawrence HJ, Shyr Y, Ye F, Li J, Nolop KB, Lee RJ, Joe AK, Ribas A (2012) Survival in BRAF V600-mutant advanced melanoma treated with vemurafenib. N Engl J Med 366(8):707–714. doi:10.1056/NEJMoa1112302
23. Flaherty KT, Infante JR, Daud A, Gonzalez R, Kefford RF, Sosman J, Hamid O, Schuchter L, Cebon J, Ibrahim N, Kudchadkar R, Burris HA 3rd, Falchook G, Algazi A, Lewis K, Long GV, Puzanov I, Lebowitz P, Singh A, Little S, Sun P, Allred A, Ouellet D, Kim KB, Patel K, Weber J (2012) Combined BRAF and MEK inhibition in melanoma with BRAF V600 mutations. N Engl J Med 367(18):1694–1703. doi:10.1056/NEJMoa1210093
24. Nijenhuis CM, Haanen JB, Schellens JH, Beijnen JH (2013) Is combination therapy the next step to overcome resistance and reduce toxicities in melanoma? Cancer Treat Rev 39(4):305–312. doi:10.1016/j.ctrv.2012.10.006
25. Kelley SK, Ashkenazi A (2004) Targeting death receptors in cancer with Apo2L/TRAIL. Curr Opin Pharmacol 4(4):333–339
26. Ashkenazi A (2002) Targeting death and decoy receptors of the tumour-necrosis factor superfamily. Nat Rev Cancer 2(6):420–430. doi:10.1038/nrc821
27. Micheau O, Shirley S, Dufour F (2013) Death receptors as targets in cancer. Br J Pharmacol 169(8):1723–1744. doi:10.1111/Bph.12238

28. Walczak H, Miller RE, Ariail K, Gliniak B, Griffith TS, Kubin M, Chin W, Jones J, Woodward A, Le T, Smith C, Smolak P, Goodwin RG, Rauch CT, Schuh JC, Lynch DH (1999) Tumoricidal activity of tumor necrosis factor-related apoptosis-inducing ligand in vivo. Nat Med 5(2):157–163
29. Herbst RS, Eckhardt SG, Kurzrock R, Ebbinghaus S, O'Dwyer PJ, Gordon MS, Novotny W, Goldwasser MA, Tohnya TM, Lum BL, Ashkenazi A, Jubb AM, Mendelson DS (2010) Phase I dose-escalation study of recombinant human Apo2L/TRAIL, a dual proapoptotic receptor agonist, in patients with advanced cancer. J Clin Oncol 28(17):2839–2846. doi:10.1200/JCO.2009.25.1991. JCO.2009.25.1991 [pii]
30. Soria JC, Mark Z, Zatloukal P, Szima B, Albert I, Juhasz E, Pujol JL, Kozielski J, Baker N, Smethurst D, Hei YJ, Ashkenazi A, Stern H, Amler L, Pan Y, Blackhall F (2011) Randomized phase II study of dulanermin in combination with paclitaxel, carboplatin, and bevacizumab in advanced non-small-cell lung cancer. J Clin Oncol 29(33):4442–4451. doi:10.1200/JCO.2011.37.2623
31. Stuckey DW, Shah K (2013) TRAIL on trial: preclinical advances in cancer therapy. Trends Mol Med 19(11):685–694. doi:10.1016/j.molmed.2013.08.007
32. Kurbanov BM, Geilen CC, Fecker LF, Orfanos CE, Eberle J (2005) Efficient TRAIL-R1/DR4-mediated apoptosis in melanoma cells by tumor necrosis factor-related apoptosis-inducing ligand (TRAIL). J Invest Dermatol 125(5):1010–1019. doi:10.1111/j.0022-202X.2005.23900.x
33. Zhang L, Fang B (2005) Mechanisms of resistance to TRAIL-induced apoptosis in cancer. Cancer Gene Ther 12(3):228–237. doi:10.1038/sj.cgt.7700792
34. Hopkins-Donaldson S, Ziegler A, Kurtz S, Bigosch C, Kandioler D, Ludwig C, Zangemeister-Wittke U, Stahel R (2003) Silencing of death receptor and caspase-8 expression in small cell lung carcinoma cell lines and tumors by DNA methylation. Cell Death Differ 10(3):356–364
35. Braun FK, Hirsch B, Al-Yacoub N, Durkop H, Assaf C, Kadin ME, Sterry W, Eberle J (2010) Resistance of cutaneous anaplastic large-cell lymphoma cells to apoptosis by death ligands is enhanced by CD30-mediated overexpression of c-FLIP. J Invest Dermatol 130(3):826–840. doi:10.1038/jid.2009.299
36. Li Y, Wang H, Wang Z, Makhija S, Buchsbaum D, LoBuglio A, Kimberly R, Zhou T (2006) Inducible resistance of tumor cells to tumor necrosis factor-related apoptosis-inducing ligand receptor 2-mediated apoptosis by generation of a blockade at the death domain function. Cancer Res 66(17):8520–8528. doi:10.1158/0008-5472.CAN-05-4364
37. Van Geelen CM, de Vries EG, de Jong S (2004) Lessons from TRAIL-resistance mechanisms in colorectal cancer cells: paving the road to patient-tailored therapy. Drug Resist Updat 7(6):345–358. doi:10.1016/j.drup.2004.11.002
38. Zhang XD, Wu JJ, Gillespie S, Borrow J, Hersey P (2006) Human melanoma cells selected for resistance to apoptosis by prolonged exposure to tumor necrosis factor-related apoptosis-inducing ligand are more vulnerable to necrotic cell death induced by cisplatin. Clin Cancer Res 12(4):1355–1364. doi:10.1158/1078-0432.CCR-05-2084
39. Kurbanov BM, Fecker LF, Geilen CC, Sterry W, Eberle J (2007) Resistance of melanoma cells to TRAIL does not result from upregulation of antiapoptotic proteins by NF-kappaB but is related to downregulation of initiator caspases and DR4. Oncogene 26(23):3364–3377
40. Berger A, Quast SA, Plotz M, Kammermeier A, Eberle J (2013) Sensitization of melanoma cells for TRAIL-induced apoptosis by BMS-345541 correlates with altered phosphorylation and activation of Bax. Cell Death Dis 4:e477. doi:10.1038/cddis.2012.198
41. Quast SA, Berger A, Buttstadt N, Friebel K, Schonherr R, Eberle J (2012) General sensitization of melanoma cells for TRAIL-induced apoptosis by the potassium channel inhibitor TRAM-34 depends on release of SMAC. PLoS One 7(6):e39290. doi:10.1371/journal.pone.0039290
42. Quast SA, Berger A, Eberle J (2013) ROS-dependent phosphorylation of Bax by wortmannin sensitizes melanoma cells for TRAIL-induced apoptosis. Cell Death Dis 4:e839. doi:10.1038/cddis.2013.344

43. Quast SA, Berger A, Plotz M, Eberle J (2014) Sensitization of melanoma cells for TRAIL-induced apoptosis by activation of mitochondrial pathways via Bax. Eur J Cell Biol 93(1–2):42–48. doi:10.1016/j.ejcb.2013.11.003
44. Zhang XD, Borrow JM, Zhang XY, Nguyen T, Hersey P (2003) Activation of ERK1/2 protects melanoma cells from TRAIL-induced apoptosis by inhibiting Smac/DIABLO release from mitochondria. Oncogene 22(19):2869–2881. doi:10.1038/sj.onc.1206427
45. Hamai A, Richon C, Meslin F, Faure F, Kauffmann A, Lecluse Y, Jalil A, Larue L, Avril MF, Chouaib S, Mehrpour M (2006) Imatinib enhances human melanoma cell susceptibility to TRAIL-induced cell death: relationship to Bcl-2 family and caspase activation. Oncogene 25(58):7618–7634. doi:10.1038/sj.onc.1209738
46. Ivanov VN, Zhou H, Partridge MA, Hei TK (2009) Inhibition of ataxia telangiectasia mutated kinase activity enhances TRAIL-mediated apoptosis in human melanoma cells. Cancer Res 69(8):3510–3519. doi:10.1158/0008-5472.CAN-08-3883
47. Gillespie SK, Zhang XD, Hersey P (2004) Ingenol 3-angelate induces dual modes of cell death and differentially regulates tumor necrosis factor-related apoptosis-inducing ligand-induced apoptosis in melanoma cells. Mol Cancer Ther 3(12):1651–1658
48. Quast SA, Steinhorst K, Plotz M, Eberle J (2015) Sensitization of melanoma cells for death ligand TRAIL is based on cell cycle arrest, ROS production, and activation of proapoptotic Bcl-2 proteins. J Invest Dermatol 135(11):2794–2804. doi:10.1038/jid.2015.250
49. Hornle M, Peters N, Thayaparasingham B, Vorsmann H, Kashkar H, Kulms D (2011) Caspase-3 cleaves XIAP in a positive feedback loop to sensitize melanoma cells to TRAIL-induced apoptosis. Oncogene 30(5):575–587. doi:10.1038/onc.2010.434
50. Zhang XD, Zhang XY, Gray CP, Nguyen T, Hersey P (2001) Tumor necrosis factor-related apoptosis-inducing ligand-induced apoptosis of human melanoma is regulated by smac/DIABLO release from mitochondria. Cancer Res 61(19):7339–7348
51. Chawla-Sarkar M, Bae SI, Reu FJ, Jacobs BS, Lindner DJ, Borden EC (2004) Downregulation of Bcl-2, FLIP or IAPs (XIAP and survivin) by siRNAs sensitizes resistant melanoma cells to Apo2L/TRAIL-induced apoptosis. Cell Death Differ 11(8):915–923. doi:10.1038/sj.cdd.4401416
52. Griffith TS, Kucaba TA, O'Donnell MA, Burns J, Benetatos C, McKinlay MA, Condon S, Chunduru S (2011) Sensitization of human bladder tumor cells to TNF-related apoptosis-inducing ligand (TRAIL)-induced apoptosis with a small molecule IAP antagonist. Apoptosis 16(1):13–26. doi:10.1007/s10495-010-0535-3
53. Vogler M, Walczak H, Stadel D, Haas TL, Genze F, Jovanovic M, Bhanot U, Hasel C, Moller P, Gschwend JE, Simmet T, Debatin KM, Fulda S (2009) Small molecule XIAP inhibitors enhance TRAIL-induced apoptosis and antitumor activity in preclinical models of pancreatic carcinoma. Cancer Res 69(6):2425–2434. doi:10.1158/0008-5472.CAN-08-2436
54. Berger A, Quast SA, Plotz M, Hein M, Kunz M, Langer P, Eberle J (2011) Sensitization of melanoma cells for death ligand-induced apoptosis by an indirubin derivative--enhancement of both extrinsic and intrinsic apoptosis pathways. Biochem Pharmacol 81(1):71–81. doi:10.1016/j.bcp.2010.09.010
55. Plotz M, Gillissen B, Quast SA, Berger A, Daniel PT, Eberle J (2013) The BH3-only protein Bim(L) overrides Bcl-2-mediated apoptosis resistance in melanoma cells. Cancer Lett 335(1):100–108. doi:10.1016/j.canlet.2013.02.005
56. Gillespie S, Borrow J, Zhang XD, Hersey P (2006) Bim plays a crucial role in synergistic induction of apoptosis by the histone deacetylase inhibitor SBHA and TRAIL in melanoma cells. Apoptosis 11(12):2251–2265. doi:10.1007/s10495-006-0283-6
57. Cartlidge RA, Thomas GR, Cagnol S, Jong KA, Molton SA, Finch AJ, McMahon M (2008) Oncogenic BRAF(V600E) inhibits BIM expression to promote melanoma cell survival. Pigment Cell Melanoma Res 21(5):534–544. doi:10.1111/j.1755-148X.2008.00491.x
58. Kim BJ, Ryu SW, Song BJ (2006) JNK- and p38 kinase-mediated phosphorylation of Bax leads to its activation and mitochondrial translocation and to apoptosis of human hepatoma HepG2 cells. J Biol Chem 281(30):21256–21265. doi:10.1074/jbc.M510644200

59. Renault TT, Manon S (2011) Bax: addressed to kill. Biochimie 93(9):1379–1391. doi:10.1016/j.biochi.2011.05.013
60. Min H, Ghatnekar GS, Ghatnekar AV, You X, Bu M, Guo X, Bu S, Shen B, Huang Q (2012) 2-Methoxyestradiol induced Bax phosphorylation and apoptosis in human retinoblastoma cells via p38 MAPK activation. Mol Carcinog 51(7):576–585. doi:10.1002/mc.20825
61. Franke JC, Plotz M, Prokop A, Geilen CC, Schmalz HG, Eberle J (2010) New caspase-independent but ROS-dependent apoptosis pathways are targeted in melanoma cells by an iron-containing cytosine analogue. Biochem Pharmacol 79(4):575–586. doi:10.1016/j.bcp.2009.09.022
62. Tochigi M, Inoue T, Suzuki-Karasaki M, Ochiai T, Ra C, Suzuki-Karasaki Y (2013) Hydrogen peroxide induces cell death in human TRAIL-resistant melanoma through intracellular superoxide generation. Int J Oncol 42(3):863–872. doi:10.3892/ijo.2013.1769

Chapter 5
Regulation of Caspase-Mediated Apoptosis by the Tumor Suppressor Par-4

James Sledziona and Vivek M. Rangnekar

Abstract The Prostate Apoptosis Response-4 gene *Par-4* encodes a tumor suppressor protein, which can act through a number of intrinsic and extrinsic apoptotic pathways. Extracellularly, Par-4 can interact with cell-surface GRP-78 and trigger apoptosis through membrane-bound GRP-78. Intracellularly, Par-4 can downgrade the activities of pro-survival pathways like NF-κB, promote translocation of Fas and FasL to the plasma membrane or inhibit topoisomerase activity.

The dual discoveries that Par-4 is secreted in response to various stimuli and can selectively induce apoptosis in tumor cells, without harming normal cells, have generated great interest in its therapeutic potential as a novel antitumor agent.

Keywords Par-4 • PAWR • Apoptosis • Fas • SAC • Death receptors • GRP-78

5.1 Introduction

Despite many decades of therapeutic research and prevention efforts, cancer remains the second leading cause of death in the USA [1]. According to the World Health Organization, 2012 saw 8.2 million cancer-related deaths and approximately 14 million new cases worldwide [2]. While therapeutic advances have significantly improved prognoses for multiple types of malignancies such as leukemia, lymphoma, and some solid tumors, overall progress remains plodding and iterative.

J. Sledziona
Graduate Center for Toxicology and Cancer Biology, University of Kentucky, 561 Biopharm Complex, 789 South Limestone St, Lexington, KY 40536, USA

V.M. Rangnekar (✉)
Graduate Center for Toxicology and Cancer Biology, University of Kentucky, 561 Biopharm Complex, 789 South Limestone St, Lexington, KY 40536, USA

Department of Radiation Medicine, University of Kentucky, Lexington, KY, USA

Department of Microbiology, Immunology and Molecular Genetics, University of Kentucky, Lexington, KY, USA

Lucille Parker Markey Cancer Center, University of Kentucky, Lexington, KY, USA
e-mail: vmrang01@email.uky.edu

O. Micheau (ed.), *TRAIL, Fas Ligand, TNF and TLR3 in Cancer*, Resistance to Targeted Anti-Cancer Therapeutics, DOI 10.1007/978-3-319-56805-8_5

Historically, treatment has focused upon some combination of surgical resection (where applicable), chemotherapy, or ionizing radiation. This approach typically generates moderate-to-severe side effects upon the patient. Discovery of useful chemotherapeutic agents was described by one researcher in 1945 as: "... almost as hard as finding some agent that will dissolve away the left ear … yet leave the right ear unharmed: so slight is the difference between the cancer cell and its normal ancestor" [3]. Despite this, improved survival rates with less harsh side effects have been achieved through application of targeted therapies.

Targeted therapies were borne of the finding that certain cancers might display increased expression or activity of specific biomarkers required for cellular proliferation, survival, or migration, compared to normal cells. These biomarkers are classified as oncogenes; commonly cited examples include EGFR, Ras, and Src. Therapeutically countering the activities of oncogenes may involve such strategies as monoclonal antibodies (e.g., herceptin/trastuzumab) against solid tumors by blocking growth factor receptor-ligand binding. Research into cancer biology also revealed that cancerous cells may also carry deletions for or downregulate a series of genes which serve to monitor or repair genetic damage, restrict cell proliferation or trigger programmed cell death (apoptosis). As cancer may result from loss of these factors, they are classified as tumor suppressors; classic examples include BRCA1/2, Retinoblastoma (Rb), and p53.

Cancer, given its huge range of types and subtypes, appropriately requires a range of therapeutic approaches. Obviously, one approach is to specifically exploit the tumor suppressors and activate the cells' apoptotic pathway. Such methods as radiation or chemotherapy, through DNA damage, enhance the intrinsic apoptotic pathway and depend upon wholly internally expressed factors. Another approach is to activate the extrinsic apoptotic pathway, which exploits externally triggered pathways- generally a receptor-ligand interaction at the cell membrane to trigger apoptosis. Classically, the membrane expressed Fas receptor (CD95), paired with its ligand, FasL (CD95L) is used by immune cells to destroy virus-infected or cancerous cells. Clinically, side effects like apoptotic liver damage have limited the therapeutic value of this pathway, and many cancers also appear highly resistant to Fas-mediated apoptosis [4]. However, research is continuing to explore Fas' utility as part of a combination therapeutic regemin [5].

5.2 Par-4

The effort to discover new tumor-suppressor genes to exploit therapeutically has led to the discovery of Prostate apoptosis response-4 (Par-4). The role of Par-4 in apoptosis was first published in 1994 by Stephen Sells [6] upon the discovery that Par-4 expression is upregulated during the apoptosis of rat prostate cells in response to androgen ablation [6]. Under normal conditions, Par-4 displays cytoplasmic localization but will translocate to the nucleus in the event of an apoptotic insult [7]. Additional experiments would demonstrate that Par-4 is not upregulated upon necrosis or growth arrest [6], further cementing its role as a tumor suppressor or apoptosis-associated gene.

As a direct indicator of the relevance of Par-4 in oncology, Par-4 has been found to be mutated and/or downregulated in renal cell carcinoma, neuroblastoma, endometrial cancer, and breast cancer [7]. In fact, Cook et al. found that 74% of renal cell carcinomas (RCCs) sampled were negative for Par-4 staining [8]. Likewise, analysis of endometrial carcinomas showed Par-4 downregulation in about 40% of samples [9]. Of these, 32% display silencing of Par-4 via promoter hypermethylation or a nonsense mutation in exon 3.

Par-4 activity is also positively correlated with cancer treatment prognosis. Alvarez et al. have found that low Par-4 expression is predictive of breast cancer recurrence and chemotherapeutic response. Recurrent breast tumors sampled were found to have significantly reduced Par-4 expression compared to primary tumors, likely rendering subsequent rounds of therapy far less effective [10]. Likewise, researchers have reported that increased Par-4 expression increases radiosensitivity and chemosensitivity of colon cancer cells [11] as well as breast tumor cells [12].

Experimentally, Par-4 knockout mice have been created and appear developmentally normal. However, they are subject to spontaneous tumors of the endometrium, lungs, liver, and bladder, resulting in significantly reduced average life spans compared to wild-type mice (19 months versus 25 months, respectively) [13].

Apoptosis involves multiple pathways and many factors; however, what makes Par-4 unique as a tumor suppressor is its ability to selectively induce apoptosis in cancer cells while leaving normal or immortalized cells unaffected. Intrinsically, Par-4 activates apoptotic pathways while concurrently suppressing cell-survival pathways. This intrinsic activity requires nuclear entry. Par-4-induced apoptosis can be p53 independent [14], rendering it of interest for treating the 50% of tumors with silenced, deleted or downregulated p53. While Par-4 certainly can act in a wholly intracellular manner, one major discovery is the fact that Par-4 can be secreted into the extracellular compartment under conditions of endoplasmic reticulum (ER) stress, p53 activation or inhibition of NF-κB transactivation potential. This finding implies that Par-4 selectively induces apoptosis in tumor cells in a paracrine and possibly autocrine manner. This novel finding is covered in greater detail later in this chapter.

5.2.1 Par-4 Structure

Human Par-4 is a 340-amino acid [15] protein of ~40 kDa that is ubiquitously expressed across most bodily tissues. This is encoded by the PAWR (*Par-4*) gene, located on human chromosome 12q21. The gene is comprised of seven exons and six introns [7].

Par-4 possesses a number of conserved functional domains (Fig. 5.1). These include two N-terminal nuclear localization sequences (NLS1 and NLS2), a C-terminal leucine zipper domain (LZ) and a C-terminal nuclear export sequence

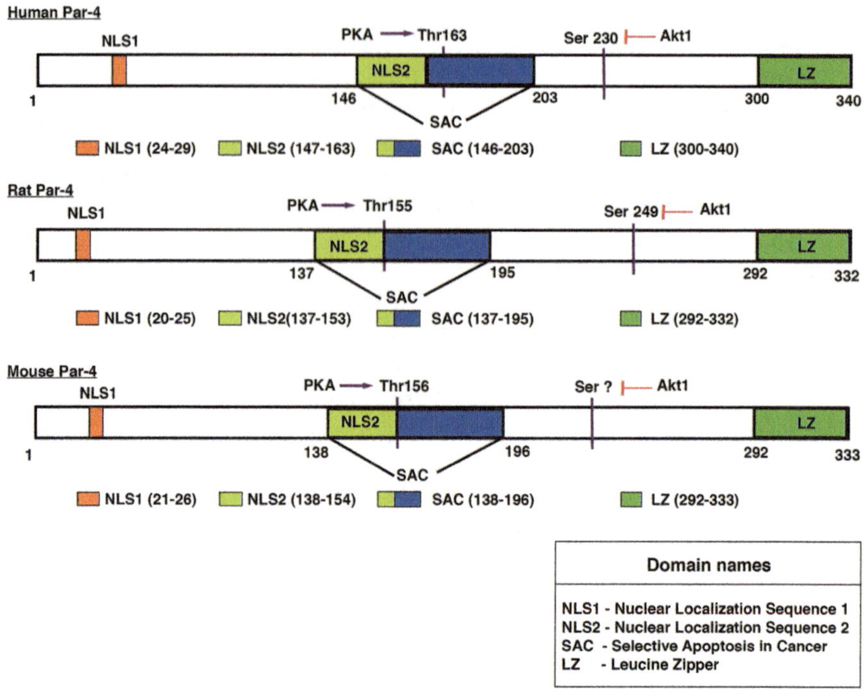

Fig. 5.1 Functional domains of human, rat, and mouse Par-4, showing the two Nuclear Localization Sequences (NLS1, and NLS2), the SAC domain, and Leucine Zipper (LZ). Source: J Cell Physiol. 2012 Dec;227(12): 3715–3721. Used with permission

(NES) [7]. Another domain is the "Selective for Apoptosis of Cancer Cells" (SAC) domain. This SAC domain has been found to be critical to Par-4-mediated apoptosis.

In addition to the functional domains, there are a number of key conserved residues which can be phosphorylated by kinases PKC, PKA, and AKT. The phosphorylation state of these residues can affect the localization and activity of Par-4 [7].

5.2.2 *The SAC Domain*

Structure–function analysis studies performed by El-Guendy et al. to evaluate the significance of Par-4's domains revealed that nuclear localization of Par-4 correlated with apoptosis induction in cancer cells. By transiently transfecting cell lines with constructs containing specific regions of rat Par-4 and observing any resultant apoptotic activity, the authors identified the core domain composed of amino acids 137–195 as the minimal functional region required for apoptosis [16].

The critical SAC domain is 59 amino acids in length. Although the starting position varies between species (Fig. 5.1), the actual sequence is fully conserved between mice, rats, and humans [7]. As it has been noted that Par-4-induced apoptosis requires both nuclear localization of Par-4 from the cytoplasm and phosphorylation of the T155 residue, it happens that the SAC domain encompasses both T155 and NLS2. This renders the SAC domain indispensable for Par-4-mediated apoptotic activity.

Phosphorylation of T155 by cAMP Activated Protein Kinase A-I (PKA type I) is a requirement of Par-4-mediated apoptosis [17]. This is evidenced by the finding that substitution of this threonine residue with alanine would fail to induce apoptosis in PC-3 prostate cancer cells. T155 resides in a phosphorylation consensus site for PKA, and inhibition of endogenous PKA activity using the inhibitory peptide PKI resulted in the significant reduction of GFP-Par-4-mediated apoptotic activity [17]. Additionally, phosphorylation of T155 and apoptotic activity mediated by Par-4 and SAC were proportional to the expression of PKA in the cell lines investigated. The significance of the SAC domain is apparent in light of evidence that expression of Type I PKA is elevated in human primary tumors as well as in experimentally transformed human cell lines. Additionally, PKA upregulation is associated with proliferative cells [18]. Cho et al. have incidentally found evidence that PKA is secreted by multiple cancer cell lines and is markedly increased in the serum of cancer patients [18]. From these studies, it is argued that Par-4 can be activated via phosphorylation as a defense mechanism against cancer-associated PKA. This in turn would partially account for the specific apoptotic activity of Par-4 in cancer cells.

5.2.3 Leucine Zipper and Nuclear Localization Sequence Domains

The leucine zipper domain of Par-4 binds to and interacts with the zinc finger (ZF) region of other proteins. One such factor is protein kinase C-zeta (ζPKC) [19]. Under stress conditions, ζPKC promotes NF-κB activity by phosphorylating the inhibitory peptide IκB—marking it for proteosomal degredation [20]. When I-κB is released, the p50 and p65 NF-κB subunits can enter the nucleus to promote gene transcription. Par-4LZ-ZF interaction with ζPKC in the cytoplasm has been found to downgrade NF-κB transcriptional activity [19]. This inhibition of NF-κB is one of the requisite steps in Par-4-mediated apoptosis. Moreover, ζPKC can phosphorylate FADD (Fas-Associated protein with Death Domain) and thereby interfere with the formation of a Fas-mediated Death-Inducing Signaling Complex or DISC [21, 22]. Thus, Par-4–ζPKC interactions may promote Fas-dependent apoptosis.

Other LZ binding partners of Par-4 include Wilms' tumor protein (WT-1) [23], THAP1, ZIP-kinase (ZIPK), and Topoisomerase I (TOPO-I). THAP1 is a nuclear proapoptotic protein component of promyelocytic nuclear bodies. While these nuclear bodies appear to recruit multiple tumor suppressor proteins, the significance of these interactions with Par-4 is unclear [24]. However, WT-1 is known to transcriptionally induce the anti-apoptotic factor Bcl-2 [25] and TOPO-1 activity is greatly increased in proliferative cell populations in order to support increased DNA replication and transcription rates (hence the use of topoisomerase I/II inhibitors in chemotherapy). However, when bound to TOPO-I through its LZ, Par-4 prevents TOPO-I DNA binding and thereby attenuates DNA replication and transcription, but this interaction does not induce apoptosis [26]. Thereby, it may be assumed that the LZ of Par-4 is not indispensable for apoptosis, but may rather have a negative regulatory role through interactions with WT-1 and ζPKC. This may explain the finding that the SAC domain can induce apoptosis against a broader range of tumor cells compared to full-length Par-4. For example: LNCaP, MDA 2b, A549, and MCF-7 cells are resistant to apoptosis in response to Par-4 overexpression but not to SAC overexpression [16].

The nuclear localization signal NLS2 is necessary for the nuclear entry of Par-4 or SAC-and is therefore necessary for Par-4-mediated apoptosis [16]. The N-terminal NLS 1 domain, by contrast does not appear to affect Par-4 nuclear localization. As deletion of this region does not affect apoptosis, its actual role is yet to be determined.

5.2.4 AKT, K-Ras, and Src—Subcellular Ruffians

Par-4 also appears to be a prerequisite for Phosphatase and Tensin Homolog (PTEN)-mediated apoptosis. The PTEN phosphatase, which is frequently missing or downregulated in cancers counters the PI3K-AKT pathway and thereby attenuates cellular proliferation. Immunoprecipitation experiments performed by Goswami et al. demonstrated that endogenous AKT1 is a binding partner of Par-4, binding and phosphorylating at serine249 in rat Par-4 (analogous to S230 in human Par-4) [27]. When AKT phosphorylates S249, Par-4 activity is reduced [27]. This AKT-dependent sequestration of Par-4 underlies reduced Par-4 activity observed in prostate cancer, for which Par-4 is not found to be downregulated, silenced or mutated [27]. Additional experiments have shown that using PI3K inhibitors or AKT1 siRNA would induce apoptosis in Par-4 wild-type PC-3 or LNCaP prostate cancer cells, but not cells transfected with Par-4 shRNA. Mechanistically, confocal microscopy indicated co-localization of GFP-Par-4 and myristoylated AKT constructs at the plasma membrane and cytoplasm—without any evidence of nuclear Par-4 [27]. This AKT-dependent cytoplasmic sequestration of Par-4 seems to be mediated by the chaperone protein 14–3-3. 14–3-3 has been previously observed binding, and sequestering AKT substrates [28]. When the Par-4 S249 residue is replaced with alanine, Par-4 and 14–3-3 are no longer associated [27]. In summary, when PTEN is depleted, AKT activity increases, Par-4 is phosphorylated, promoting binding between Par-4 and 14–3-3, and subsequent cytoplasmic sequestration of Par-4 (Fig. 5.2).

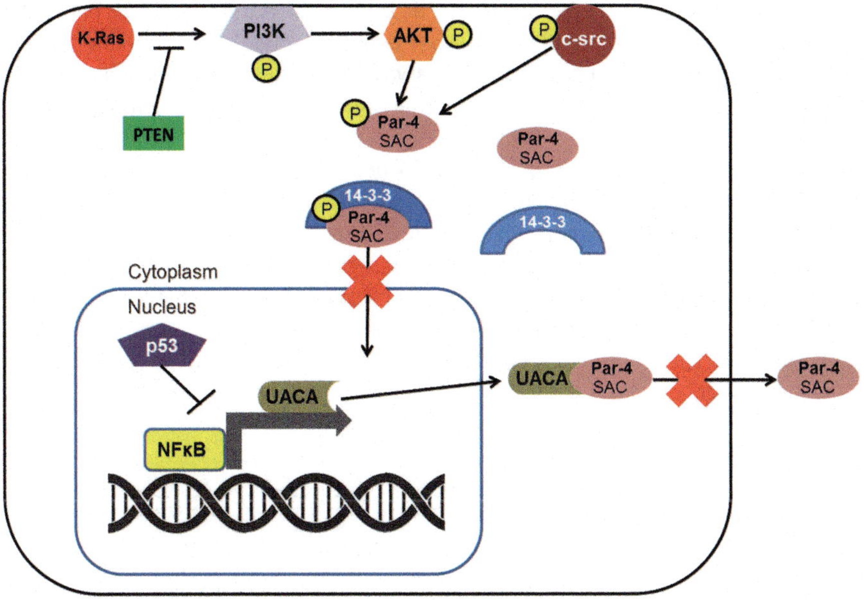

Fig. 5.2 Downregulation of Par-4 activity. Oncogenic Ras (KRas) can increase AKT kinase activity. When Par-4 is phosphorylated by AKT or c-src, it becomes a target for binding by 14–3-3, preventing Par-4 nuclear translocation. Also, active NFκB increases transcription of UACA, which binds Par-4, preventing secretion of Par-4. This activity can however be countered by p53

Besides mutational or epigenetic changes, Par-4 is downregulated by major oncogenes like *k-RAS* and *src*. The *c-src* proto-oncogene has been found to co-immunoprecipitate with Par-4, phosphorylates Par-4 and promotes binding to 14–3-3 to prevent nuclear translocation. These experiments however did not conclude whether this activity was AKT dependent [29].

The Ras family of small GTPases is responsible for the regulation of a wide array of cellular processes, including cell growth, proliferation, migration, and apoptosis. Consequently, Ras mutations may be highly oncogenic and transformative. In fact, about 30% of human tumors screened have been found to carry some form of Ras mutation. In particular, oncogenic *K-Ras* mutations were found in 25–30% of screened tumor samples [30]. This oncogenic Ras promotes growth and prevents apoptosis predominantly through activation of the PI3K/AKT signaling axis as well as downstream MAP kinases MEK and ERK. Furthermore, oncogenic Ras will also activate the pro-survival transcription factor NFκB. Experimentally, transformation of epithelial cells can be achieved through activation of the MAPK pathway. This pathway activates the DNA methyltransferase DNMT1, which has been found to hypermethylate and silence the Par-4 promoter, leading to transformation [31].

Experiments by Qiu et al. found that the transformation of fibroblasts with Ras or activating an inducible oncogenic H-Ras construct would result in greatly reduced levels of Par-4 protein and *Par-4* RNA compared to controls. Experiments focusing upon inhibition of the PI3K-AKT and the Raf-MEK-ERK pathways indicated that this downregulation of Par-4 expression is likely due to the actions of ERK2 (although not necessarily exclusive) [32]. One possible mechanism for this was found by Pruitt et al.; methylation-specific PCR showed hypermethylation of the Par-4 promoter in Ras transformed cells. An additional experiment demonstrated that adminstration of the DNA methyltransferase inhibitor azadeoxycytidine to Ras transformed RIE-1 cells restored Par-4 RNA and protein expression levels. The implication is that Ras-mediated Par-4 downregulation may be attributed to the hypermethylation of the Par-4 promoter [31]. While Par-4 is downregulated by oncogenic Ras, further observations show that restoration of Par-4 levels via addition of ectopic Par-4 was able to prevent oncogenic Ras-mediated foci. Therefore, Par-4 downregulation is a prerequisite for cellular transformation by oncogenic Ras [32].

5.3 Par-4 and Death Receptors

One of the earliest mechanisms by which Par-4 was found to trigger apoptosis, was the finding that it can interact with surface death receptors, triggering an extrinsic apoptotic cascade [33]. Briefly, this pathway is characterized by the oligomerization of such surface death receptors as Fas/CD95 or TNFα-R. These receptor complexes recruit adaptor proteins like FADD and TRADD, resulting in the activation of caspase-8. This combination of receptor, FADD, and caspase 8 form a Death-Inducing Signalling Complex, or DISC. Caspase 8 can then cleave caspase 3 and/or cleave the Bcl-2 family protein Bid. This culminates in the release of mitochondrial cytochrome-c and formation of the apoptosome [34, 35]. Of particular relevance to Par-4 is the role of Fas.

Chakraborty, et al. discovered that Par-4 overexpression through transfection of prostate cancer cell lines can trigger translocation of Fas/ FasL to the cancer cell surface [36] as demonstrated through Western blotting of surface membrane fractions and immunocytostaining. Inhibition of the classical secretory pathway through addition of brefeldin-A (BFA) was found to prevent this translocation. However, this Par-4-mediated translocation is not universal as, thus far, it has only been observed in the androgen-independent prostate cancer cell lines PC-3, and DU-145 [36]. By contrast, neither the androgen-independent prostate tumor line LNCaP nor normal prostate epithelial cells undergo Fas/ FasL surface translocation and apoptosis in response to Par-4 overexpression. In further support of this, Chakraborty et al., injected PC-3 prostate cells into the flanks of nude mice to generate solid tumors. Injection of a Par-4 containing adenoviral construct caused regression of the tumors. Immunostaining of the tumor sections showed that Fas was highly expressed at the cell membranes of the tumors transduced by Par-4 containing adenoviruses. However, xenografts generated from PC-3 cells overexpressing p65 did not undergo regression.

Par-4 can also affect Fas activity via a secondary mechanism. ζPKC interferes with FasL-induced apoptosis by interfering with the formation of the DISC and downstream caspose-8 processing [21]. As Par-4 binds to ζPKC with its LZ, Par-4 can sequester ζPKC and protect the Fas pathway from the inhibitory effects [16].

In addition to the translocation of Fas, there has been found a concurrent down-regulation of NF-κB by Par-4 which reduces transcription of anti-apoptotic products [36]. Nuclear translocation of Par-4 has been found to be necessary for this activity [37]. The authors conclude that the inhibition of p65 (an NFκB transcription factor)-dependent transcription is necessary but insufficient by itself to trigger Par-4-mediated apoptosis in prostate cancer cells. Experimental abrogation of the Fas signaling pathway in PC-3 and DU-145 cells resulted in inhibition of Par-4-inducible apoptosis. Thereby, the concurrent Fas/FasL translocation and NF-κB downregulation appear to be necessary for Par-4-mediated tumor regression [36].

5.3.1 Par-4 Secretion and GRP-78

While the relationship between Par-4 and Fas/FasL is certainly important in the context of extrinsic apoptotic activity, there has been an abundance of interest regarding Par-4 as an extracellular signaling protein. Burikhanov et al. noted that induction of endoplasmic reticulum (ER) stress in PC-3 cells using tunicamycin or thapsigargin resulted in extracellular secretion of Par-4 and subsequent apoptotic response in a BFA-dependent manner. The Par-4 secretory response was subsequently replicated in diverse cell lines. Excitingly, conditioned medium collected from PC-3 cells transfected with Par-4 constructs were able to induce apoptosis in nontransfected control PC-3 cells [38]. As this effect was neutralized with co-addition of anti-Par-4 antibodies, it is demonstrably Par-4 dependent.

Subsequent pulldown experiments using GST-tagged-Par-4 against PC-3 cell lysates showed that Par-4 had a 78-kDa binding partner that was identified as GRP-78 [38]. This was further verified through immunoprecipitation experiments. Subsequent co-immunoprecipitation experiments demonstrated that Par-4 interacts with GRP-78 at the SAC domain and GRP-78 would co-immunoprecipitate with SAC-GFP constructs, further highlighting the critical nature of SAC. Moreover, Par-4 and GRP-78 co-localize at the cell surface, as well as in the ER [38].

GRP-78 (also referred to in the literature as BiP) is a chaperone protein which is described as a central regulator for managing ER stress and the unfolded protein response (UFP) [39]. GRP-78 can be transcriptionally activated by ER stress brought on by misfolded protein accumulation, or calcium ion efflux. While GRP-78 is normally found in the ER lumen, it is sometimes found to be expressed on the cell surface. Cell surface expression of GRP-78 is particularly noticeable after exposure to ER stressing agents [40] and intriguingly, basal surface GRP-78 expression is specific to tumor cells [41, 42], and not to the surrounding normal cells or tissue. The cancer-specific surface expression of GRP-78 further explains how extracellular Par-4 specifically targets tumor cells for apoptosis. Therapeutic evidence for this comes from induction of apoptosis in triple-negative breast cancer by pharmacologically inducing cell-surface expression of GRP-78. The investigators were able to prevent apoptosis by blocking with an anti-GRP-78 antibody, lending additional credence to this hypothesis [40]. By contrast, cell lines lacking surface GRP-78, such as A549 lung adenoma cells, are resistant to extracellular Par-4 or SAC.

Later experiments by the same group have found that Par-4 secretion can be induced through treatment with the IKK inhibitor PS1145 (leading to NF-κB inhibition) [43], or the addition of Nutlin-3a, a compound which stabilizes p53 by blocking MDM2 [44]. Hypothesizing that Par-4 may have a binding partner which prevents its secretion (as opposed to the aforementioned 14–3-3 that prevents nuclear translocation), yeast-two hybrid and co-IP studies, identified the 163 kDa protein UACA as a binding partner. UACA is transcriptionally upregulated by NFκB [43], and secretion of Par-4 and GRP-78 was observed to be tightly associated with NFκB activity. This mechanism would be extended to include p53. The coding region for UACA has a p53 binding site, and chromatin immunoprecipitation confirmed that p53 activation with Nutlin-3a promotes binding of p53 to the UACA sequence, with correspondingly reduced UACA expression. This inhibition was found to be NFκB independent. Thus, NF-κB and/or p53 could transcriptionally promote or inhibit UACA and vary Par-4 mediated apoptotic acivity by modulating sequestration of Par-4 and GRP-78 in the cytoplasm (Fig. 5.2).

To summarize the mechanism, Par-4 colocalizes at the SAC domain with GRP78 in the ER, but under stress conditions, the paired proteins are relocated to the membrane, where Par-4 is released but GRP-78 is left at the surface. When circulating Par-4 binds the membrane GRP-78, the complex is believed to recruit FADD, which in turn recruits and cleaves procaspase 8, cleaving in turn caspase 3, and triggering an apoptotic cascade (Fig. 5.3).

5.3.2 Par-4 and TRAIL

TRAIL (TNF-Related Apoptosis Inducing Ligand) is a secreted death ligand that has been investigated for its antitumor potential. TRAIL can be secreted by most cells in the body in response to such signals as interferon or retinoic acid [45, 46]. Binding of trimeric TRAIL to the membrane-bound receptors TRAIL-R1 and -R2 induces receptor trimerization and DISC formation. Like Fas, this complex will recruit and activate caspases-8 and -10 to promote the classical extrinsic apoptotic pathway [47].

Although, to date, TRAIL has not been successfully exploited in clinical trials, it may be linked to other useful pathways. Treatment of PC-3 cells with TRAIL has been found by Burikhanov et al. to promote secretion of Par-4 via a BFA-sensitive pathway [38]. Additional experiments demonstrated that TRAIL would induce intracellular and plasma membrane expression of GRP-78. Co-treatment of PC-3

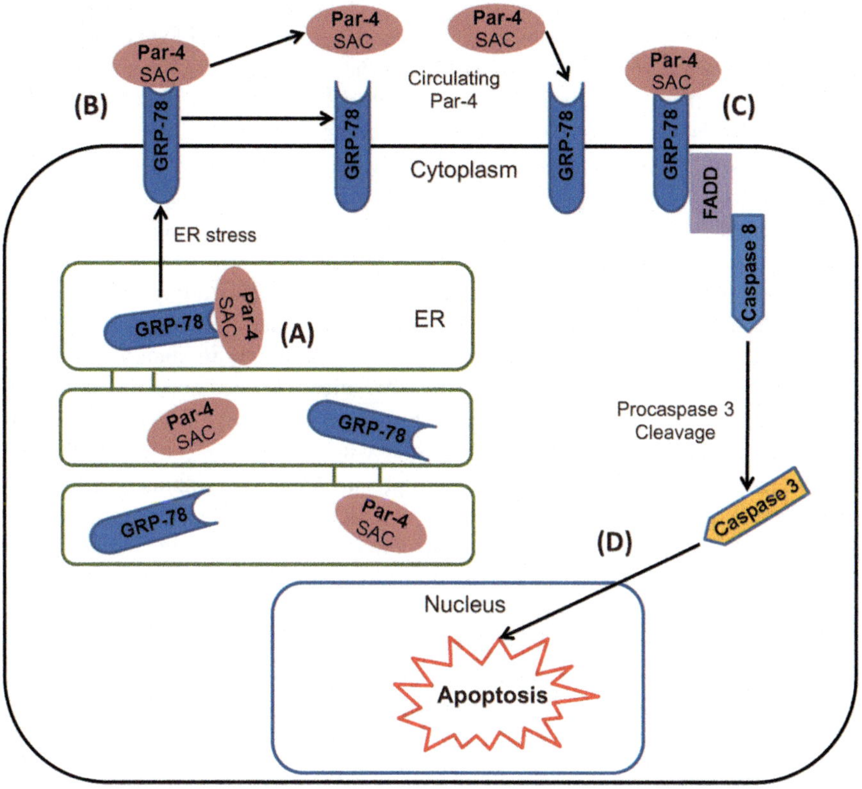

Fig. 5.3 Par-4 colocalizes at the SAC domain with GRP78 in the ER (**a**), Under stress conditions, the paired proteins are relocated to the plasma membrane, where Par-4 is released, leaving GRP-78 at the surface (**B**), When circulating Par-4 binds the membrane GRP-78, the complex (**C**), Recruits FADD, which in turn recruits and cleaves procaspase 8, cleaving in turn procaspase 3, and triggering an apoptotic cascade (**D**)

cells with TRAIL and neutralizing antibodies for either Par-4 or GRP-78, inhibited TRAIL-mediated apoptosis. These observations indicated that Par-4 secretion is necessary for TRAIL-mediated apoptosis [38].

5.4 SAC Transgenic Mice

As the SAC domain of Par-4 lacks the negative regulatory LZ region, apoptotic activity is not downgraded by WT, ζPKC, or AKT. In vitro, SAC overexpression proved highly effective at apoptotis induction with a wide variety of tumor cells. Zhao and colleagues tried to replicate this in vivo. This group cloned a construct containing GFP-tagged SAC domain of rat Par-4 into a pCAGGS vector. This vector contained both a β-actin promoter and a CMV enhancer. The new SAC constructs were injected into the pronuclei of B6C3F1 mouse embryos and allowed to develop. The resulting animals ubiquitously expressed the SAC-GFP transgene and exhibited normal fertility, viability, and aging [39]. Primary fibroblasts grown from these embryos (MEFs), as well as GFP transgene control littermates were transfected with constructs containing c-Myc or oncogenic Ras in an attempt to transform the MEFs. The SAC expressing MEFs were found to be highly resistant to transformation as demonstrated by lack of foci in culture and underwent apoptosis at a rate nearly ten times that of the control MEFs.

However, these effects were not limited to culture, as the resulting animal turned out to be essentially a tumor-resistant mouse. B6C3F1 mice are known to spontaneously develop lymphoma and liver tumors. While these tumors manifested in the GFP control mice at around 18 months, the SAC mice remained normal and necropsies showed normal hepatic and splenic architecture, highly resistant to spontaneous tumor formation [37]. Crossing the SAC mice with prostate-cancer prone TRAMP mice significantly reduced the likelihood of prostatic adenocarcinoma formation. A subsequent experiment in which Lewis-Lung Carcinoma (LLC) cells were injected into the flanks of SAC-transgenic and control mice also demonstrated a high degree of resistance to tumor formation in SAC transgenic mice [48].

This cancer resistant phenotype has been found to be transferable. By transplanting bone marrow from the SAC-overexpressing mice to irradiated control mice, serum samples obtained would induce apoptosis in cultured LLC cells. By contrast, this effect was not observed through administration of serum from control mice. As this suggested that the resistant phenotype was due to circulating SAC, the investigators proceeded to a metastasis model. Wild type mice were first injected with LLC1 cells (which are expected to generate lung tumors), followed by recombinant Par-4 protein, recombinant SAC protein or protein tag. While Par-4 treated animals exhibited a significantly reduced tumor load in the lungs upon sacrifice, SAC-treated mice would show an even greater reduction. This series of experiments indicate further therapeutic potential for Par-4 or SAC against tumors.

5.5 Future Directions

Par-4 represents an endogenous factor which can be secreted and specifically induces apoptosis in cancer cells, while leaving normal cells unaffected. This makes Par-4 an ideal candidate for development against cancer.

Baseline secretion of Par-4 is insufficient to promote widespread apoptosis of tumor cells, therefore, it would be useful to elevate circulating Par-4 concentrations—at least as an adjuvant to conventional therapies. Nutlin-3 and PS1145 have already been mentioned for their in vitro effects. Based upon the structure of Nutlin-3, Burikhanov et al. synthesized and screened a library of chemical compounds bearing halogenated aromatic rings for their ability to induce secretion of Par-4. The group found that fluorinated 3-arylquinolines were particularly effective in this regard, and focused upon a compound designated Arylquin-1. Administration of Arylquin-1 was able to induce Par-4 secretion in vitro, with subsequent specific apoptosis of tumor cells, in a BFA-dependent manner. Administration of this compound to mice led to a fivefold increase in plasma Par-4 levels compared to baseline concentrations. Taking this one step further, serum from mice treated with Alylquin-1, but not vehicle treated animals, were also able to induce ex vivo cancer cell apoptosis. As this effect is abrogated through the addition of anti-Par-4 antibody, it is Par-4-dependent [49]. Discovery of such secretagogues is an area of active investigation.

Besides promoting extracellular secretion of Par-4, it would be useful to induce Par-4 to act intracellularly to increase Fas signaling or inhibit TOPO-1 activity. One possibility is to test methyltransferase inhibitors to prevent silencing of the *Par-4* promoter. This would be a topic for future research.

5.6 Summary

- Par-4 is a tumor suppressor that can act through intracellular and extracellular pathways.
- Intracellularly, Par-4 can act through inhibition of NF-κB dependent transactivation and TOPO-1.
- Intracellularly, Par-4 activity requires nuclear translocation and inhibition of NF-κB dependent transactivation.
- Extracellularly, Par-4 stimulates translocation of Fas to the cell surface.
- Par-4 secretion can be induced through ER stress, p53 activation, or NF-κB inhibition.
- The SAC domain of Par-4 is the minimal region required for Par-4 to induce apoptosis.
- Inducing secretion of Par-4 and/or SAC show therapeutic promise.

References

1. FastStats—Leading causes of death
2. WHO cancer
3. EiC May 2008—Feature—Fighting cancer—the early years
4. Peter ME, Hadji A, Murmann AE, Brockway S, Putzbach W, Pattanayak A, Ceppi P (2015) The role of CD95 and CD95 ligand in cancer. Cell Death Differ 22(4):549–559. doi:10.1038/cdd.2015.1033
5. Symes JC, Kurin M, Fleshner NE, Medin JA (2008) Fas-mediated killing of primary prostate cancer cells is increased by mitoxantrone and docetaxel. Mol Cancer Ther 7(9):3018–3028. doi:10.1158/1535-7163.MCT-3008-0335
6. Sells SF, Wood DP, Joshi-Barve SS, Muthukumar S, Jacob RJ, Crist SA, Humphreys S, Rangnekar VM (1994) Commonality of the gene programs induced by effectors of apoptosis in androgen-dependent and -independent prostate cells. Cell Growth Differ 5(4):457–466

7. Shrestha-Bhattarai T, Rangnekar VM (2010) Cancer-selective apoptotic effects of extracellular and intracellular Par-4. Oncogene 29(27):3873–3880. doi:10.1038/onc.2010.141
8. Cook J, Krishnan S, Ananth S, Sells SF, Shi Y, Walther MM, Linehan WM, Sukhatme VP, Weinstein MH, Rangnekar VM (1999) Decreased expression of the pro-apoptotic protein Par-4 in renal cell carcinoma. Oncogene 18(5):1205–1208. doi:10.1038/sj.onc.1202416
9. Moreno-Bueno G, Fernandez-Marcos PJ, Collado M, Tendero MJ, Rodriguez-Pinilla SM, Garcia-Cao I, Hardisson D, Diaz-Meco MT, Moscat J, Serrano M, Palacios J (2007) Inactivation of the candidate tumor suppressor Par-4 in endometrial cancer. Cancer Res 67(5):1927–1934. doi:10.1158/0008-5472.CAN-06-2687
10. Alvarez JV, Pan T-C, Ruth J, Feng Y, Zhou A, Pant D, Grimley JS, Wandless TJ, Demichele A, Chodosh LA (2013) Par-4 downregulation promotes breast cancer recurrence by preventing multinucleation following targeted therapy. Cancer Cell 24(1):30–44. doi:10.1016/j.ccr.2013.05.007
11. Contract D, Mackley H, Irby RB (2011) Par-4 sensitizes human colon cancer cells to chemoradiotherapy. J Cancer Ther 2:542–547. doi:10.4236/jct.2011.24074
12. Pereira MC, de Bessa-Garcia SA, Burikhanov R, Pavanelli AC, Antunes L, Rangnekar VM, Nagai MA (2013) Prostate apoptosis response-4 is involved in the apoptosis response to docetaxel in MCF-7 breast cancer cells. Int J Oncol 43(2):531–538
13. Garcıa-Cao I, Duran A, Collado M, Carrascosa MJ, MartÃın-Caballero J, Flores JM, Diaz-Meco MT, Moscat J, Serrano M (2005) Tumour-suppression activity of the proapoptotic regulator Par4. EMBO Rep 6(6):577–583. doi:10.1038/sj.embor.7400421
14. Rangnekar VM (1998) Apoptosis mediated by a novel leucine zipper protein Par-4. Apoptosis 3(2):61–66
15. Chaudhry P, Singh M, Parent S, Asselin E (2012) Prostate apoptosis response 4 (Par-4), a novel substrate of caspase-3 during apoptosis activation. Mol Cell Biol 32(4):826–839. doi:10.1128/MCB.06321-11
16. El-Guendy N, Zhao Y, Gurumurthy S, Burikhanov R, Rangnekar VM (2003) Identification of a unique core domain of Par-4 sufficient for selective apoptosis induction in cancer cells. Mol Cell Biol 23(16):5516–5525
17. Gurumurthy S, Goswami A, Vasudevan KM, Rangnekar VM (2005) Phosphorylation of Par-4 by protein kinase a is critical for apoptosis. Mol Cell Biol 25(3):1146–1161. doi:10.1128/MCB.25.3.1146-1161.2005
18. Cho YS, Park YG, Lee YN, Kim MK, Bates S, Tan L, Cho-Chung YS (2000) Extracellular protein kinase a as a cancer biomarker: its expression by tumor cells and reversal by a myristate-lacking Calpha and RIIbeta subunit overexpression. Proc Natl Acad Sci U S A 97(2):835–840
19. Sanz-Navares E, Fernandez N, Kazanietz MG, Rotenberg SA (2001) Atypical protein kinase Czeta suppresses migration of mouse melanoma cells. Cell Growth Differ 12(10):517–524
20. Moscat J, Rennert P, Diaz-Meco MT (2006) PKCzeta at the crossroad of NF-kappaB and Jak1/Stat6 signaling pathways. Cell Death Differ 13(5):702–711. doi:10.1038/sj.cdd.4401823
21. Leroy I, de Thonel A, Laurent G, Quillet-Mary A (2005) Protein kinase C zeta associates with death inducing signaling complex and regulates Fas ligand-induced apoptosis. Cell Signal 17(9):1149–1157. doi:10.1016/j.cellsig.2004.12.013
22. Zhang J, Zhang D, Hua Z (2004) FADD and its phosphorylation. IUBMB Life 56(7):395–401. doi:10.1080/15216540400008929
23. Johnstone RW, See RH, Sells SF, Wang J, Muthukkumar S, Englert C, Haber DA, Licht JD, Sugrue SP, Roberts T, Rangnekar VM, Shi Y (1996) A novel repressor, Par-4, modulates transcription and growth suppression functions of the Wilms' tumor suppressor WT1. Mol Cell Biol 16(12):6945–6956
24. Roussigne M, Cayrol C, Clouaire T, Amalric F, Girard J-P (2003) THAP1 is a nuclear proapoptotic factor that links prostate-apoptosis-response-4 (Par-4) to PML nuclear bodies. Oncogene 22:2432–2442. doi:10.1038/sj.onc.1206271
25. Cheema SK, Mishra SK, Rangnekar VM, Tari AM, Kumar R, Lopez-Berestein G (2003) Par-4 transcriptionally regulates Bcl-2 through a WT1-binding site on the bcl-2 promoter. J Biol Chem 278(22):19995–20005. doi:10.1074/jbc.M205865200

26. Goswami A, Qiu S, Dexheimer TS, Ranganathan P, Burikhanov R, Pommier Y, Rangnekar VM (2008) Par-4 binds to topoisomerase 1 and attenuates its DNA relaxation activity. Cancer Res 68(15):6190–6198. doi:10.1158/0008-5472.CAN-08-0831
27. Goswami A, Burikhanov R, de Thonel A, Fujita N, Goswami M, Zhao Y, Eriksson JE, Tsuruo T, Rangnekar VM (2005) Binding and phosphorylation of Par-4 by akt is essential for cancer cell survival. Mol Cell 20(1):33–44. doi:10.1016/j.molcel.2005.08.016
28. Brunet A, Bonni A, Zigmond MJ, Lin MZ, Juo P, Hu LS, Anderson MJ, Arden KC, Blenis J, Greenberg ME (1999) Akt promotes cell survival by phosphorylating and inhibiting a forkhead transcription factor. Cell 96(6):857–868. doi:10.1016/S0092-8674(1000)80595-80594
29. Kline CLB, Irby RB (2011) The pro-apoptotic protein prostate apoptosis response protein-4 (Par-4) can be activated in colon cancer cells by treatment with Src inhibitor and 5-FU. Apoptosis 16(12):1285–1294. doi:10.1007/s10495-011-0648-3
30. Fernandez-Medarde A, Santos E (2011) Ras in cancer and developmental diseases. Genes Cancer 2(3):344–358. doi:10.1177/1947601911411084
31. Pruitt K, Ülkü AS, Frantz K, Rojas RJ, Muniz-Medina VM, Rangnekar VM, Der CJ, Shields JM (2005) Ras-mediated loss of the pro-apoptotic response protein Par-4 is mediated by DNA hypermethylation through Raf-independent and Raf-dependent signaling cascades in epithelial cells. J Biol Chem 280(24):23363–23370. doi:10.1074/jbc.M503083200
32. Qiu SG, Krishnan S, el-Guendy N, Rangnekar VM (1999) Negative regulation of Par-4 by oncogenic Ras is essential for cellular transformation. Oncogene 18(50):7115–7123. doi:10.1038/sj.onc.1203199
33. Zhao Y, Rangnekar VM (2008) Apoptosis and tumor resistance conferred by Par-4. Cancer Biol Ther 7(12):1867–1874
34. Beere HM (2005) Death versus survival: functional interaction between the apoptotic and stress-inducible heat shock protein pathways. J Clin Invest 115(10):2633–2639. doi:10.1172/JCI26471
35. Kaufmann T, Strasser A, Jost PJ (2012) Fas death receptor signalling: roles of bid and XIAP. Cell Death Differ 19(1):42–50. doi:10.1038/cdd.2011.121
36. Chakraborty M, Qiu SG, Vasudevan KM, Rangnekar VM (2001) Par-4 drives trafficking and activation of Fas and FasL to induce prostate cancer cell apoptosis and tumor regression. Cancer Res 61(19):7255–7263
37. Zhao Y, Burikhanov R, Qiu S, Lele SM, Jennings CD, Bondada S, Spear B, Rangnekar VM (2007) Cancer resistance in transgenic mice expressing the SAC module of Par-4. Cancer Res 67(19):9276–9285. doi:10.1158/0008-5472.CAN-07-2124
38. Burikhanov R, Zhao Y, Goswami A, Qiu S, Schwarze SR, Rangnekar VM (2009) The tumor suppressor Par-4 activates an extrinsic pathway for apoptosis. Cell 138(2):377–388. doi:10.1016/j.cell.2009.05.022
39. Lee AS (2005) The ER chaperone and signaling regulator GRP78/BiP as a monitor of endoplasmic reticulum stress. Methods 35(4):373–381. doi:10.1016/j.ymeth.2004.10.010
40. Raiter A, Yerushalmi R, Hardy B (2014) Pharmacological induction of cell surface GRP78 contributes to apoptosis in triple negative breast cancer cells. Oncotarget 5(22):11452–11463. doi:10.18632/oncotarget.2576
41. Arap MA, Lahdenranta J, Mintz PJ, Hajitou A, Sarkis AS, Arap W, Pasqualini R (2004) Cell surface expression of the stress response chaperone GRP78 enables tumor targeting by circulating ligands. Cancer Cell 6(3):275–284. doi:10.1016/j.ccr.2004.1008.1018
42. Zhang Y, Liu R, Ni M, Gill P, Lee AS (2010) Cell surface relocalization of the endoplasmic reticulum chaperone and unfolded protein response regulator GRP78/BiP. J Biol Chem 285(20):15065–15075. doi:10.1074/jbc.M109.087445
43. Burikhanov R, Shrestha-Bhattarai T, Qiu S, Shukla N, Hebbar N, Lele SM, Horbinski C, Rangnekar VM (2013) Novel mechanism of apoptosis resistance in cancer mediated by extracellular PAR-4. Cancer Res 73(2):1011–1019. doi:10.1158/0008-5472.CAN-12-3212
44. Burikhanov R, Shrestha-Bhattarai T, Hebbar N, Qiu S, Zhao Y, Zambetti GP, Rangnekar VM (2014) Paracrine apoptotic effect of p53 mediated by tumor suppressor Par-4. Cell Rep 6(2):271–277. doi:10.1016/j.celrep.2013.12.020

45. Dhandapani L, Yue P, Ramalingam SS, Khuri FR, Sun S-Y (2011) Retinoic acid enhances TRAIL-induced apoptosis in cancer cells by upregulating TRAIL receptor 1 expression. Cancer Res 71(15):5245–5254. doi:10.1158/0008-5472.CAN-10-4180
46. Miura Y, Tsujioka T, Nishimura Y, Sakaguchi H, Maeda M, Hayashi H, Dong M, Hyodoh F, Yata K-I, Wada H, Sugihara T, Otsuki T (2006) TRAIL expression up-regulated by interferon-gamma via phosphorylation of STAT1 induces myeloma cell death. Anticancer Res 26(6B):4115–4124
47. Lemke J, von Karstedt S, Zinngrebe J, Walczak H (2014) Getting TRAIL back on track for cancer therapy. Cell Death Differ 21(9):1350–1364. doi:10.1038/cdd.2014.81
48. Zhao Y, Burikhanov R, Brandon J, Qiu S, Shelton BJ, Spear B, Bondada S, Bryson S, Rangnekar VM (2011) Systemic Par-4 inhibits non-autochthonous tumor growth. Cancer Biol Ther 12(2):152–157
49. Burikhanov R, Sviripa VM, Hebbar N, Zhang W, Layton WJ, Hamza A, Zhan C-G, Watt DS, Liu C, Rangnekar VM (2014) Arylquins target vimentin to trigger Par-4 secretion for tumor cell apoptosis. Nat Chem Biol 10(11):924–926. doi:10.1038/nchembio.1631

Chapter 6
Stem Cell Regulation by Death Ligands and Their Use in Cell Therapy

Andrea Mohr and Ralf Zwacka

Abstract Stem cells are an essential to repair damaged tissues. Their functions, proliferation and differentiation need to be tightly controlled, as impairments can lead to various diseases including cancer. Induction of apoptosis is one way to control the number of stem cells and to eliminate rogue and/or precancerous cells. One way of triggering apoptosis, and probably the physiologically most important one, is via binding of death ligand to their cognate receptors. The death receptor–ligand family encompasses five pairs: FAS/FASL; TNF-R1/TNF; DR3/TL1A and TWEAK; DR4 and DR5/TRAIL; and DR6/unknown ligand. Of these, FASL and TRAIL and to a lesser extent TNF are strong inducers of apoptosis, whereas the others possess relative weak cell-death-inducing activity. Interestingly, these death receptors and ligands also have non-canonical functions and in specific cellular and molecular contexts can regulate cell proliferation, differentiation, chemokine production and inflammatory responses. Some of these non-apoptotic functions have been shown to be of relevance in stem and progenitor cells.

Stem cells have also been used as part of cell therapies in connection with delivery of death ligands to target their respective receptors, in particular in experimental anti-cancer therapies. Stem cells, at least some types, are attractive in these approaches because they are capable to infiltrate certain tissues including tumours to deliver their therapeutic payload. This way of cellular delivery can be more efficacious and specific compared to recombinant proteins or direct gene therapy.

This chapter summarises our current understanding of stem cell regulation by death receptor–ligand signalling and in the second part how certain types of stem cells have been used to deliver death-ligand gene therapies in the laboratory and increasingly in clinical trials.

A. Mohr (✉) • R. Zwacka (✉)
Cancer and Stem Cell Biology Group, School of Biological Sciences, University of Essex, Colchester CO4 3SQ, UK
e-mail: amohr@essex.ac.uk; rzwacka@essex.ac.uk

O. Micheau (ed.), *TRAIL, Fas Ligand, TNF and TLR3 in Cancer*, Resistance to Targeted Anti-Cancer Therapeutics, DOI 10.1007/978-3-319-56805-8_6

Keywords Stem cells • Death receptor • Non-apoptotic function • TRAIL • MSCs • Cell therapy • Cancer

6.1 Introduction

Apoptosis can be distinguished into two different forms, intrinsic or stress-induced apoptosis and extrinsic cell death, respectively. The latter is triggered by activation of death receptors including FAS (CD95), TNF-RI (TNFR55), DR3 (TRAMP), DR4 (TRAIL-R1), DR5 (TRAIL-R2) and DR6 (CD353) by their respective ligands [1]. Death receptors are members of the tumour necrosis factor receptor superfamily (TNFRSF) characterised by a ligand specific ectodomain and a cytoplasmic part known as death domain that is essential for conveying signals from the outside of a cell to the intracellular apoptosis machinery. Death receptors are activated by binding of their cognate ligands (ligand–receptor: FASL/FAS [2–4], TNF/TNF-R1 [5–7], TL1A and TWEAK/DR3 [8–10], TRAIL/DR4 and DR5 [11–13], unknown/DR6 [14]). These ligands belong to the tumour necrosis factor superfamily (TNFSF). While FASL, TRAIL and to a lesser extent TNF are potent inducers of programmed cell death, the others have at best weak apoptosis-triggering activity. The death ligands initiate signalling via receptor oligomerisation, which firstly leads to the recruitment of specialised adaptor proteins (TRADD and/or FADD), followed by the initiator caspase, caspase-8. Within this death-inducing signalling complex (DISC) caspase-8 is activated though oligomerisation and autocatalysis. Activated caspase-8 gives rise to apoptosis via two parallel pathways. It can then either directly cleave and activate caspase-3, or process Bid, a pro-apoptotic BH3-only protein of the Bcl-2 family, to truncated Bid (tBid). The tBid protein translocates to the mitochondria, inducing the release of pro-apoptotic factors such as cytochrome c and Smac/DIABLO into the cytosol, leading to sequential activation of caspases-9 and -3 and/or blocking of the anti-apoptotic protein XIAP, respectively. However, more recent results point to additional, non-apoptosis signalling pathways that are controlled by death receptors and its ligands, including cell proliferation and differentiation, chemokine production, inflammatory responses and tumour-promoting activities.

As stem cells are an essential source for new cells needed to repair damaged tissues and replace worn-out cells, these death receptor–ligand-mediated biological mechanisms have potential roles in the regulation of their activities and functions. At the same time some of the characteristics of stem cells, such as their potential to home to certain tissues even when exogenously administered, make them attractive cell therapy vehicle for the treatment of degenerative diseases as well as cancer. Therefore, this chapter starts with a summary of our current understanding of stem cell regulation by death receptor–ligand signalling and reviews in the second part how certain types of stem cells have been used to deliver death-ligand gene therapies in the laboratory and increasingly in clinical trials.

6.2 Regulation of Stem Cell Activity

Stem cells are defined by the capacity to self-renew and the ability to produce differentiated cells. They can generate either identical daughter cells (self-renewal) or give rise to progeny with restricted potential to further differentiate with very specific functions (differentiated cells). Generally, we distinguish between pluripotent embryonic stem cells (ESCs) and usually multipotent adult stem cells. ESCs are essential for the development of multicellular organisms. In the 3- to 5-day-old embryo, called a blastocyst, the cells of the inner cell mass, from which ESCs are derived, give rise to all adult tissues, including all of the many specialised cell types and organs such as the heart, lungs, skin, sperm, eggs and other tissues. Adult stem cells such as haematopoietic stem cells (HSCs) are undifferentiated cells with a more limited differentiation range, found in many tissues or organs. Aside from being able to self-renew, these adult stem cells are believed to differentiate to yield some or all of the major specialised cell types of the tissue or organ they reside in. Thus, their main role is to maintain and repair the tissue in which they are found. In some organs, such as the gut and bone marrow (BM), stem cells regularly divide to repair and replace exhausted or damaged cells. In other organs, however, such as the pancreas and the heart, stem cells only divide under special conditions. However, some types of adult stem cells can be mobilised from their regular sites of residence and infiltrate distal tissues where they assist in repair and regeneration processes. In these different environments, milieus and contexts stem cells encounter members of the TNFSF family including death ligands that regulate the fate of differentiated cells. Given their value it is thought that stem cells are resistant to the apoptosis-inducing activities of these factors. However, worn-out stem cells might need to be removed and apoptosis might be a clean and elegant way to achieve this. Furthermore, there are other biological processes such as proliferation or differentiation that can be controlled by death ligands and members of the wider TNFSF family. As stem cells offer new approaches for treating diseases such as diabetes and heart diseases it is of relevance to understand such regulatory pathways in stem cells in order to optimise their application in regenerative medicine. Additionally, as there is an increasing body of evidence that some stem cells types have utility in cancer treatment owing to their recruitment to tumour tissues it is important to identify, which death ligands/TNFSFs can be safely and efficaciously be used in such approaches.

6.2.1 Regulation by TNF

Most stem cells, including haematopoietic stem cells (HSCs), are considered to be resistant to the apoptosis-inducing effects of death ligands under normal physiological conditions. Various mechanisms account for this resistance and include lack of death receptor expression and/or expression of apoptosis-inhibiting factors such as the caspase-8 splice variant caspase-8 L [15]. However, there are other pathways that can be affected. In particular, TNF has been shown in many different cellular contexts to possess non-apoptotic functions. TNF is the first identified member of the TNF family. TNF exerts its effects by interacting with two different receptors: TNF-R1 and TNF-R2, of which TNF-R1 is able to initiate apoptosis pathways, while TNF-R2 is only able to convey to non-apoptotic signals [16].

Multipotent self-renewing HSCs are needed for reconstitution of all blood cell lineages. Thus, the survival of HSCs is a requisite for life, but uncontrolled expansion of HSCs might enhance the propensity for leukaemia development. Early studies implicated TNF signalling through TNF-R1 in reduced maintenance of murine and human HSCs in vitro and in vivo [17–19]. Zhang et al. found that the number of murine primitive HSCs ($Lin^{-}Sca\text{-}1^{+}$ $c\text{-}kit^{+}$) was significantly increased in TNF-R1 deficient mice compared to wild-type mice without affecting the overall BM cellularity. In several in vitro assays, TNF was able to block the proliferation of wild-type mouse-derived HSCs in response to a combination of stimulatory growth factors (G-CSF plus SCF or IL-3 plus SCF). It also gave rise to a G0/G1-S-phase arrest in stimulated HSCs. In contrast, TNF failed to affect growth and cell cycle progression of HSCs from TNF-R1 knock-out mice suggesting that TNF-α, via signalling through TNF-R1, is an important regulator of haematopoiesis by inhibiting the growth of both primitive stem and more committed $Lin^{-}Sca\text{-}1^{-}c\text{-}kit^{+}$ progenitor cells [19].

In human HSCs ($CD34^{+}$ $CD38^{-}$), derived from cord blood and adult bone marrow, it was shown that they were capable of proliferation in the presence of TNF before ultimately becoming sensitive to TNF-induced growth inhibition [18]. Furthermore, cycling human HSCs exposed to TNF were severely compromised in their ability to reconstitute NOD-SCID mice and long term cultures. These effects were limited to cycling HSCs as cells cultured in the presence of thrombopoietin (TPO) alone, which promotes survival rather than proliferation under the specific experimental culturing conditions, were not adversely affected by TNF. Using TNF-mutants that were specific for TNF-R1 or TNF-R2 revealed that the inhibition was affected by signalling through TNF-R1 with little or no contribution from TNF-R2. Apoptosis measurements and addition of FASL neutralising antibodies showed that the effects of TNF were not caused by cell death induction nor were they triggered indirectly via induced production of FASL and subsequent engagement of its receptor FAS. Furthermore, TNF did not alter the cell cycle distribution of cultured human HSCs. However, TNF appeared to stimulate myeloid differentiation and might therefore regulate HSC fate by promoting their differentiation rather than self-renewal [18]. Interestingly, despite the lack of a role for induced FASL in TNF-treated HSC cultures, the same group reported that murine $Lin^{-}Sca\text{-}1^{+}c\text{-}kit^{+}$ stem cells, which were induced to undergo self-renewal by c-kit ligand, IL-3 and IL-6 acquired high FAS expression levels in the presence of TNF. Consequently, colony formation was inhibited in these cells when additionally treated with the FAS agonistic antibody Jo2 [17]. In summary, HSCs constitutively express little or no FAS, and only enforced cycling in combination with TNF leads to FAS expression rendering them susceptible to FAS-mediated suppression. As there is ample evidence for an involvement of excessive TNF and FAS activities in various BM failure syndromes and graft-versus-host disease (GvHD) [20, 21], these findings indicate that self-renewing HSCs are likely targets for TNF- and FAS-induced BM suppression.

6.2.2 Regulation by FASL

FAS signalling has been linked to normal stem cells and is identified as a candidate stem cell marker (similar to other well-established stem cell markers such as Lin28, Oct4, Nanog and Sox2) in a serial analysis of gene expression (SAGE) profiling of human embryonic stem cells [22].

In one of the studies linking FAS signalling to regenerative activity and thereby stem cell functions, it was shown that partial hepatectomy, not only protected mice against the lethal effects of FAS-specific antibodies and prevented hepatocyte apoptosis, but also accelerated liver regeneration. Mutant lpr mice that have decreased cell surface expression of FAS exhibited delayed liver regeneration, whereas regeneration was not affected in lpr-cg mutant mice, which harbour a FAS mutation that prevents apoptosis but not FAS-dependent growth stimulation. These results point to a role for FAS in (stem) cells that are involved in regenerating or healing tissues [23].

Further functional evidence of a prosurvival function of FAS signalling in stem cells came from studies that showed that the stimulation of FAS signalling in neuronal stem cells did not lead to cell death, but rather increased the survival of neuronal stem cells. These effects were mediated by the activation of the Src/PI3K/AKT/mTOR pathway, ultimately giving rise to an increase in protein translation. While lack of hippocampal FAS resulted in a reduction in neurogenesis and working memory deficits, forced expression of FASL in the adult subventricular zone had the opposite effect. Induction of neurogenesis by FAS was further confirmed in the ischaemic CA1 region, in the naive dentate gyrus and following global ischaemia, after which FAS-mediated brain repair rescued behavioural impairment [24].

As normal stem cells are often the origin of cancer stem cells (CSCs), these data were suggestive that FAS may also have a non-apoptotic function in CSCs. To this end, it was recently demonstrated that FAS is required for the survival of CSCs and allows new CSCs to emerge [25]. This reprogramming or retro-differentiation activity of FAS was independent of its apoptosis-inducing function and CSCs derived from highly apoptosis-sensitive cancer cells became resistant to FAS-mediated apoptosis. Overall, stimulation of FAS not only increased the number of cancer cells with stem cell traits but also prevented differentiation of CSCs, suggesting that FAS expression on cancer cells maintains the CSC pool [25]. A similar connection between FAS and CSCs was also recently reported in pancreatic cancer, in which FAS expression strongly correlated with stemness and EMT markers. Consequently, inhibition of FASL decreased tumour growth and metastasis development [26].

In the context of mesenchymal stem cells (MSCs), cells that were selected by FACS for high FASL expression showed remarkable inhibitory effects on multiple myeloma (MM) growth and dissemination in an MM mouse model. The injected MSCs were able to extend the mouse survival rate and inhibit tumour growth, bone resorption in the lumbus and collum femoris, as well as reduce MM cell metastasis to lungs and kidneys. Thus, these results suggest that FAS/FASL-induced apoptosis in MM cells plays a crucial role in the observed MSC-based inhibition of MM growth [27, 28], and also offer new directions for therapeutic interventions [29]. To this end, it is noteworthy that it was recently reported that licochalcone A, which can be isolated from the roots of *Glycyrrhiza glabra* (liquorice), up-regulated FASL in MSCs and strengthened bone formation and increased bone mass [30]. This effect was mediated by ERK phosphorylation, leading to GSK-3β inactivation and consequent β-catenin stabilisation in MSCs giving rise to enhanced or recovered function of osteogenic differentiation of damaged cells both in vivo and in vitro.

FASL was also found to promote proliferation of MSCs in vitro and to inhibit their differentiation into adipocytes. MSCs treated with low concentrations of FASL proliferated more rapidly than untreated cells without apoptosis, inducing ERK1/2 that was phosphorylated and upregulating survivin in these cells. When MSCs were cultured in adipogenic medium, FASL reversibly prevented differentiation into fat cells by modulating peroxisome proliferator-activated receptor gamma (PPARγ) and expression of the adipocyte binding protein FABP4/aP2 [31]. These results demonstrate that the FASL/FAS system has a potential role in MSC biology via regulation of both proliferation and adipogenesis, and may have clinical importance because circulating FASL levels decline with age and several age-related conditions, including osteoporosis, that are characterised by adipocyte accumulation in the bone marrow.

On MSC-derived pre-osteoblasts FASL appeared to have a conventional apoptosis-inducing activity owing to increased FAS levels, whereas differentiating adipocytes underwent a reduction in FAS expression and became resistant to FASL-induced cell death [32]. As MSC cell death and consequent loss of cells post-implantation is seen as a major obstacle to the utility in regenerative medicine, the authors assessed the effect of the growth factor EGF, and in particular EGF tethered onto a two-dimensional surface (tEGF), on responses of MSCs. They found that tEGF gave rise to sustained activation of EGFR and promoted survival from FASL-induced cell death pointing to a possible approach to assist MSCs to survive in the inflammatory wound milieu and increase their regenerative potential.

Another role for FASL was described in liver transplantation in a mouse model. Infusion of MSCs markedly ameliorated liver graft injury and improved survival post-transplantation and suppressed Kupffer cell apoptosis, Th1/Th17 immune responses, chemokine expression, and inflammatory cell infiltration. In vitro, PGE2 secreted by MSCs inhibited Kupffer cell apoptosis via regulation of the TLR4-ERK1/2-FAS/FASL-caspase-3 axis [33]. This study points to a potential option for the clinical application of MSC administration to protect liver grafts and prolong post-transplant survival in the future.

6.2.3 Regulation by TRAIL

CD34⁺ HSCs cells do not express TRAIL-receptors and are protected from TRAIL-induced apoptosis [34–36]. However, there is accumulating evidence that points to a role for TRAIL in the BM in the pathophysiology of a number of haematological disorders including aplastic anaemia, Fanconi anaemia, and myelodysplastic syndromes. Very severe aplastic anaemia (vSAA) is characterised by a hypoplastic BM due to destruction of $CD34^+$ stem cells by autoreactive T cells. Investigation of the pathomechanism by patient-specific gene expression analysis revealed that the apoptosis-inducing death ligand TRAIL was strongly up-regulated in $CD34^+$ cells of patients with vSAA [37]. However, $CD34^+$ cells from vSAA patients showed no changes in the expression of TRAIL-R1 and -R2 when compared to healthy controls. In contrast, TRAIL-R3 was up-regulated in $CD34^+$ cells of vSAA patients. TRAIL-R3 lacks the cytoplasmic region that contains the death-inducing protein domain and is not capable of triggering apoptosis. It is understood to act as a decoy receptor and protects cells from TRAIL-induced cytotoxicity by competing with other TRAIL receptors for ligand binding. The authors of this study speculated that up-regulation of a decoy receptor for TRAIL ligand may enable $CD34^+$ stem cells from vSAA patients to kill infiltrating effector lymphocytes through TRAIL while remaining resistant themselves. This resembles protective mechanisms found in some solid tumours that induce massive death of cytotoxic T cells by producing soluble and membrane-bound TRAIL [38–41]. TRAIL may also participate in the pathological suppression of erythropoiesis in SAA patients, since immature erythroblasts are sensitive to TRAIL owing to the expression of TRAIL-R1 and TRAIL-R2 [42]. Therefore, these precursors might be depleted leading to reduced numbers of mature erythrocytes. In addition, elevated TRAIL levels in the BM may also play a key role in other BM failure syndromes, such as Fanconi anaemia and myelodysplastic syndrome [43, 44].

In the context of survival, expansion and differentiation of erythroid progenitors it was discovered that the Bruton's tyrosine kinase (Btk) was phosphorylated by SCF also known as Kit-ligand, a factor that together with erythropoietin (EPO) is essential in the control of afore mentioned biological processes. Phosphorylation of Btk causes association with TRAIL-R1 and in the absence of Btk, erythroid progenitors are hypersensitive to TRAIL. Thus, Btk regulated signalling in erythroid progenitors that enhances survival and expansion of these cells which is, in part, afforded by providing resistance to TRAIL [45]. Interestingly, in patients with chronic lymphocytic leukaemia developing resistance to Btk-inhibition with Ibrutinib, a haplo-insufficiency of TRAIL-R was discovered. This is a consequence of del(8p) observed in 3 out of 5 patients, resulting in TRAIL insensitivity, which in turn may contribute to Ibrutinib resistance [46].

In summary, TRAIL and its receptors are either not detectable or expressed at very low levels in human haematopoietic progenitors under steady-state conditions; therefore, these cells are largely unaffected by this signalling pathway [34]. This is supported by results from infusion studies of recombinant TRAIL into rodents that did not show any gross abnormalities in haematopoiesis [47]. The only part of haematopoiesis that appeared affected when TRAIL was administered, not to rodents, but to nonhuman primates, was erythropoiesis evident by the mild anaemia that developed in these animals [69].

6.3 Use of Stem Cells to Deliver Death Ligands

While there are many different stem cell types there are only a few for which utility as cell therapeutic vehicle has been demonstrated. Most of the studies have been conducted with MSCs, while far fewer have tested other types such as HSCs and induced pluripotent stem (iPS)-derived stem cells.

6.3.1 Mesenchymal Stem Cells

MSCs are non-haematopoietic cell precursors initially found in the bone marrow, but actually present in many other tissues such as umbilical cord blood, placenta or adipose tissue. The International Society of Cellular Therapy (ISCT) used three criteria to define MSCs [48]. Firstly, MSCs can adhere to plastic under standard culture conditions; secondly, MSCs express cell surface markers including CD105, CD73 and CD90 with no expression of other contaminating endothelial, haematopoietic, or immunological cell markers such as CD45, CD34, CD14, CD11b, CD79α, CD19 and HLA-DR; thirdly, MSCs have the ability to differentiate into osteoblasts, adipocytes and chondroblasts when exposed to the appropriate stimuli [49]. Studies have shown that MSCs from different sources may vary in their differentiation capacity even if cultured under exactly the same conditions. BM-derived MSCs have the highest degree of lineage plasticity as they are capable of giving rise to virtually all cell types after being implanted into early blastocysts [50, 51]. The capacity of MSCs to differentiate into various cell lineages and proliferate in vitro makes them attractive targets for regenerative medicine applications [52]. Moreover, MSCs can be readily transduced by a variety of vectors such as adenovirus, lentivirus and adeno-associated virus and can maintain transgene expression after in vivo differentiation [53]. MSCs are also immune-privileged owing to the lack of co-stimulatory molecules present on the cell surface including B7–1, B7–2, CD40 and CD40 ligand [54]. MSCs also secrete prostaglandin E2 (PGE2), transforming growth factor ß (TGF-ß) and hepatocyte growth factor (HGF), which regulate the immune response of T cells to novel antigens, thereby decreasing the chances of a cytotoxic T cell response to the transduced MSCs. In addition to suppressing cytotoxic T cell functions, MSCs are also able to inhibit the differentiation of dendritic cells and regulate the production of proinflammatory cytokines [55–57]. All these features are important in protecting MSCs from immune responses. Therefore, MSCs possess immune-regulatory functions. Another well-established function of

MSCs is the ability to migrate to damaged tissues, ischaemia and tumour microenvironments. Also, MSCs are capable of extravasating towards tumours when introduced into the organism via the local blood stream [58]. Although the mechanisms behind the migration of MSCs are still not fully understood, studies have shown that the migration is regulated by various cytokines and their corresponding receptors, i.e., SDF-1/CXCR4, HGF/c-Met, VEGF/VEGFR, PDGF/PDGFR, MCP-1/CCR2, and HMGB1/RAGE [59]. In summary, the fact that MSCs can be easily transduced, have immune-regulatory properties, and their capacity for tumour-directed migration, makes MSC therapy a promising new approach for the treatment of cancer.

6.3.2 *Targeting Death Receptors with MSCs*

Currently, an innovative strategy in tumour therapy is the activation of apoptosis through the binding of death ligands to their corresponding death receptors and to have the ligands delivered by stem cells. Signalling through death receptors is one way to directly induce apoptosis, thereby circumventing chemotherapeutic resistance. Integration of the TNF in such stem cell systems has been tested using MSC-mediated delivery and showed a strong suppressive effect on gastric tumour growth in immune-deficient nude mice [60]. However, it is generally recognised that TNF as a (cancer) therapeutic agent has limited therapeutic efficacy and substantial side effects, and can only be applied in very restricted circumstances such as the treatment of metastases from melanoma and sarcoma by hyperthermic-isolated limb perfusion [61]. Therefore, the focus turned to other members of the TNF superfamily. LIGHT is another member of this family, which is naturally expressed on immature dendritic cells (DCs) and activated T cells [62]. LIGHT normally binds to two functional receptors, HVEM and lymphotoxin β receptor (LTβR); the former is broadly expressed on the surface of T cells, NK cells, and monocytes while the latter is mainly expressed on stromal cells and monocyte cells [62]. Owing to its regulatory activity on immune cells, LIGHT has a priming role in anti-tumour immunity and has therefore attracted considerable attention as it could be an important element in tumour immune therapies [62, 63]. In one study, MSC delivery of LIGHT enhanced T cells infiltrating into tumours and reversed the local suppressive environment and resulted in tumour regression [64]. Similarly, MSCs expressing LIGHT possessed an obvious anti-tumour effect in a gastric tumour xenograft mouse model [65]. Thus, therapeutic strategies centred on LIGHT signalling hold great promise, but the complexity of this system makes therapeutic inhibition strategies less straightforward than for other inhibitory receptors or ligands such as PD1/PDL1 or CTLA4/CD80 and CD86 (also called B7–1 and B7–2, respectively).

Among the different TNF members, the most promising one appears to be TRAIL for adoption to a stem cell delivery system, and in fact a clinical trial has been initiated with the goal to treat lung cancer patients with MSCs that express TRAIL at University College London. TRAIL is a type 2 transmembrane protein and is composed of 281 amino acids [66]. It can induce apoptosis in cancer cells while sparing normal cells although the molecular basis for the tumour-selective activity of TRAIL remains to be fully defined [67]. In addition, unlike conventional chemotherapeutics, TRAIL can induce apoptosis in a p53-independent manner. Since p53 is frequently inactivated in human tumours, TRAIL may have the ability to induce apoptosis in those cancer cells. These features make TRAIL a promising agent for anti-cancer therapy. Although TRAIL is a very promising anti-tumour agent, there are a number of limitations to its use as a recombinant protein including the resistance of various human cancers, especially some highly malignant tumours, to this death receptor pathway [66]. Moreover, repeated application of TRAIL can result in selection and expansion of TRAIL-resistant cells leading to acquired resistance [68]. The success of TRAIL treatments can also be hampered by the short half-life and instability in vivo [69]. While not all of these issues can be addressed by stem cell-based delivery, in particular MSC engineered to express TRAIL (MSC-TRAIL) have been shown to overcome some of the described limitations. To this end, a number of studies have shown the therapeutic efficacy of such MSCs in various cancer models and treatment schedules both in vitro or in vivo (Table 6.1) [70–81]. For example, MSCs with expression of TRAIL exert apoptosis-inducing activity in vitro, including cervical carcinoma, pancreatic cancer and colon cancer [75]. MSC-TRAIL were able also to inhibit the growth of glioma in nude mice and prolong the survival of glioma-bearing mice compared with controls after intratumoural injection [71, 72]. In addition, delivery of MSC-TRAIL could inhibit lung tumour growth and even eliminate lung tumour metastases [73, 76]. Most of the earlier MSC-TRAIL studies used full-length TRAIL (aa1-aa281) which is expressed as a membrane-bound protein restricting the apoptosis-inducing activity to neighbouring cancer cells. Since then a number of improvements have been made to increase the reach of the MSC-produced TRAIL and its cancer cell-killing activity. This was achieved by engineering and using an expression cassette of soluble and trimeric form of TRAIL (sTRAIL) [82, 83]. Using sTRAIL (aa114-aa281) instead of full-length membrane bound TRAIL, enables TRAIL to also on act distant cells. This independency from MSC-tumour-cell interaction increases the efficiency of MSC-TRAIL-based therapies as it principally requires a lower number of TRAIL expressing MSCs in the tumour tissue. Furthermore, forcing trimerisation of secreted TRAIL by inclusion of an isoleucine zipper in the sTRAIL expression cassette has been shown to increase the potency compared to full-length TRAIL [71, 76, 84, 85]. Another approach was to include specific point mutations in the TRAIL sequence to render them TRAIL receptor-specific [86–89]. These TRAIL variants were designed by computer modelling and specifically target TRAIL-R1 or TRAIL-R2 and have shown improved anti-tumour effects in vitro and in vivo as recombinant protein [90–94] as well as when delivered by MSCs [84].

Notwithstanding, some tumours remain insensitive to TRAIL-induced apoptosis [95, 96] and MSC expressing TRAIL alone may be ineffective. Therefore, combinations of MSCs expressing TRAIL with other approaches like chemotherapeutic agents, irradiation, down-regulation of anti-apoptotic protein or co-expressed with other proteins have been tested and shown to overcome resistance and to enhance efficacy (Table 6.2) [75–77, 79, 81, 84, 97, 98]. Such combined approaches are

Table 6.1 Selected MSC-TRAIL experimental studies (in chronological order of publication)

MSCs sources	Transduction vectors	Outcome/summary	Citations
Human bone marrow	Adenoviral vector	MSCs-TRAIL inhibited the tumour growth of lung cancer model in vivo	[70]
Human umbilical cord blood	Adenoviral vector	MSCs-TRAIL inhibited tumour growth and prolonged the survival of glioma-bearing mouse.	[71]
Human bone marrow	Lentiviral vector	MSC-sTRAIL have anti-tumour effects on both malignant and invasive primary gliomas in vivo	[72]
Human bone marrow	Lentiviral vector	MSC-TRAIL can reduce breast tumour cells growth and eliminate metastases in vivo	[73]
Human bone marrow	rAAV vector	MSC-TRAIL can prolong the survival of brainstem glioma-bearing mouse	[74]
Human adipose	Retroviral vector	MSC-TRAIL can induce apoptosis in various cancer cells in vitro and reduce tumour growth of cervical carcinoma in vivo	[75]
Mouse bone marrow	Adenoviral vector	MSC-TRAIL combined with silencing of XIAP resulted in tumour regression and inhibition of metastasis of pancreatic cancer in vivo	[76]
Human umbilical cord blood	Adenoviral vector	MSC-TRAIL combined with irradiation synergistically inhibited tumour growth in a xenograft glioma mice model	[77]
Human bone marrow	Lentiviral vector	MSC-TRAIL inhibited the growth of selected TRAIL-resistant colorectal carcinoma cells both in vitro and in vivo	[78]
Human adipose	Retroviral vector	MSC-TRAIL can induce apoptosis in multiple myeloma cells in vitro	[79]
Human pancreas	Plasmid	MSC-TRAIL inhibit the growth of pancreatic cancer cells in vitro	[80]
Human bone marrow	Adenoviral vector	MSC-TRAIL in combination with lipoxygenase inhibitor MK886 resulted in prolonged delivery of TRAIL both in vitro and in vivo, and resulted in significantly enhanced apoptosis orthotopic mouse models of glioma	[81]

mostly based on results obtained with recombinant TRAIL over the last 15 years. TRAIL has been administered together with a variety of agents and several of these co-treatments could sensitise otherwise resistant tumour cells to TRAIL-induced apoptosis. For example, Doxorubicin, 5-Fluorouracil, Etoposide and irradiation have been shown to up-regulate DR4 and/or DR5 and synergise with TRAIL [98–101]. Down-regulation of c-FLIP levels can also enhance the sensitivity to TRAIL in various cancer cells [102, 103]. In some cells, the process of apoptosis is subjected to the regulation of Bcl-2 family members. Various agents have been used in combination with TRAIL to overcome resistance through modulation of Bcl-2 family members. For example, topoisomerase I inhibitor CPT-11 in combination with TRAIL increased Bax and reduced Bcl-XL expression and resulted in a synergistic cytotoxic effect [104]. Bortezombib, a proteasome inhibitor, was shown to enhance TRAIL

Table 6.2 Selected combination MSC-TRAIL studies

Approaches	Effects	Citations
MSC were engineered to co-express herpes simplex virus thymidine kinase (HSV-TK) with TRAIL	MSC delivery of both HSV-TK and TRAIL exerted stronger apoptotic response than MSC expressing HSV-TK or TRAIL alone in renal cancer cells both in vitro and in vivo	[97]
Down-regulation of XIAP	MSC-TRAIL together with XIAP down-regulation suppresses metastatic growth of pancreatic carcinoma	[76]
Irradiation	Irradiation enhance the MSC-TRAIL induced apoptosis in xenograft glioma mice model	[77]
Proteasome inhibitor bortezomib	Combination use of MSC-TRAIL with Bortezomib significantly increases apoptosis in TRAIL-resistant breast cancer cells	[75]
Lipoxygenase inhibitor MK886	Lipoxygenase inhibitor MK886 combined with MSC-TRAIL significantly enhanced apoptosis and prolonged delivery of TRAIL both in vitro and in orthotopic mouse models of glioma	[81]
Proteasome inhibitor bortezomib	MSC-TRAIL in combination with bortezomib significantly induced more apoptosis in myeloma cells	[79]
Histone-deacetylase inhibitor MS-275	MSC-TRAIL combined with MS-275 could overcome TRAIL-resistant in medulloblastomas both in vitro and in vivo	[98]
5-FU	MSC-TRAIL combined with 5-FU induced more apoptosis in colorectal cancer cells both in vitro and in vivo	[84]

apoptosis-inducing activity through decreasing Bcl-2 and Bcl-XL levels in vitro [105]. To date, several Bcl-2 inhibitors are being tested in clinical trials and the results are promising [106]. For example, the small molecular Bcl-2 inhibitor HA14–1 was able to restore TRAIL-induced apoptosis in colon cancer cells with high Bcl-2 expression levels [107, 108]. ABT-737 (A-779024, Abbott Laboratories) is a small molecule BH3 mimetic that binds to and antagonises Bcl-2/Bcl-XL, thereby promoting Bax and Bak oligomerisation and apoptosis [109]. ABT-737 could enhance TRAIL-induced apoptosis in human pancreatic cancer cells and glioblastoma cells through the augmentation of intrinsic pathway activation [110, 112]. Interestingly, ABT-737 could also up-regulate DR5 thereby increasing apoptosis through the extrinsic pathway induced by TRAIL in renal, prostate, and lung cancer cells [112].

XIAP is a potent and broad inhibitor of cell death. XIAP inhibitors have been extensively studied in combination with TRAIL or TRAIL receptor agonists in various cancer cells. XIAP inhibitors were shown to synergise with TRAIL to induce apoptosis in breast cancer cells and leukaemic T cells [113, 114]. Pancreatic cancer cells that have high expression levels of XIAP often show resistance to TRAIL. Silencing of XIAP in combination with TRAIL can overcome this resistance and suppress carcinoma growth both in vivo and in vitro [115, 116]. Our group also showed that apoptosis induced by TRAIL was significantly increased with concomitant knockdown of XIAP by RNAi in pancreatic cancer cells both in vitro and in vivo [76]. TRAIL receptor agonistic antibodies also cooperate with XIAP inhibitors to induce apoptosis in pancreatic carcinoma cells [117]. Moreover, IAP inhibitor enhanced the anti-tumour effect of TRAIL in a human malignant glioma xenograft model in vivo and, although XIAP inhibitors do not sensitise Cholangiocarcinoma (CCA) cells to apoptosis, they reduce TRAIL-stimulated invasion and metastasis [118, 119]. Taken together, combination with IAP inhibitors may be a good option to increase the efficacy of TRAIL therapy.

TRAIL signalling does not only activate the apoptotic pathways but also non-apoptotic cellular signalling pathways like NF-κB and PKB/Akt that could in turn affect the TRAIL sensitivity [120]. Agents such as 17-AAG (17-allylamino-17-demethoxygeldanamycin) can enhance TRAIL-induced apoptosis through inhibition of NF-κB [120]. The NF-κB specific inhibitors PS-1145 or AS602868 have been found to sensitise TRAIL-induced apoptosis in pancreatic cancer cells and myeloma [121, 122]. PKB/Akt is a PI3-kinase activated protein kinase that belongs to the cAMP-dependent protein kinase (AGC) superfamily [123]. Inhibition of PKB/Akt could sensitise human umbilical vein endothelial cells to TRAIL-mediated apoptosis [124]. Perifosine, an inhibitor of Akt, could synergise with TRAIL to induce apoptosis in acute myelogenous leukaemia (AML) cells [125]. Another Akt inhibitor named Triciribine could also sensitise prostate tumour cells to TRAIL-induced apoptosis [126]. The Myc pathway also appears to be able to affect TRAIL sensitivity. Myc was found to sensitise cells to TRAIL-induced apoptosis by interfering with the TRAIL-dependent NF-κB-induced expression of anti-apoptotic genes such as Mcl-1 and cIAP2 [127]. HDAC inhibition (HDACi) is an apoptosis-inducing strategy that can activate both extrinsic and intrinsic pathways [128]. The combined use of HDACi and TRAIL exhibited strongly enhanced apoptosis-inducing activity in haematological and solid tumours both in vitro and in vivo [129, 130].

Thus, stem cell-based treatments might eventually become part of targeted combination treatments, in which more conventional treatment types such as chemotherapeutic drugs or radiation are used to render cancer cells vulnerable followed by stem cells effectively delivering a therapeutic payload to exploit such induced "Achilles' heels".

6.3.3 Targeting Death Receptors with Other Stem Cell Types (HSCs, ESCs)

In one study, the full-length mouse TRAIL (mTRAIL) gene was transduced into mouse BM cells by retroviral transduction in vitro, and these cells were then transplanted into lethally irradiated mice of the same strain. It was found that the transgenic TRAIL expression was limited to the haematopoietic cells of the BM recipient mice. This has several advantages in that the major cell population overexpressing

TRAIL, namely haematopoietic cells, including immune cells and other leukocytes, are known to infiltrate tumour tissues and are seen as the major cellular force in anti-tumour activity in the body. Indeed, the overexpression of TRAIL could significantly inhibit the growth of EMT6.5 and 4 T1.2 syngeneic tumours in BALB/c mice without causing a toxic effect on normal tissues in vivo [131]. The authors of this study commented that although tumour inhibition was clearly seen in TRAIL-transduced mice, these animals still succumbed to their tumours eventually suggesting that TRAIL could only partially inhibit tumour growth. Combining TRAIL with other antitumor agents may be more effective than using TRAIL alone; for example, increasing TRAIL expression combined with inhibition of angiogenesis might be a more effective approach to tumour inhibition.

In a model of glioma, a usually very aggressive and difficult to treat type of brain tumour, researchers tested the ability of ESCs to deliver TRAIL. For this, malignant glioma A172 cells were used to establish heterotopic xenografts in nude mice. Subsequently, ESC-derived astrocytes conditionally expressing TRAIL were injected into the xenografts. Following external gene induction, a significant reduction in tumour volume was detected in the experimental groups. Terminal dUTP nick end labelling (TUNEL) revealed apoptotic responses in tumour cells in the TRAIL treated cohort. Seven days after injection, the tumours showed signs of severe necrosis, with only scattered residual tumour cells at the periphery [132]. These results suggest that ESC derived astrocytes expressing TRAIL should be considered as potential delivery vehicle for the treatment of glioma.

Thus, while MSCs are currently the preferred stem cell type to deliver death receptor targeting therapies, other stem cell types might offer specific advantages in particular neoplastic diseases and will have to undergo further analysis. Going forward, stem cells derived from iPS cells might be able to replace the often difficult to source stem cell types. For example, induced MSCs (iMSCs) are transpiring as an attractive source for MSCs because they offer autologous cells for treatment and could be considered as an inexhaustible source of MSCs that could be used to meet the unmet clinical needs [133, 134].

References

1. Guicciardi ME, Gores GJ (2009) Life and death by death receptors. FASEB J 23(6):1625–1637. doi:10.1096/fj.08-111005
2. Itoh N, Nagata S (1993) A novel protein domain required for apoptosis. Mutational analysis of human Fas antigen. J Biol Chem 268(15):10932–10937
3. Suda T, Takahashi T, Golstein P, Nagata S (1993) Molecular cloning and expression of the Fas ligand, a novel member of the tumor necrosis factor family. Cell 75(6):1169–1178
4. Trauth BC, Klas C, Peters AM, Matzku S, Moller P, Falk W, Debatin KM, Krammer PH (1989) Monoclonal antibody-mediated tumor regression by induction of apoptosis. Science 245(4915):301–305
5. Beutler B, Greenwald D, Hulmes JD, Chang M, Pan YC, Mathison J, Ulevitch R, Cerami A (1985) Identity of tumour necrosis factor and the macrophage-secreted factor cachectin. Nature 316(6028):552–554

6. Loetscher H, Pan YC, Lahm HW, Gentz R, Brockhaus M, Tabuchi H, Lesslauer W (1990) Molecular cloning and expression of the human 55 kd tumor necrosis factor receptor. Cell 61(2):351–359
7. Schall TJ, Lewis M, Koller KJ, Lee A, Rice GC, Wong GH, Gatanaga T, Granger GA, Lentz R, Raab H et al (1990) Molecular cloning and expression of a receptor for human tumor necrosis factor. Cell 61(2):361–370
8. Chicheportiche Y, Bourdon PR, Xu H, Hsu YM, Scott H, Hession C, Garcia I, Browning JL (1997) TWEAK, a new secreted ligand in the tumor necrosis factor family that weakly induces apoptosis. J Biol Chem 272(51):32401–32410
9. Marsters SA, Sheridan JP, Donahue CJ, Pitti RM, Gray CL, Goddard AD, Bauer KD, Ashkenazi A (1996) Apo-3, a new member of the tumor necrosis factor receptor family, contains a death domain and activates apoptosis and NF-kappa B. Curr Biol 6(12):1669–1676
10. Wang EC (2012) On death receptor 3 and its ligands. Immunology 137(1):114–116. doi:10.1111/j.1365-2567.2012.03606.x
11. Walczak H, Degli-Esposti MA, Johnson RS, Smolak PJ, Waugh JY, Boiani N, Timour MS, Gerhart MJ, Schooley KA, Smith CA, Goodwin RG, Rauch CT (1997) TRAIL-R2: a novel apoptosis-mediating receptor for TRAIL. EMBO J 16(17):5386–5397
12. Pan G, O'Rourke K, Chinnaiyan AM, Gentz R, Ebner R, Ni J, Dixit VM (1997) The receptor for the cytotoxic ligand TRAIL. Science 276(5309):111–113
13. Wiley SR, Schooley K, Smolak PJ, Din WS, Huang CP, Nicholl JK, Sutherland GR, Smith TD, Rauch C, Smith CA et al (1995) Identification and characterization of a new member of the TNF family that induces apoptosis. Immunity 3(6):673–682
14. Pan G, Bauer JH, Haridas V, Wang S, Liu D, Yu G, Vincenz C, Aggarwal BB, Ni J, Dixit VM (1998) Identification and functional characterization of DR6, a novel death domain-containing TNF receptor. FEBS Lett 431(3):351–356
15. Mohr A, Zwacka RM, Jarmy G, Buneker C, Schrezenmeier H, Dohner K, Beltinger C, Wiesneth M, Debatin KM, Stahnke K (2005) Caspase-8L expression protects CD34+ hematopoietic progenitor cells and leukemic cells from CD95-mediated apoptosis. Oncogene 24(14):2421–2429
16. Aggarwal BB (2003) Signalling pathways of the TNF superfamily: a double-edged sword. Nat Rev Immunol 3(9):745–756
17. Bryder D, Ramsfjell V, Dybedal I, Theilgaard-Monch K, Hogerkorp CM, Adolfsson J, Borge OJ, Jacobsen SE (2001) Self-renewal of multipotent long-term repopulating hematopoietic stem cells is negatively regulated by Fas and tumor necrosis factor receptor activation. J Exp Med 194(7):941–952
18. Dybedal I, Bryder D, Fossum A, Rusten LS, Jacobsen SE (2001) Tumor necrosis factor (TNF)-mediated activation of the p55 TNF receptor negatively regulates maintenance of cycling reconstituting human hematopoietic stem cells. Blood 98(6):1782–1791
19. Zhang Y, Harada A, Bluethmann H, Wang JB, Nakao S, Mukaida N, Matsushima K (1995) Tumor necrosis factor (TNF) is a physiologic regulator of hematopoietic progenitor cells: increase of early hematopoietic progenitor cells in TNF receptor p55-deficient mice in vivo and potent inhibition of progenitor cell proliferation by TNF alpha in vitro. Blood 86(8):2930–2937
20. Mori T, Nishimura T, Ikeda Y, Hotta T, Yagita H, Ando K (1998) Involvement of Fas-mediated apoptosis in the hematopoietic progenitor cells of graft-versus-host reaction-associated myelosuppression. Blood 92(1):101–107
21. Vinci G, Chouaib S, Autran B, Vernant JP (1991) Evidence that residual host cells surviving the conditioning regimen to allogeneic bone marrow transplantation inhibit donor hematopoiesis in vitro—the role of TNF-alpha. Transplantation 52(3):406–411
22. Richards M, Tan SP, Tan JH, Chan WK, Bongso A (2004) The transcriptome profile of human embryonic stem cells as defined by SAGE. Stem Cells 22(1):51–64. doi:10.1634/stemcells.22-1-51

23. Desbarats J, Newell MK (2000) Fas engagement accelerates liver regeneration after partial hepatectomy. Nat Med 6(8):920–923. doi:10.1038/78688
24. Corsini NS, Sancho-Martinez I, Laudenklos S, Glagow D, Kumar S, Letellier E, Koch P, Teodorczyk M, Kleber S, Klussmann S, Wiestler B, Brustle O, Mueller W, Gieffers C, Hill O, Thiemann M, Seedorf M, Gretz N, Sprengel R, Celikel T, Martin-Villalba A (2009) The death receptor CD95 activates adult neural stem cells for working memory formation and brain repair. Cell Stem Cell 5(2):178–190. doi:10.1016/j.stem.2009.05.004
25. Ceppi P, Hadji A, Kohlhapp FJ, Pattanayak A, Hau A, Liu X, Liu H, Murmann AE, Peter ME (2014) CD95 and CD95L promote and protect cancer stem cells. Nat Commun 5:5238. doi:10.1038/ncomms6238
26. Teodorczyk M, Kleber S, Wollny D, Sefrin JP, Aykut B, Mateos A, Herhaus P, Sancho-Martinez I, Hill O, Gieffers C, Sykora J, Weichert W, Eisen C, Trumpp A, Sprick MR, Bergmann F, Welsch T, Martin-Villalba A (2015) CD95 promotes metastatic spread via Sck in pancreatic ductal adenocarcinoma. Cell Death Differ 22(7):1192–1202. doi:10.1038/cdd.2014.217
27. Li X, Ling W, Khan S, Yaccoby S (2012) Therapeutic effects of intrabone and systemic mesenchymal stem cell cytotherapy on myeloma bone disease and tumor growth. J Bone Miner Res 27(8):1635–1648. doi:10.1002/jbmr.1620
28. Li X, Ling W, Pennisi A, Wang Y, Khan S, Heidaran M, Pal A, Zhang X, He S, Zeitlin A, Abbot S, Faleck H, Hariri R, Shaughnessy JD Jr, van Rhee F, Nair B, Barlogie B, Epstein J, Yaccoby S (2011) Human placenta-derived adherent cells prevent bone loss, stimulate bone formation, and suppress growth of multiple myeloma in bone. Stem Cells 29(2):263–273. doi:10.1002/stem.572
29. Atsuta I, Liu S, Miura Y, Akiyama K, Chen C, An Y, Shi S, Chen FM (2013) Mesenchymal stem cells inhibit multiple myeloma cells via the Fas/Fas ligand pathway. Stem Cell Res Ther 4(5):111. doi:10.1186/scrt322
30. Ming L, Jin F, Huang P, Luo H, Liu W, Zhang L, Yuan W, Zhang Y, Jin Y (2014) Licochalcone a up-regulates of FasL in mesenchymal stem cells to strengthen bone formation and increase bone mass. Sci Rep 4:7209. doi:10.1038/srep07209
31. Rippo MR, Babini L, Prattichizzo F, Graciotti L, Fulgenzi G, Tomassoni Ardori F, Olivieri F, Borghetti G, Cinti S, Poloni A, Fazioli F, Procopio AD (2013) Low FasL levels promote proliferation of human bone marrow-derived mesenchymal stem cells, higher levels inhibit their differentiation into adipocytes. Cell Death Dis 4:e594. doi:10.1038/cddis.2013.115
32. Rodrigues M, Blair H, Stockdale L, Griffith L, Wells A (2013) Surface tethered epidermal growth factor protects proliferating and differentiating multipotential stromal cells from FasL-induced apoptosis. Stem Cells 31(1):104–116. doi:10.1002/stem.1215
33. Tian Y, Wang J, Wang W, Ding Y, Sun Z, Zhang Q, Wang Y, Xie H, Yan S, Zheng S (2016) Mesenchymal stem cells improve mouse non-heart-beating liver graft survival by inhibiting Kupffer cell apoptosis via TLR4-ERK1/2-Fas/FasL-caspase3 pathway regulation. Stem Cell Res Ther 7(1):157. doi:10.1186/s13287-016-0416-y
34. Mizrahi K, Stein J, Pearl-Yafe M, Kaplan O, Yaniv I, Askenasy N (2010) Regulatory functions of TRAIL in hematopoietic progenitors: human umbilical cord blood and murine bone marrow transplantation. Leukemia 24(7):1325–1334. doi:10.1038/leu.2010.97
35. Tao W, Hangoc G, Hawes JW, Si Y, Cooper S, Broxmeyer HE (2003) Profiling of differentially expressed apoptosis-related genes by cDNA arrays in human cord blood CD34+ cells treated with etoposide. Exp Hematol 31(3):251–260
36. Zauli G, Secchiero P (2006) The role of the TRAIL/TRAIL receptors system in hematopoiesis and endothelial cell biology. Cytokine Growth Factor Rev 17(4):245–257. doi:10.1016/j.cytogfr.2006.04.002
37. Fischer U, Ruckert C, Hubner B, Eckermann O, Binder V, Bakchoul T, Schuster FR, Merk S, Klein HU, Fuhrer M, Dugas M, Borkhardt A (2012) CD34+ gene expression profiling of individual children with very severe aplastic anemia indicates a pathogenic role of integ-

rin receptors and the proapoptotic death ligand TRAIL. Haematologica 97(9):1304–1311. doi:10.3324/haematol.2011.056705
38. Giovarelli M, Musiani P, Garotta G, Ebner R, Di Carlo E, Kim Y, Cappello P, Rigamonti L, Bernabei P, Novelli F, Modesti A, Coletti A, Ferrie AK, Lollini PL, Ruben S, Salcedo T, Forni G (1999) A "stealth effect": adenocarcinoma cells engineered to express TRAIL elude tumor-specific and allogeneic T cell reactions. J Immunol 163(9):4886–4893
39. Grimm M, Kim M, Rosenwald A, von Raden BH, Tsaur I, Meier E, Heemann U, Germer CT, Gasser M, Waaga-Gasser AM (2010) Tumour-mediated TRAIL-receptor expression indicates effective apoptotic depletion of infiltrating CD8+ immune cells in clinical colorectal cancer. Eur J Cancer 46(12):2314–2323. doi:10.1016/j.ejca.2010.05.025
40. Shiraki K, Yamanaka T, Inoue H, Kawakita T, Enokimura N, Okano H, Sugimoto K, Murata K, Nakano T (2005) Expression of TNF-related apoptosis-inducing ligand in human hepatocellular carcinoma. Int J Oncol 26(5):1273–1281
41. Zhao S, Asgary Z, Wang Y, Goodwin R, Andreeff M, Younes A (1999) Functional expression of TRAIL by lymphoid and myeloid tumour cells. Br J Haematol 106(3):827–832
42. Secchiero P, Melloni E, Heikinheimo M, Mannisto S, Di Pietro R, Iacone A, Zauli G (2004) TRAIL regulates normal erythroid maturation through an ERK-dependent pathway. Blood 103(2):517–522
43. Campioni D, Secchiero P, Corallini F, Melloni E, Capitani S, Lanza F, Zauli G (2005) Evidence for a role of TNF-related apoptosis-inducing ligand (TRAIL) in the anemia of myelodysplastic syndromes. Am J Pathol 166(2):557–563. doi:10.1016/S0002-9440(10)62277-8
44. Pigullo S, Ferretti E, Lanciotti M, Bruschi M, Candiano G, Svahn J, Haneline L, Dufour C, Pistoia V, Corcione A (2007) Human Fanconi a cells are susceptible to TRAIL-induced apoptosis. Br J Haematol 136(2):315–318. doi:10.1111/j.1365-2141.2006.06432.x
45. Schmidt U, van den Akker E, Parren-van Amelsvoort M, Litos G, de Bruijn M, Gutierrez L, Hendriks RW, Ellmeier W, Lowenberg B, Beug H, von Lindern M (2004) Btk is required for an efficient response to erythropoietin and for SCF-controlled protection against TRAIL in erythroid progenitors. J Exp Med 199(6):785–795. doi:10.1084/jem.20031109. jem.20031109 [pii]
46. Burger JA, Landau DA, Taylor-Weiner A, Bozic I, Zhang H, Sarosiek K, Wang L, Stewart C, Fan J, Hoellenriegel J, Sivina M, Dubuc AM, Fraser C, Han Y, Li S, Livak KJ, Zou L, Wan Y, Konoplev S, Sougnez C, Brown JR, Abruzzo LV, Carter SL, Keating MJ, Davids MS, Wierda WG, Cibulskis K, Zenz T, Werner L, Dal Cin P, Kharchencko P, Neuberg D, Kantarjian H, Lander E, Gabriel S, O'Brien S, Letai A, Weitz DA, Nowak MA, Getz G, Wu CJ (2016) Clonal evolution in patients with chronic lymphocytic leukaemia developing resistance to BTK inhibition. Nat Commun 7:11589. doi:10.1038/ncomms11589
47. Walczak H, Miller RE, Ariail K, Gliniak B, Griffith TS, Kubin M, Chin W, Jones J, Woodward A, Le T, Smith C, Smolak P, Goodwin RG, Rauch CT, Schuh JC, Lynch DH (1999) Tumoricidal activity of tumor necrosis factor-related apoptosis-inducing ligand in vivo. Nat Med 5(2):157–163
48. Dominici M, Le Blanc K, Mueller I, Slaper-Cortenbach I, Marini F, Krause D, Deans R, Keating A, Prockop D, Horwitz E (2006) Minimal criteria for defining multipotent mesenchymal stromal cells. The International Society for Cellular Therapy position statement. Cytotherapy 8(4):315–317
49. Pittenger MF, Mackay AM, Beck SC, Jaiswal RK, Douglas R, Mosca JD, Moorman MA, Simonetti DW, Craig S, Marshak DR (1999) Multilineage potential of adult human mesenchymal stem cells. Science 284(5411):143–147
50. Jiang Y, Jahagirdar BN, Reinhardt RL, Schwartz RE, Keene CD, Ortiz-Gonzalez XR, Reyes M, Lenvik T, Lund T, Blackstad M, Du J, Aldrich S, Lisberg A, Low WC, Largaespada DA, Verfaillie CM (2002) Pluripotency of mesenchymal stem cells derived from adult marrow. Nature 418(6893):41–49. doi:10.1038/nature00870. nature00870 [pii]

51. Orlic D, Kajstura J, Chimenti S, Jakoniuk I, Anderson SM, Li B, Pickel J, McKay R, Nadal-Ginard B, Bodine DM, Leri A, Anversa P (2001) Bone marrow cells regenerate infarcted myocardium. Nature 410(6829):701–705. doi:10.1038/35070587. 35070587 [pii]
52. Prockop DJ (2017) The exciting prospects of new therapies with mesenchymal stromal cells. Cytotherapy 19(1):1–8. doi:10.1016/j.jcyt.2016.09.008
53. Roelants V, Labar D, de Meester C, Havaux X, Tabilio A, Gambhir SS, Di Ianni M, Bol A, Bertrand L, Vanoverschelde JL (2008) Comparison between adenoviral and retroviral vectors for the transduction of the thymidine kinase PET reporter gene in rat mesenchymal stem cells. J Nucl Med 49(11):1836–1844. doi:10.2967/jnumed.108.052175. 49/11/1836 [pii]
54. Rasmusson I (2006) Immune modulation by mesenchymal stem cells. Exp Cell Res 312(12):2169–2179. doi:10.1016/j.yexcr.2006.03.019. S0014-4827(06)00122-4 [pii]
55. Le Blanc K, Tammik L, Sundberg B, Haynesworth SE, Ringden O (2003) Mesenchymal stem cells inhibit and stimulate mixed lymphocyte cultures and mitogenic responses independently of the major histocompatibility complex. Scand J Immunol 57(1):11–20. doi:1176 [pii]
56. Zhang W, Ge W, Li C, You S, Liao L, Han Q, Deng W, Zhao RC (2004) Effects of mesenchymal stem cells on differentiation, maturation, and function of human monocyte-derived dendritic cells. Stem Cells Dev 13(3):263–271. doi:10.1089/154732804323099190
57. Chen X, Armstrong MA, Li G (2006) Mesenchymal stem cells in immunoregulation. Immunol Cell Biol 84(5):413–421. doi:10.1111/j.1440-1711.2006.01458.x. ICB1458 [pii]
58. Caplan AI (2007) Adult mesenchymal stem cells for tissue engineering versus regenerative medicine. J Cell Physiol 213(2):341–347. doi:10.1002/jcp.21200
59. Momin EN, Vela G, Zaidi HA, Quinones-Hinojosa A (2010) The oncogenic potential of Mesenchymal stem cells in the treatment of cancer: directions for future research. Curr Immunol Rev 6(2):137–148. doi:10.2174/157339510791111718
60. Mao W, Zhu X, Tang D, Zhao Y, Zhao B, Ma G, Zhang X, An G, Li Y (2012) TNF-alpha expression in the UCB-MSCs as stable source inhibits gastric cancers growth in nude mice. Cancer Invest 30(6):463–472. doi:10.3109/07357907.2012.675385
61. Roberts NJ, Zhou S, Diaz LA Jr, Holdhoff M (2011) Systemic use of tumor necrosis factor alpha as an anticancer agent. Oncotarget 2(10):739–751. doi:10.18632/oncotarget.344
62. Yu P, Fu YX (2008) Targeting tumors with LIGHT to generate metastasis-clearing immunity. Cytokine Growth Factor Rev 19(3–4):285–294. doi:10.1016/j.cytogfr.2008.04.004
63. Ward-Kavanagh LK, Lin WW, Sedy JR, Ware CF (2016) The TNF receptor superfamily in co-stimulating and co-inhibitory responses. Immunity 44(5):1005–1019. doi:10.1016/j.immuni.2016.04.019
64. Zou W, Zheng H, He TC, Chang J, Fu YX, Fan W (2012) LIGHT delivery to tumors by mesenchymal stem cells mobilizes an effective antitumor immune response. Cancer Res 72(12):2980–2989. doi:10.1158/0008-5472.CAN-11-4216. 0008-5472.CAN-11-4216 [pii]
65. Zhu X, Su D, Xuan S, Ma G, Dai Z, Liu T, Tang D, Mao W, Dong C (2012) Gene therapy of gastric cancer using LIGHT-secreting human umbilical cord blood-derived mesenchymal stem cells. Gastric Cancer. doi:10.1007/s10120-012-0166-1
66. Gonzalvez F, Ashkenazi A (2010) New insights into apoptosis signaling by Apo2L/TRAIL. Oncogene 29(34):4752–4765. doi:10.1038/onc.2010.221
67. Ashkenazi A (2008) Directing cancer cells to self-destruct with pro-apoptotic receptor agonists. Nat Rev Drug Discov 7(12):1001–1012. doi:10.1038/nrd2637. nrd2637 [pii]
68. Zhang L, Gu J, Lin T, Huang X, Roth JA, Fang B (2002) Mechanisms involved in development of resistance to adenovirus-mediated proapoptotic gene therapy in DLD1 human colon cancer cell line. Gene Ther 9(18):1262–1270
69. Ashkenazi A, Pai RC, Fong S, Leung S, Lawrence DA, Marsters SA, Blackie C, Chang L, McMurtrey AE, Hebert A, DeForge L, Koumenis IL, Lewis D, Harris L, Bussiere J, Koeppen H, Shahrokh Z, Schwall RH (1999) Safety and antitumor activity of recombinant soluble Apo2 ligand. J Clin Invest 104(2):155–162

70. Mohr A, Lyons M, Deedigan L, Harte T, Shaw G, Howard L, Barry F, O'Brien T, Zwacka R (2008) Mesenchymal stem cells expressing TRAIL lead to tumour growth inhibition in an experimental lung cancer model. J Cell Mol Med 12(6B):2628–2643. doi:10.1111/j.1582-4934.2008.00317.x
71. Kim SM, Lim JY, Park SI, Jeong CH, Oh JH, Jeong M, Oh W, Park SH, Sung YC, Jeun SS (2008) Gene therapy using TRAIL-secreting human umbilical cord blood-derived mesenchymal stem cells against intracranial glioma. Cancer Res 68(23):9614–9623. doi:10.1158/0008-5472.CAN-08-0451
72. Sasportas LS, Kasmieh R, Wakimoto H, Hingtgen S, van de Water JA, Mohapatra G, Figueiredo JL, Martuza RL, Weissleder R, Shah K (2009) Assessment of therapeutic efficacy and fate of engineered human mesenchymal stem cells for cancer therapy. Proc Natl Acad Sci U S A 106(12):4822–4827. doi:10.1073/pnas.0806647106. 0806647106 [pii]
73. Loebinger MR, Eddaoudi A, Davies D, Janes SM (2009) Mesenchymal stem cell delivery of TRAIL can eliminate metastatic cancer. Cancer Res 69(10):4134–4142. doi:10.1158/0008-5472.CAN-08-4698. 0008-5472.CAN-08-4698 [pii]
74. Yang B, Wu X, Mao Y, Bao W, Gao L, Zhou P, Xie R, Zhou L, Zhu J (2009) Dual-targeted antitumor effects against brainstem glioma by intravenous delivery of tumor necrosis factor-related, apoptosis-inducing, ligand-engineered human mesenchymal stem cells. Neurosurgery 65 (3):610–624.; discussion 624. doi:10.1227/01.NEU.0000350227.61132.A7
75. Grisendi G, Bussolari R, Cafarelli L, Petak I, Rasini V, Veronesi E, De Santis G, Spano C, Tagliazzucchi M, Barti-Juhasz H, Scarabelli L, Bambi F, Frassoldati A, Rossi G, Casali C, Morandi U, Horwitz EM, Paolucci P, Conte P, Dominici M (2010) Adipose-derived mesenchymal stem cells as stable source of tumor necrosis factor-related apoptosis-inducing ligand delivery for cancer therapy. Cancer Res 70(9):3718–3729. doi:10.1158/0008-5472.CAN-09-1865. 0008-5472.CAN-09-1865 [pii]
76. Mohr A, Albarenque SM, Deedigan L, Yu R, Reidy M, Fulda S, Zwacka RM (2010) Targeting of XIAP combined with systemic mesenchymal stem cell-mediated delivery of sTRAIL ligand inhibits metastatic growth of pancreatic carcinoma cells. Stem Cells 28(11):2109–2120
77. Kim SM, Oh JH, Park SA, Ryu CH, Lim JY, Kim DS, Chang JW, Oh W, Jeun SS (2010) Irradiation enhances the tumor tropism and therapeutic potential of tumor necrosis factor-related apoptosis-inducing ligand-secreting human umbilical cord blood-derived mesenchymal stem cells in glioma therapy. Stem Cells 28(12):2217–2228. doi:10.1002/stem.543
78. Mueller LP, Luetzkendorf J, Widder M, Nerger K, Caysa H, Mueller T (2011) TRAIL-transduced multipotent mesenchymal stromal cells (TRAIL-MSC) overcome TRAIL resistance in selected CRC cell lines in vitro and in vivo. Cancer Gene Ther 18(4):229–239. doi:10.1038/cgt.2010.68. cgt201068 [pii]
79. Ciavarella S, Grisendi G, Dominici M, Tucci M, Brunetti O, Dammacco F, Silvestris F (2012) In vitro anti-myeloma activity of TRAIL-expressing adipose-derived mesenchymal stem cells. Br J Haematol 157(5):586–598. doi:10.1111/j.1365-2141.2012.09082.x
80. Moniri MR, Sun XY, Rayat J, Dai D, Ao Z, He Z, Verchere CB, Dai LJ, Warnock GL (2012) TRAIL-engineered pancreas-derived mesenchymal stem cells: characterization and cytotoxic effects on pancreatic cancer cells. Cancer Gene Ther 19(9):652–658. doi:10.1038/cgt.2012.46. cgt201246 [pii]
81. Kim SM, Woo JS, Jeong CH, Ryu CH, Lim JY, Jeun SS (2012) Effective combination therapy for malignant glioma with TRAIL-secreting mesenchymal stem cells and lipoxygenase inhibitor MK886. Cancer Res 72(18):4807–4817. doi:10.1158/0008-5472.CAN-12-0123. 0008-5472.CAN-12-0123 [pii]
82. Kim CY, Jeong M, Mushiake H, Kim BM, Kim WB, Ko JP, Kim MH, Kim M, Kim TH, Robbins PD, Billiar TR, Seol DW (2006) Cancer gene therapy using a novel secretable trimeric TRAIL. Gene Ther 13(4):330–338
83. Kim MH, Billiar TR, Seol DW (2004) The secretable form of trimeric TRAIL, a potent inducer of apoptosis. Biochem Biophys Res Commun 321(4):930–935. doi:10.1016/j.bbrc.2004.07.046

84. Yu R, Deedigan L, Albarenque SM, Mohr A, Zwacka RM (2013) Delivery of sTRAIL variants by MSCs in combination with cytotoxic drug treatment leads to p53-independent enhanced antitumor effects. Cell Death Dis 4:e503. doi:10.1038/cddis.2013.19. cddis201319 [pii]
85. Menon LG, Kelly K, Yang HW, Kim SK, Black PM, Carroll RS (2009) Human bone marrow-derived mesenchymal stromal cells expressing S-TRAIL as a cellular delivery vehicle for human glioma therapy. Stem Cells 27(9):2320–2330. doi:10.1002/stem.136
86. van der Sloot AM, Tur V, Szegezdi E, Mullally MM, Cool RH, Samali A, Serrano L, Quax WJ (2006) Designed tumor necrosis factor-related apoptosis-inducing ligand variants initiating apoptosis exclusively via the DR5 receptor. Proc Natl Acad Sci U S A 103(23):8634–8639
87. Kelley RF, Totpal K, Lindstrom SH, Mathieu M, Billeci K, DeForge L, Pai R, Hymowitz SG, Ashkenazi A (2005) Receptor-selective mutants of apoptosis-inducing ligand 2/tumor necrosis factor-related apoptosis-inducing ligand reveal a greater contribution of death receptor (DR) 5 than DR4 to apoptosis signaling. J Biol Chem 280(3):2205–2212
88. MacFarlane M, Kohlhaas SL, Sutcliffe MJ, Dyer MJ, Cohen GM (2005) TRAIL receptor-selective mutants signal to apoptosis via TRAIL-R1 in primary lymphoid malignancies. Cancer Res 65(24):11265–11270
89. Tur V, van der Sloot AM, Reis CR, Szegezdi E, Cool RH, Samali A, Serrano L, Quax WJ (2008) DR4-selective tumor necrosis factor-related apoptosis-inducing ligand (TRAIL) variants obtained by structure-based design. J Biol Chem 283(29):20560–20568
90. Duiker EW, de Vries EG, Mahalingam D, Meersma GJ, Boersma-van Ek W, Hollema H, Lub-de Hooge MN, van Dam GM, Cool RH, Quax WJ, Samali A, van der Zee AG, de Jong S (2009) Enhanced antitumor efficacy of a DR5-specific TRAIL variant over recombinant human TRAIL in a bioluminescent ovarian cancer xenograft model. Clin Cancer Res 15(6):2048–2057
91. Reis CR, van der Sloot AM, Natoni A, Szegezdi E, Setroikromo R, Meijer M, Sjollema K, Stricher F, Cool RH, Samali A, Serrano L, Quax WJ (2010) Rapid and efficient cancer cell killing mediated by high-affinity death receptor homotrimerizing TRAIL variants. Cell Death Dis 1:e83
92. Szegezdi E, Reis CR, van der Sloot AM, Natoni A, O'Reilly A, Reeve J, Cool RH, O'Dwyer M, Knapper S, Serrano L, Quax WJ, Samali A (2011) Targeting AML through DR4 with a novel variant of rhTRAIL. J Cell Mol Med 15(10):2216–2231. doi:10.1111/j.1582-4934.2010.01211.x
93. van Geelen CM, Pennarun B, Le PT, de Vries EG, de Jong S (2011) Modulation of TRAIL resistance in colon carcinoma cells: different contributions of DR4 and DR5. BMC Cancer 11:39. doi:10.1186/1471-2407-11-39
94. Yu R, Albarenque SM, Cool RH, Quax WJ, Mohr A, Zwacka RM (2014) DR4 specific TRAIL variants are more efficacious than wild-type TRAIL in pancreatic cancer. Cancer Biol Ther 15(12):1658–1666. doi:10.4161/15384047.2014.972183
95. Kurbanov BM, Fecker LF, Geilen CC, Sterry W, Eberle J (2007) Resistance of melanoma cells to TRAIL does not result from upregulation of antiapoptotic proteins by NF-kappaB but is related to downregulation of initiator caspases and DR4. Oncogene 26(23):3364–3377
96. Dyer MJ, MacFarlane M, Cohen GM (2007) Barriers to effective TRAIL-targeted therapy of malignancy. J Clin Oncol 25(28):4505–4506. doi:10.1200/JCO.2007.13.1011. 25/28/4505 [pii]
97. Kim SW, Kim SJ, Park SH, Yang HG, Kang MC, Choi YW, Kim SM, Jeun SS, Sung YC (2013) Complete regression of metastatic renal cell carcinoma by multiple injections of engineered Mesenchymal stem cells expressing Dodecameric TRAIL and HSV-TK. Clin Cancer Res 19(2):415–427. doi:10.1158/1078-0432.CCR-12-1568. 1078-0432.CCR-12-1568 [pii]
98. Nesterenko I, Wanningen S, Bagci-Onder T, Anderegg M, Shah K (2012) Evaluating the effect of therapeutic stem cells on TRAIL resistant and sensitive medulloblastomas. PLoS One 7(11):e49219. doi:10.1371/journal.pone.0049219. PONE-D-12-07471 [pii]

99. Keane MM, Ettenberg SA, Nau MM, Russell EK, Lipkowitz S (1999) Chemotherapy augments TRAIL-induced apoptosis in breast cell lines. Cancer Res 59(3):734–741
100. Gibson SB, Oyer R, Spalding AC, Anderson SM, Johnson GL (2000) Increased expression of death receptors 4 and 5 synergizes the apoptosis response to combined treatment with etoposide and TRAIL. Mol Cell Biol 20(1):205–212
101. Wu XX, Kakehi Y, Mizutani Y, Nishiyama H, Kamoto T, Megumi Y, Ito N, Ogawa O (2003) Enhancement of TRAIL/Apo2L-mediated apoptosis by adriamycin through inducing DR4 and DR5 in renal cell carcinoma cells. Int J Cancer 104(4):409–417. doi:10.1002/ijc.10948
102. Cheung HH, Mahoney DJ, Lacasse EC, Korneluk RG (2009) Down-regulation of c-FLIP enhances death of cancer cells by smac mimetic compound. Cancer Res 69(19):7729–7738. doi:10.1158/0008-5472.CAN-09-1794
103. Ge R, Wang Z, Zeng Q, Xu X, Olumi AF (2011) F-box protein 10, an NF-kappaB-dependent anti-apoptotic protein, regulates TRAIL-induced apoptosis through modulating c-Fos/c-FLIP pathway. Cell Death Differ 18(7):1184–1195. doi:10.1038/cdd.2010.185
104. Ray S, Almasan A (2003) Apoptosis induction in prostate cancer cells and xenografts by combined treatment with Apo2 ligand/tumor necrosis factor-related apoptosis-inducing ligand and CPT-11. Cancer Res 63(15):4713–4723
105. Yin D, Zhou H, Kumagai T, Liu G, Ong JM, Black KL, Koeffler HP (2005) Proteasome inhibitor PS-341 causes cell growth arrest and apoptosis in human glioblastoma multiforme (GBM). Oncogene 24(3):344–354. doi:10.1038/sj.onc.1208225. 1208225 [pii]
106. Kang MH, Reynolds CP (2009) Bcl-2 inhibitors: targeting mitochondrial apoptotic pathways in cancer therapy. Clin Cancer Res 15(4):1126–1132. doi:10.1158/1078-0432.CCR-08-0144. 15/4/1126 [pii]
107. Wang JL, Liu D, Zhang ZJ, Shan S, Han X, Srinivasula SM, Croce CM, Alnemri ES, Huang Z (2000) Structure-based discovery of an organic compound that binds Bcl-2 protein and induces apoptosis of tumor cells. Proc Natl Acad Sci U S A 97(13):7124–7129. doi:97/13/7124 [pii]
108. Sinicrope FA, Penington RC, Tang XM (2004) Tumor necrosis factor-related apoptosis-inducing ligand-induced apoptosis is inhibited by Bcl-2 but restored by the small molecule Bcl-2 inhibitor, HA 14-1, in human colon cancer cells. Clin Cancer Res 10(24):8284–8292. doi:10.1158/1078-0432.CCR-04-1289. 10/24/8284 [pii]
109. Oltersdorf T, Elmore SW, Shoemaker AR, Armstrong RC, Augeri DJ, Belli BA, Bruncko M, Deckwerth TL, Dinges J, Hajduk PJ, Joseph MK, Kitada S, Korsmeyer SJ, Kunzer AR, Letai A, Li C, Mitten MJ, Nettesheim DG, Ng S, Nimmer PM, O'Connor JM, Oleksijew A, Petros AM, Reed JC, Shen W, Tahir SK, Thompson CB, Tomaselli KJ, Wang B, Wendt MD, Zhang H, Fesik SW, Rosenberg SH (2005) An inhibitor of Bcl-2 family proteins induces regression of solid tumours. Nature 435(7042):677–681
110. Cristofanon S, Fulda S (2012) ABT-737 promotes tBid mitochondrial accumulation to enhance TRAIL-induced apoptosis in glioblastoma cells. Cell Death Dis 3:e432. doi:10.1038/cddis.2012.163. cddis2012163 [pii]
111. Huang S, Sinicrope FA (2008) BH3 mimetic ABT-737 potentiates TRAIL-mediated apoptotic signaling by unsequestering Bim and Bak in human pancreatic cancer cells. Cancer Res 68(8):2944–2951. doi:10.1158/0008-5472.CAN-07-2508. 68/8/2944 [pii]
112. Song JH, Kandasamy K, Kraft AS (2008) ABT-737 induces expression of the death receptor 5 and sensitizes human cancer cells to TRAIL-induced apoptosis. J Biol Chem 283(36):25003–25013. doi:10.1074/jbc.M802511200
113. Bockbrader KM, Tan M, Sun Y (2005) A small molecule Smac-mimic compound induces apoptosis and sensitizes TRAIL- and etoposide-induced apoptosis in breast cancer cells. Oncogene 24(49):7381–7388. doi:10.1038/sj.onc.1208888
114. Guo F, Nimmanapalli R, Paranawithana S, Wittman S, Griffin D, Bali P, O'Bryan E, Fumero C, Wang HG, Bhalla K (2002) Ectopic overexpression of second mitochondria-derived activator of caspases (Smac/DIABLO) or cotreatment with N-terminus of Smac/DIABLO

peptide potentiates epothilone B derivative-(BMS 247550) and Apo-2L/TRAIL-induced apoptosis. Blood 99(9):3419–3426
115. Braeuer SJ, Buneker C, Mohr A, Zwacka RM (2006) Constitutively activated nuclear factor-kappaB, but not induced NF-kappaB, leads to TRAIL resistance by up-regulation of X-linked inhibitor of apoptosis protein in human cancer cells. Mol Cancer Res 4(10):715–728. doi:10.1158/1541-7786.MCR-05-0231
116. Vogler M, Walczak H, Stadel D, Haas TL, Genze F, Jovanovic M, Bhanot U, Hasel C, Moller P, Gschwend JE, Simmet T, Debatin KM, Fulda S (2009) Small molecule XIAP inhibitors enhance TRAIL-induced apoptosis and antitumor activity in preclinical models of pancreatic carcinoma. Cancer Res 69(6):2425–2434
117. Stadel D, Mohr A, Ref C, MacFarlane M, Zhou S, Humphreys R, Bachem M, Cohen G, Moller P, Zwacka RM, Debatin KM, Fulda S (2010) TRAIL-induced apoptosis is preferentially mediated via TRAIL receptor 1 in pancreatic carcinoma cells and profoundly enhanced by XIAP inhibitors. Clin Cancer Res 16(23):5734–5749. doi:10.1158/1078-0432.CCR-10-0985. 1078-0432.CCR-10-0985 [pii]
118. Fulda S, Wick W, Weller M, Debatin KM (2002) Smac agonists sensitize for Apo2L/TRAIL- or anticancer drug-induced apoptosis and induce regression of malignant glioma in vivo. Nat Med 8(8):808–815
119. Fingas CD, Blechacz BR, Smoot RL, Guicciardi ME, Mott J, Bronk SF, Werneburg NW, Sirica AE, Gores GJ (2010) A smac mimetic reduces TNF related apoptosis inducing ligand (TRAIL)-induced invasion and metastasis of cholangiocarcinoma cells. Hepatology 52(2):550–561. doi:10.1002/hep.23729
120. Fulda S, Debatin KM (2004) Modulation of TRAIL signaling for cancer therapy. Vitam Horm 67:275–290. doi:10.1016/S0083-6729(04)67015-4. S0083672904670154 [pii]
121. Khanbolooki S, Nawrocki ST, Arumugam T, Andtbacka R, Pino MS, Kurzrock R, Logsdon CD, Abbruzzese JL, McConkey DJ (2006) Nuclear factor-kappaB maintains TRAIL resistance in human pancreatic cancer cells. Mol Cancer Ther 5(9):2251–2260. doi:10.1158/1535-7163.MCT-06-0075. 5/9/2251 [pii]
122. Romagnoli M, Desplanques G, Maiga S, Legouill S, Dreano M, Bataille R, Barille-Nion S (2007) Canonical nuclear factor kappaB pathway inhibition blocks myeloma cell growth and induces apoptosis in strong synergy with TRAIL. Clin Cancer Res 13(20):6010–6018. doi:10.1158/1078-0432.CCR-07-0140. 13/20/6010 [pii]
123. Song G, Ouyang G, Bao S (2005) The activation of Akt/PKB signaling pathway and cell survival. J Cell Mol Med 9(1):59–71. doi:009.001.07 [pii]
124. Secchiero P, Gonelli A, Carnevale E, Milani D, Pandolfi A, Zella D, Zauli G (2003) TRAIL promotes the survival and proliferation of primary human vascular endothelial cells by activating the Akt and ERK pathways. Circulation 107(17):2250–2256
125. Tazzari PL, Tabellini G, Ricci F, Papa V, Bortul R, Chiarini F, Evangelisti C, Martinelli G, Bontadini A, Cocco L, McCubrey JA, Martelli AM (2008) Synergistic proapoptotic activity of recombinant TRAIL plus the Akt inhibitor Perifosine in acute myelogenous leukemia cells. Cancer Res 68(22):9394–9403. doi:10.1158/0008-5472.CAN-08-2815. 68/22/9394 [pii]
126. Dieterle A, Orth R, Daubrawa M, Grotemeier A, Alers S, Ullrich S, Lammers R, Wesselborg S, Stork B (2009) The Akt inhibitor triciribine sensitizes prostate carcinoma cells to TRAIL-induced apoptosis. Int J Cancer 125(4):932–941. doi:10.1002/ijc.24374
127. Ricci MS, Kim SH, Ogi K, Plastaras JP, Ling J, Wang W, Jin Z, Liu YY, Dicker DT, Chiao PJ, Flaherty KT, Smith CD, El-Deiry WS (2007) Reduction of TRAIL-induced mcl-1 and cIAP2 by c-Myc or sorafenib sensitizes resistant human cancer cells to TRAIL-induced death. Cancer Cell 12(1):66–80
128. Kruyt FA (2008) TRAIL and cancer therapy. Cancer Lett 263(1):14–25. doi:10.1016/j.canlet.2008.02.003. S0304-3835(08)00084-0 [pii]
129. Rosato RR, Almenara JA, Dai Y, Grant S (2003) Simultaneous activation of the intrinsic and extrinsic pathways by histone deacetylase (HDAC) inhibitors and tumor necrosis

factor-related apoptosis-inducing ligand (TRAIL) synergistically induces mitochondrial damage and apoptosis in human leukemia cells. Mol Cancer Ther 2(12):1273–1284
130. Zopf S, Neureiter D, Bouralexis S, Abt T, Glaser KB, Okamoto K, Ganslmayer M, Hahn EG, Herold C, Ocker M (2007) Differential response of p53 and p21 on HDAC inhibitor-mediated apoptosis in HCT116 colon cancer cells in vitro and in vivo. Int J Oncol 31(6):1391–1402
131. Song K, Benhaga N, Anderson RL, Khosravi-Far R (2006) Transduction of tumor necrosis factor-related apoptosis-inducing ligand into hematopoietic cells leads to inhibition of syngeneic tumor growth in vivo. Cancer Res 66(12):6304–6311
132. Uzzaman M, Keller G, Germano IM (2009) In vivo gene delivery by embryonic-stem-cell-derived astrocytes for malignant gliomas. Neuro Oncol 11(2):102–108. doi:10.1215/15228517-2008-056
133. Sabapathy V, Kumar S (2016) hiPSC-derived iMSCs: NextGen MSCs as an advanced therapeutically active cell resource for regenerative medicine. J Cell Mol Med 20(8):1571–1588. doi:10.1111/jcmm.12839
134. Zhao Q, Gregory CA, Lee RH, Reger RL, Qin L, Hai B, Park MS, Yoon N, Clough B, McNeill E, Prockop DJ, Liu F (2015) MSCs derived from iPSCs with a modified protocol are tumor-tropic but have much less potential to promote tumors than bone marrow MSCs. Proc Natl Acad Sci U S A 112(2):530–535. doi:10.1073/pnas.1423008112

Chapter 7
Atypical Immune Functions of CD95/CD95L

Amanda Poissonnier and Patrick Legembre

Abstract The receptor CD95 (also named Fas or APO-1) is a member of the tumor necrosis factor receptor (TNF-R) superfamily. Its cognate ligand, CD95L, is implicated in immune homeostasis and immune surveillance. Mutations of this receptor or its ligand lead to autoimmune disorders such as systemic lupus erythematosus (SLE) and to cancers; hence, CD95 and CD95L were initially classified as having a tumor suppressor role. However, more recent data indicate that, in different pathophysiological contexts, CD95 can evoke nonapoptotic signals, promote inflammation, and contribute to carcinogenesis. We show that, because CD95L can exist in two different forms, a transmembrane and a soluble metalloprotease-cleaved ligand (cl-CD95L), CD95 can implement apoptotic or nonapoptotic signalling pathways, respectively. In this chapter, we discuss the roles of CD95 on the modulation of immune functions.

Keywords Carcinogenesis • Cytokine • Dendritic cell • Fas • Inflammation • T-cell

7.1 Introduction

The immune system consists of specialized cells protecting the body from infection and cell transformation. Antigen (Ag)-presenting cells (APCs) survey tissues for non-self-Ags. They capture pathogenic agents, process Ags, and present them at the cell surface in the context of major histocompatibility complex (MHC) molecules. Like macrophages and B-lymphocytes, dendritic cells (DCs) are professional APCs. APCs present Ags within MHC class II molecules, and these cells not only participate in activating non-self-Ag-recognizing T-cells, but also contribute to the elimination of immune cells recognizing self-Ags with a too strong affinity, a process called peripheral tolerance. The variability of the αβ T-cell receptor (TCR) expressed

A. Poissonnier • P. Legembre (✉)
Centre Eugène Marquis, INSERM U1242-COSS Equipe Labellisée Ligue Contre Le Cancer, Rue Bataille Flandres Dunkerque, 35042 Rennes, France

Université de Rennes-1, 2 av. du Prof. Léon Bernard, 35043 Rennes, France
e-mail: patrick.legembre@inserm.fr

O. Micheau (ed.), *TRAIL, Fas Ligand, TNF and TLR3 in Cancer*, Resistance to Targeted Anti-Cancer Therapeutics, DOI 10.1007/978-3-319-56805-8_7

by T-cells assures that a small subset of activated T-cells will exhibit high affinity towards antigenic peptides and differentiate and proliferate to eliminate Ag-expressing cells. Defining two distinct immune functions, αβ T-cells display either CD4 or CD8 on their surface. While CD4$^+$ helper T-cells (Th) bind Ag presented in the context of MHC class II molecules expressed by professional APCs and produce cytokines structuring the immune response, CD8$^+$ lymphocytes recognize antigenic peptides presented by MHC class I molecules expressed at the surface of all cells (apart from some transformed or infected cells) and this interaction leads to the elimination of these target cells.

The list of Th subset lineages being discovered is growing continuously, showing the complexity of the mechanisms developed by the immune system to respond to the diversity of infections and cancers. Polarization of these CD4$^+$ subsets occurs through external stimuli inducing the expression of different transcription factors such as STAT1, STAT4, and T-bet for Th1 cells, STAT6 and GATA-3 for Th2 cells, FoxP3 for regulatory T-cells (Tregs), Bcl6 for follicular T-helper cells (TFH) [1], RORγt, RORα, and STAT3 for Th17 cells, T-bet and AhR for Th22 cells [2], and PU-1 for Th9 cells (Fig. 7.1) [3]. These T-cells will express a set of cytokines that will organize the whole immune system (innate and adaptive immune cells) to respond adequately or not to infection and transformation. Accordingly, identification of the immune architecture cannot only serve as a prognostic marker to evaluate the risk of disease progression but can also help clinicians to predict the efficiency or failure of chemotherapeutic/radiotherapeutic treatments.

On the other hand, CD8$^+$ cytotoxic lymphocytes destroy target cells and spare bystanders. For a long time, because TCR aggregation was shown to implement CD95L expression by CD8$^+$ lymphocytes, this ligand was only seen as a weapon at the disposal of these cells to kill target cells [4–6]. Based on recent data, CD95 is in fact a non-apoptotic receptor with pro-inflammatory functions and the role of the CD95–CD95L pair appears to be definitively more complex than expected. This review discusses the emerging roles of CD95/CD95L in the immune response.

To simplify, APCs present Ags to CD4$^+$ Th cells, which in turn orchestrate the activation of the immune response through a cellular (Th1/Th17) or humoral (Th2) response or by down-regulating the intensity/kinetics of the adaptive immune response by promoting the differentiation of Tregs. Once the immune function has been achieved, effector T-cells have to be eliminated through molecular mechanisms relying on death receptors (DRs) or BH3-only factors (i.e., BIM) according to the affinity with which cells have been stimulated by the Ags (low vs. high affinity) [7] while some Ag-specific memory T-cells persist.

CD4$^+$ Th cells are the conductors of the adaptive immune response requiring the use of a variety of CD4$^+$ Th subsets including Th1, Th2, Th9, and Th17 cells and Tregs to finely tune the response to a variety of infections and cancer cells. In addition, the efficiency of the immune response relies on the ability of these cells to cross blood vessels and migrate within the inflamed or transformed tissue to reach the target. Selectins, integrins, and chemokine receptors have a central role in T-cell

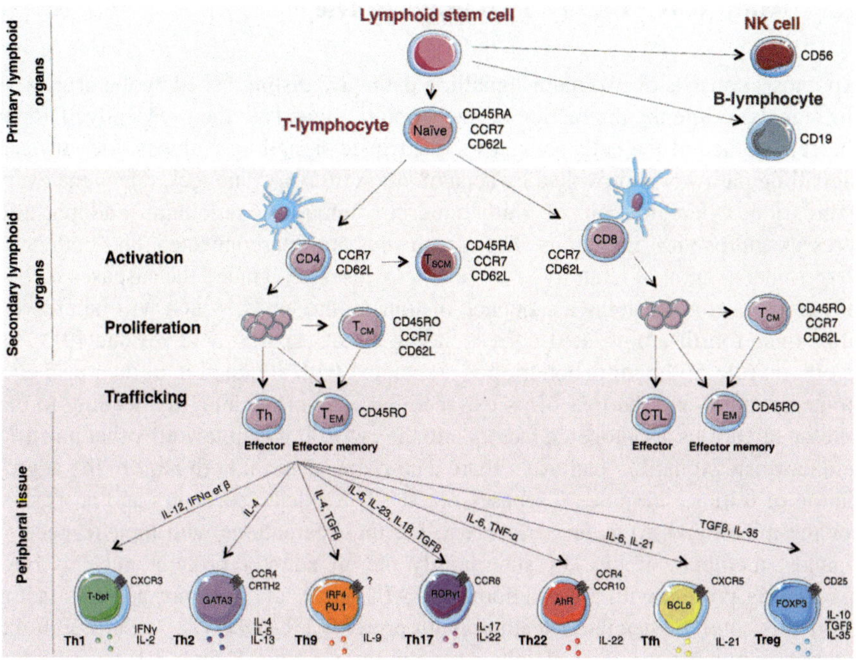

Fig. 7.1 Development of T lymphocytes. -presenting cells (APCs) present antigens (Ags) to naïve T-cells. T-lymphocytes proliferate and differentiate into effector and memory T-cells. Effector T-cells, both CD8 (cytotoxic T lymphocytes or CTL) and CD4 (T helper cells or Th) traffic to peripheral tissues where they mount the immune response. Memory T-cells can develop into effector memory cells (TEM) migrating to peripheral tissues or central memory T-cells (TCM) that flow through lymphoid organs. Activated CD4^{+} T-cells differentiate into different phenotypes according to the cytokine cocktail present in the microenvironment. These CD4 subsets are discriminated based on the expression of cell surface markers, the expression of different cytokines and the activation of different transcription factors. *NK* natural killer cell, *TSCM* stem memory T-cell

extravasation involving different steps including cell arrest, spreading, crawling, and transendothelial migration. Our recent data demonstrate that CD95/CD95L can participate in this cellular process to fuel inflammation in lupus patients [8]. Therefore, deregulation of T-cell differentiation, proliferation, transmigration, or death will be responsible for chronic inflammatory and autoimmune disorders.

Lpr (for lymphoproliferation) and gld (for generalized lymphoproliferative disease) mice harboring mutations in the *CD95* and *CD95L* genes, respectively, have provided valuable insights into the pivotal role played by the CD95–CD95L pair in lymphocyte homeostasis. However, it is noteworthy that most, if not all, of the studies using these mice focused on the consequence of apoptotic deregulation and neglected the nonapoptotic signalling pathways induced by this receptor–ligand pair.

7.2 Apoptosis: Mainly Two Ways to Die

Apoptosis consists of two main signalling pathways distinguished by the origins of the signals. While the interaction of the apoptotic ligands to their respective DRs at the cell surface of the cells activates the extrinsic signalling pathway, the intrinsic signalling pathway is provoked by accumulation of DNA damages, oncogene overexpressions, deregulation of mitochondrial functions, reticulum endoplasmic stresses and/or viral infections. These pathways are interconnected, and both converge on activation of a family of cysteine proteases designated the caspases recognizing in a set of proteins a sequence of four amino acids, which will be cleaved after their fourth amino acid corresponding to an aspartic acid residue [9]. The apoptotic role of the mitochondrion is associated with a reduction in its transmembrane potential and the loss of its extracellular membrane integrity, leading to the release of various apoptogenic factors into the cytosol. It is noteworthy that intrinsic and extrinsic signalling pathways share a common feature; both require the aggregation of initiator caspases (caspases-8 and -10 for death receptors and caspase-9 for the mitochondria) as an early event. During interactions with their respective ligands, members of the DR superfamily recruit adaptor proteins such as Fas-associating protein with a death domain (FADD) [10, 11] or tumor necrosis factor (TNF) receptor 1-associated death domain protein (TRADD) [12], resulting in the aggregation and activation of initiator caspases (caspase-8 and -10) to form the death-inducing signalling complex (DISC) [13]. In a similar manner, the release of cytochrome c and ATP from the mitochondria promotes the formation of the apoptosome (along with cytosolic APAF-1) [14], resulting in the aggregation and activation of the initiator caspase-9, which in turn cleaves caspase-3 [15].

The DRs CD95 [16], TNFR1 [17], DR4 [18], DR5 [19], and DR6 [20] were all originally cloned based on their ability to elicit apoptosis. The latter statement is important to keep in mind in order to understand why some of these receptors are still considered as pure death receptors despite the fact that this is not the case [21–24]. Although soon after these genes were cloned, they were also found to be involved in nonapoptotic functions [25, 26], most if not all studies on these proteins have been performed to characterize the molecular events leading to cell death. Revealingly, several agonistic molecules were developed to kill cancer cells and none achieved satisfactory results in clinical trials. For instance, a recombinant CD95L (APO010) exhibiting a hexameric stoichiometry killed tumor cell lines and reduced tumor growth in animal models [27, 28] but a phase I clinical trial planned in 2007 in patients with solid tumors has never been carried out. Meanwhile, new concepts emerged suggesting that the use of CD95 antagonists could be attractive therapeutic options to treat certain cancers and patients affected by chronic inflammatory disorders such as lupus. For instance, a combination of an antagonist of CD95 with radiotherapy in patients affected by glioma showed promising results in a Phase II clinical trial [29]. The unique vision of CD95 as a DR has therefore changed as evidence has accumulated showing that DR-mediated nonapoptotic signalling pathways contribute to the progression of chronic inflammatory disorders and carcinogenesis.

In the late eighties, Krammer's laboratory identified a monoclonal antibody, they named "anti-apoptosis antigen 1 (APO-1)," able to bind a plasma membrane receptor and trigger an apoptotic signalling pathway leading to the death of tumor cells [30]. Nagata's team cloned Fas as the receptor recognized by APO-1 in 1991 [16], and its ligand FasL in 1993 [31]. Based on the antitumor assay that identified APO-1, most of the future studies on CD95 focused on (1) understanding the molecular ordering of the apoptotic signal, (2) deciphering if the concentration of this receptor–ligand pair was deregulated in tumor and inflammatory disorders or if some mutations could prevent the implementation of the apoptotic signal in patients affected by inflammatory disorders or cancers and (3) developing therapeutic molecules to activate this receptor to kill tumor cells. The latter approach remains a huge disappointment in terms of clinical trials (as aforementioned) probably due to the fact that CD95 is not per se a DR and that its inhibition instead of its activation corresponds to a more attractive therapeutic option to cure patients suffering from certain cancers and chronic inflammatory disorders.

CD95 simultaneously implements apoptotic and nonapoptotic signalling pathways, and, although the molecular ordering of the apoptotic signal is well understood, it remains to be determined how CD95 implements the nonapoptotic signalling pathways (i.e., NFκB, MAPK, PI3K). For instance, a crucial question that has to be addressed is if these pathways stem from the death domain (DD) or if they rely on different regions in CD95 to be initiated. In the latter option, it will be possible to engineer inhibitors selective of the nonapoptotic signalling pathways that thereby may prevent the implementation of the pro-inflammatory/oncogenic cues without affecting the apoptotic signalling pathway contributing to the antitumor and anti-infectious responses [7].

Unlike membrane-bound (i.e., transmembrane) CD95L, its metalloprotease-cleaved counterpart fails to trigger cell death but induces the PI3K signalling pathway [32, 33]. We hypothesize that a difference in the kinetics of the CD95 aggregation, internalization, and membrane distribution processes may account for the induction of one signalling pathway being favored over the other. This difference could be the result of ligand stoichiometry; the metalloprotease-processed CD95L is mainly found as a homotrimer [34] while its membrane-bound counterpart is detected multi-aggregated and polarized at the membrane of cells in the process of killing [35].

It is noteworthy that we did not observe any correlation between the intensity of the nonapoptotic signalling pathways and the resistance of the cells to the apoptotic signal, ruling out that the CD95-mediated nonapoptotic signalling pathway counteracts its apoptotic counterpart [36]. In agreement with this initial observation, Martin Seamus and colleagues showed that, in cells undergoing apoptosis in the presence of membrane-bound (cytotoxic) CD95L, induction of the nonapoptotic signalling pathway causes the production of cytokines including MCP-1 and IL-8 that recruit phagocytes through a cellular inhibitor of apoptosis (cIAP)-1- and cIAP-2-driven molecular mechanism [37]. This interplay between apoptotic and nonapoptotic signalling pathways promotes the accumulation of macrophages and phagocytes that engulf dying cells, eliciting an adaptive immune response.

7.3 TNF Receptor Family

The DRs TNFR1, CD95, DR3, DR4, DR5, and DR6 belong to the TNF receptor (TNFR) superfamily. These type I transmembrane proteins share common features including extracellular amino-terminal cysteine-rich domains (CRDs) [38, 39] contributing to both ligand specificity [40] and receptor pre-association [41–43], and the DD, a conserved 80-amino acid sequence located in the cytoplasmic tail, which implements the apoptotic signal through protein protein interactions (PPIs) [44, 45]. Receptors of the TNFR superfamily do not possess any enzymatic activity on their own, and therefore rely on PPI formation for signalling. Among the adaptor proteins interacting with DD, TRADD and FADD are instrumental in the implementation of cell death processes [10–13].

An important feature of TNF family members is that these ligands can be processed by metalloproteases and released into the bloodstream as soluble ligands [21]. Due to the difference in their stoichiometry (a homotrimeric soluble ligand versus a multi-aggregated homotrimeric membrane-bound counterpart), these ligands are able to implement different signalling pathways upon binding to their receptor [21]. TNF-α is synthesized as a 26-kDa transmembrane type II protein (m-TNF-α) of 233 amino acids [46], which can be cleaved by the metalloprotease TACE [47, 48] to release the 17 kDa soluble form of the cytokine (sTNF-α). Whereas sTNF-α only activates TNFR1, m-TNF-α can bind and activate both TNFR1 and TNFR2 [49]. Activation of TNFR1 induces cellular processes ranging from cell death (apoptosis or necroptosis) to cell proliferation, migration, and differentiation; the implementation of these cellular responses reflects the dynamic formation of molecular complexes following receptor activation [50].

The transmembrane CD95L (CD178/FasL) is mainly expressed at the surface of activated lymphocytes [51] and natural killer (NK) cells [52], where it is involved in the elimination of transformed and infected cells. However, CD95L can also be detected on the surface of neurons [53], corneal epithelia and endothelia [54, 55], and Sertoli cells [56], where it can prevent the infiltration of immune cells and thereby inhibit the spread of inflammation in sensitive organs (i.e., brain, eyes, and testis, respectively), commonly referred to as "immune-privileged" sites. Of note, the graft of CD95L-expressing colon carcinoma cells (i.e., CT-26 cells) leads to a more rapid rejection than parental cells because of a massive accumulation of neutrophils in the transplanted area [57]. Interestingly, the presence of TGFβ in this microenvironment prevents tumor rejection [57] strongly supporting that the cytokine cocktail present in the organ modulates the CD95L-driven immunologic tolerance.

Following the description of its role in the immune privilege, two groups independently described that CD95L can be overexpressed by malignant cells and that this ligand contributes to the elimination of infiltrating T-lymphocytes, thus establishing what they call a "tumor counterattack" [58, 59]. Nonetheless, these observations are controversial. Firstly, because other experiments revealed, using ectopic expression of CD95L in allogeneic transplant of β-islets [60, 61] and in tumor cell lines [57], an accelerated elimination of these cells relative to control cells, at least in part due to increased infiltration of neutrophils and macrophages endowed with antitumor activity; and secondly, because all anti-CD95L antibodies used in the immunohistochemical analyses in the original studies have since been reported to be nonspecific and thus cannot allow us to conclude with certainty that CD95L is present in these tissues [62]. Also, contrary to the concept of "immune counterattack," CD95L-expressing cells can supply T-cells with a survival signal [63]. Indeed, CD95L-expressing β-islets enhance $CD8^+$ activation that leads to organ damage and NOD mice backcrossed with $MRL^{lpr/lpr}$ mice, exhibiting a loss of CD95 (see below), do not develop diabetes [64]. Although accumulating evidence emphasize that CD95L can behave as a chemoattractant for neutrophils, macrophages [57, 61, 65], T lymphocytes [33], and malignant cells in which the CD95-mediated apoptotic signal is nonproductive [66, 67], the biological role of this soluble CD95L must be further clarified.

7.4 Two Different CD95Ls Able to Trigger Different Signalling Pathways

CD95L is a transmembrane cytokine whose ectodomain can be processed close to the plasma membrane by metalloproteases such as MMP3 [68], MMP7 [69], MMP9 [70], and ADAM-10 [71, 72], and then released into the bloodstream as a soluble ligand (Fig. 7.2). Based on data showing that hexameric CD95L represents the minimal level of self-association required to signal apoptosis [73], and that cleavage by metalloproteases releases a homotrimeric ligand [34, 73], this soluble ligand has long been considered to be an inert molecule only competing with its membrane-bound counterpart to antagonize the death signal [34, 74]. However, recent work demonstrated that this metalloprotease-cleaved CD95L (cl-CD95L) actively aggravates inflammation and autoimmunity in patients affected by systemic lupus erythematosus (SLE) by inducing NF-κB and PI3K [33, 75] signalling pathways (Fig. 7.3). Unlike transmembrane CD95L whose interaction with CD95 leads to formation of the apoptotic complex DISC, cl-CD95L leads to the formation of a molecular complex devoid of FADD and caspase-8 that instead recruits and activates the src kinase c-yes by the presence of NADPH oxidase 3 and ROS production [33, 67]; this unconventional receptosome was designated the motility-inducing signalling complex (MISC) [32, 33]. Although we do not detect any trace of caspase-8 in the MISC, this enzyme participates in cell migration. Indeed, the protease activity of caspase-8 can be abrogated by its phosphorylation at tyrosine 380 (Y380) by src kinase [76] and this phosphorylation allows the recruitment of the PI3K adaptor p85 alpha subunit inducing the activation of the PI3K signalling pathway [77]. Nonetheless, it is noteworthy that CD95-induced migration and invasion seem to occur through a DD-independent mechanism (reviewed in [78]), suggesting that a caspase-8-independent mode of cell migration exists in cells exposed to CD95L. Because tyrosine kinase receptor (RTK) EGFR can induce the tyrosine

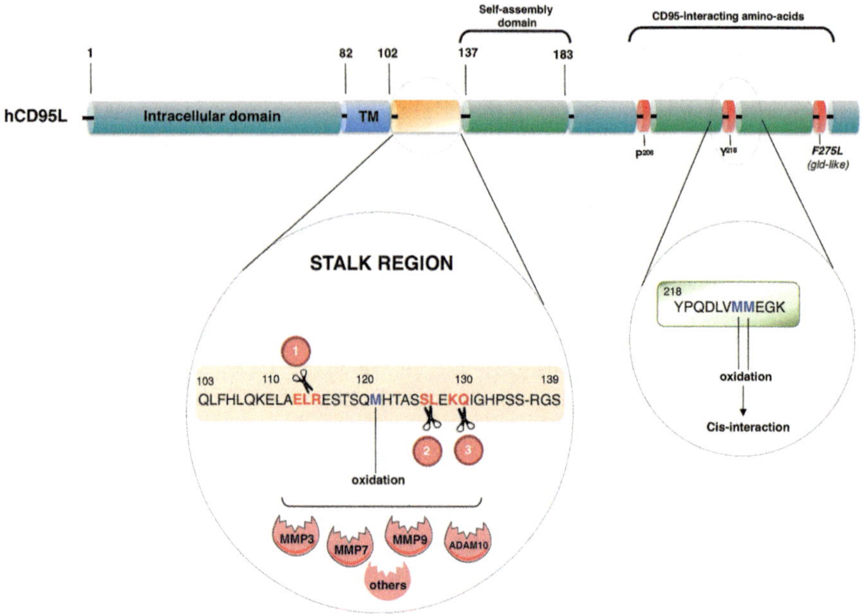

Fig. 7.2 Diagram of human CD95L protein (hCD95L). CD95L is a type II transmembrane molecule of 281 amino acids. The transmembrane region encompasses amino acids 82–102. Amino acids involved in the interaction with CD95 are indicated. Three different metalloprotease cleavage sites (indicated in *red*) have been described in CD95L, inside its juxtamembrane region (called the stalk region). The region responsible for CD95L self-assembly is depicted. Oxidation of methionine residues (indicated in *blue*) in positions 224 and 225 increases the aggregation level of CD95L, and at methionine 121 inhibits the metalloprotease-mediated cleavage of CD95L

phosphorylation of caspase-8 and this RTK is recruited by CD95 in triple-negative breast cancer cells stimulated with cl-CD95L, we hypothesize that Y380 phosphorylation of caspase-8 may prime certain cancer cells to become unresponsive to the apoptotic signal triggered by cytotoxic CD95L, and meanwhile promotes cell migration, an essential step in cancer cell metastasis. In triple-negative breast cancer cells exposed to cl-CD95L, we observed a CD95-driven recruitment of EGFR, which in combination with c-yes promotes MISC formation, and this RTK orchestrates the activation of PI3K in an EGF-independent manner. These data are in accordance with a recent study showing that another RTK, PDGFR-β is recruited by CD95 in colon cancer cells exposed to CD95L to trigger cancer cell metastasis [79]. These findings emphasize that RTK recruitment by CD95 corresponds to an ordinary process that simultaneously inhibits the apoptotic signal by phosphorylating caspase-8, and promotes cell motility by activating the PI3K signalling pathway.

Different forms of soluble CD95L exist. Although the soluble form of CD95L generated by MMP7 (by cleavage inside the ^{113}ELR^{115} sequence of the CD95L stalk region) induces apoptosis [69], its counterpart cleaved between serine 126 and leucine 127 does not [33, 34, 75]. We speculate that different quaternary structures can

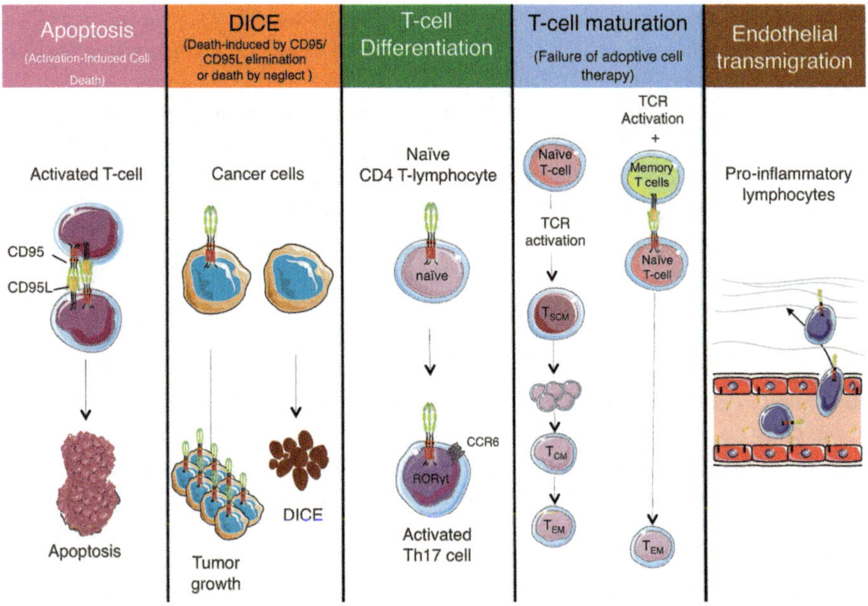

Fig. 7.3 Immunological roles of CD95–CD95L pair. The presence or absence of CD95 can implement pro-apoptotic or pro-survival signalling pathways, depending on CD95L (membrane-bound or soluble), the cell, and/or the microenvironment. CD95 triggers apoptosis. A death by neglect exists and is designated Death-induced by CD95/CD95L. This observation indicates that CD95 expression implements cell survival signals and thereby the loss of the receptor induces a death by neglect. CD95 also orchestrates the differentiation of Th17 lymphocytes and the maturation of memory T-cells. The metalloprotease-cleaved CD95L can promote trafficking of IL17-expressing cells in inflamed organs of systemic lupus erythematosus patients. *TSCM* stem memory T-cell, *TEM* effector memory T-cell, *TCM* central memory T-cell

exist for the naturally processed CD95L molecules, which can account for the induction of opposite signalling complexes. Consistent with this notion, soluble CD95L incubated in the bronchoalveolar lavage (BAL) fluid of patients suffering from acute respiratory distress syndrome (ARDS) undergoes oxidation at methionines 224 and 225, promoting aggregation of the soluble ligand and boosting its cytotoxic activity [80]. The same study found that the stalk region of CD95L, corresponding to amino acids 103–136 and encompassing all metalloprotease cleavage sites described in the literature (Fig. 7.2), participates in CD95L multimerization, accounting for the damage to the lung epithelium that is observed in ARDS patients [80]. Of note, in ARDS BAL fluid, additional oxidation occurs at methionine 121, preventing the cleavage of CD95L by MMP7, and thereby potentially explains why this cytotoxic ligand keeps its stalk region and contributes to the pathology [80]. Nonetheless, preservation of this region in soluble CD95L raises the question of whether an yet unidentified MMP7-independent cleavage site exists in the juxtamembrane region of CD95L, near the plasma membrane, or whether the ligand detected in ARDS patients corresponded in fact to the full-length form of CD95L embedded in exosomes [81, 82]. Indeed, exosome-bound CD95L can be expressed by human prostate cancer cells (i.e., the LNCaP cell line), and it evokes apoptosis in activated T-lymphocytes [83].

Overall, these findings emphasize the importance of finely characterizing the quaternary structure of naturally processed CD95L from the sera of patients affected by cancers or chronic/acute inflammatory disorders. Such investigations will improve our understanding of the molecular mechanisms set in motion by this ligand, and thus our appreciation of its downstream biological functions.

Transmembrane CD95L is a pivotal weapon at the disposal of immune cells to eliminate pre-tumor cells. Therefore, pre-tumor cells that escape immune surveillance will tend to be selected according to their ability to resist the CD95-mediated apoptotic signalling pathway, a process termed immunoediting [84]. Accordingly, most tumor cells are resistant to the CD95-induced apoptotic signalling pathway but these cells do not lose expression of the receptor [85]. This observation suggests that the remaining wild-type CD95 allele contributes to carcinogenesis. Indeed, tumor cells resistant to the CD95-mediated apoptotic signal can still migrate in the presence of CD95L [66] confirming that CD95 can behave as an oncogene. Also, patients suffering from an autoimmune disorder called autoimmune lymphoproliferative syndrome (ALPS) type Ia exhibit a mutation in their CD95 gene associated with a loss of the apoptotic function [86–88], but most of them retain a wild-type CD95 allele [89]. Similarly to cancers, we showed that, although the remaining wild-type CD95 allele failed to implement the apoptotic signalling pathway, its presence was sufficient and necessary to trigger the nonapoptotic signalling pathways [90]. These data strongly support that the activation threshold of the CD95-mediated nonapoptotic signalling pathway is lower than that necessary to trigger an apoptotic cue. In keeping with this, different studies have demonstrated that it is not only the default of apoptosis that is responsible for the progression of the pathology in autoimmune disorders such as lupus but also the chronic activation of the CD95 nonapoptotic signalling pathways, which contribute to fueling inflammation in these patients [33, 75].

In summary, although the CD95–CD95L interaction can eliminate malignant cells by promoting formation of the DISC, it can also promote carcinogenesis by sustaining inflammation and/or inducing metastatic dissemination [33, 65–67, 75, 91, 92]. The molecular mechanisms underlying the switch between these different signalling pathways remain enigmatic. An important question to be addressed is how the magnitude of CD95 aggregation regulates the formation of "Death"- versus "Motility"-ISCs. Answering these questions will lead to the development of new therapeutic agents with the ability to prevent the spread and chronicity of inflammation or to impinge on carcinogenesis, at least in pathologies associated with increased soluble CD95L, such as cancers (e.g., pancreatic cancer [93], large granular lymphocytic leukemia, breast cancer [94], and NK-cell lymphoma [95]) or autoimmune disorders (e.g., rheumatoid arthritis and osteoarthritis [96], and graft-versus-host disease [97, 98] or SLE [33, 99]).

7.5 CD95 and CD95L: Cell Signalling Pathways

Similar to the TNFR [100], CD95 is pre-associated at the plasma membrane as a homotrimer, and this quaternary structure is mandatory for transmission of apoptotic signals in the presence of CD95L [42, 43]. Homotrimerization of CD95 occurs mainly through homotypic interactions involving the CRD1 [41–43]. Binding of CD95L or agonistic anti-CD95 mAbs to CD95 alters the receptor's conformation and the extent to which the receptor is multimerized at the plasma membrane [101]. The intracellular region of CD95 DD consists of six antiparallel α-helices [102]. Upon addition of CD95L, CD95 undergoes conformational modification of the DD, inducing a shift of helix 6 and fusion with helix 5, promoting both oligomerization of the receptor and recruitment of the adaptor protein FADD [103]. One consequence of the opening of the globular structure of CD95 is that the receptor becomes connected through this helix bridge, which increases the extent of its homo-aggregation. This long helix allows stabilization of the complex by recruitment of FADD. The CD95-DD:FADD-DD crystal structure provides several insights into the formation of the large CD95 clusters observed by imaging or biochemical methods in cells stimulated with CD95L. In addition, the structure also confirms that alteration in the conformation of CD95 plays an instrumental role in signal induction [103]. However, the idea of an elongated C-terminal α-helix favoring the *cis*-dimerization of CD95-DD was challenged by Driscoll et al., who did not observe the fusion of the last two helices at a more neutral pH (pH 6.2) than the acidic conditions (pH 4) used by Scott et al. in the study that initially resolved the CD95-DD:FADD-DD structure [103]. At pH 6.2, association of CD95 predominantly interacts with FADD in a 5:5 complex via a polymerization mechanism that involves three types of asymmetric interactions, but without major alteration of the DD globular structure [104, 105]. It is likely that the low pH conditions used by Scott et al. altered the conformation of CD95, resulting in the formation of nonphysiological CD95:FADD oligomers [103]. Nonetheless, we cannot rule out the possibility that a local decrease in intracellular pH affects the initial steps of the CD95 signalling pathway in vivo, for example, by promoting the opening of the CD95-DD and eventually contributing to formation of a complex that elicits a sequence of events distinct from that occurring at physiologic pH. We recently observed that, in the presence of cl-CD95L, CD95 activates the Na^+/H^+ exchanger 1 (NHE1) through an Akt and RhoA-driven molecular mechanism [106]. NHE1 is a pH regulator that can extrude proton outside the cell and thereby modulates pH at the plasma membrane [106]. While the presence of cl-CD95L activates NHE1, no such modulation is observed in cells stimulated with a cytotoxic, multi-aggregated CD95L, suggesting that an acid pH may surround the intracellular region of CD95 in cells stimulated with cytotoxic CD95L as compared to CD95 in cells exposed to cl-CD95L [106]. This observation is a plausible explanation for an alteration in pH close to CD95 favoring a receptor conformation that promotes or prevents implementation of the apoptotic signalling pathway.

Once docked onto CD95-DD, FADD self-associates [107], and binds procaspases-8 and -10, which are autoprocessed and released in the cytosol as active caspases.

Activated caspases cleave many substrates, ultimately leading to the execution of the apoptotic program and cell death. The CD95/FADD/caspase-8/-10 complex is the so-called DISC [13]. Due to the importance of DISC formation to cell fate, it is not surprising that numerous cellular and viral proteins have evolved to hamper the formation of this structure; for example, both FLIP [108, 109] and PED/PEA-15 [110] interfere with the recruitment of caspase-8/-10.

7.6 What Mouse Models Can Teach Us

Three mouse models exist in which either CD95L affinity for CD95 is reduced (due to the germline mutation F273L in CD95L, which decreases CD95L binding to CD95, referred to as gld (for generalized lymphoproliferative disease) mice [51, 111]; the level of CD95 expression is down-regulated (due to an insertion of a retrotransposon in intron 2 of the receptor gene, referred to as lpr (for lymphoproliferation) mice [112–114]), or DISC formation is hampered (due to a spontaneous mutation inside the CD95 DD replacing valine 238 by asparagine, referred to as lpr^{cg} (for *lpr* gene complementing *gld*) mice [115].

These mice harboring mutation in CD95 and CD95L, respectively, develop lupus-like symptoms and they have provided valuable insights into the pivotal role played by CD95–CD95L pair lupus pathogenesis by modulating the homeostasis of different immune cells. Nonetheless, it is noteworthy that most, if not all, of the studies using these mice focused on the consequence of the apoptotic deregulation and neglected the nonapoptotic signalling pathways induced by this couple.

These mice have provided valuable insights into the pivotal role played by CD95 and CD95L in immune surveillance and immune tolerance [7]. In an attempt to simplify, some authors associated the phenotypes observed in these lpr, lpr^{cg}, or gld mice with the complete loss of CD95 or CD95L [116]. However, conclusions must be drawn with caution. Indeed, the interpretation of the clinical signs in lpr^{cg} mice can be rendered complex because DD mutation in these mice does not totally abrogate FADD recruitment but merely reduces it [117]. Furthermore, CD95 can still interact with CD95L harboring the *gld* mutation, albeit somewhat more weakly than wild-type CD95L [118]. Finally, lpr, lpr^{cg}, and *gld* mice overexpress CD95L relative to their wild-type counterparts [4]. Using T-lymphocytes from ALPS type Ia patients or lpr mice, we observed that far less intact CD95 is required to activate NF-κB than to induce apoptosis; therefore, although a single wild-type allele cannot restore cell death induction in these cells, it is sufficient to transduce NF-κB and MAPK cues [36, 90]. Overall, these observations support the notion that the biological roles ascribed to the CD95–CD95L pair, based on the analysis of these patients and mouse models, correspond to the additive effects of the receptor's inability to induce cell death and its tendency to implement nonapoptotic signals.

In agreement with the notion that the maintain of a wild type allele is pivotal in the pathogenesis of cancers and chronic inflammatory disorders, elimination of the remaining CD95 allele leads to the induction of a cell death program called "death induced by CD95R/L elimination" (DICE) (Fig. 7.3) [119]. These data highlight that stimulating DICE by eliminating CD95 expression, is a novel and promising approach to killing tumor cells and more specifically cancer stem cells, which are defined as resistant to the classical cell death programs. However, how DICE is induced and the identity of the molecules contributing to this signal remains to be addressed. Nonetheless, because DICE is not affected by inhibitors of several types of cell death (autophagy, necroptosis, and apoptosis), downregulating CD95 in cancer patients may be an attractive therapeutic approach.

7.7 Immune Cells and CD95/CD95L

7.7.1 CD95L Is a Chemoattractant for Immune Cells

Although initially there was some expectation that transplanted organs could be protected by making them express CD95L, seminal experiments with β-islet cells [61] and colon cancer cells [57] revealed that ectopic expression of this ligand enhanced the pace with which the cells were rejected, mainly through the attraction of host neutrophils. Similarly, injection of DCs engineered to express CD95L induces an inflammatory response involving granulocytes, Th1 cells and cytotoxic $CD8^+$ T-lymphocytes [120]. Indeed, these CD95L-expressing DCs cause severe lung granulomatous vasculitis sharing many features of human Wegener granulomatosis [120]. In these studies, the authors did not evaluate whether the accumulation of activated neutrophils in transplanted tissues was due to the presence of metalloproteases responsible for the generation of cl-CD95L, or whether the presence of its membrane-bound counterpart killed cells such as fibroblasts in the transplanted microenvironment, which in dying secrete soluble chemoattractant factors. Indeed, recent data show that, in parallel to the apoptotic signal, dying tumor cells exposed to cytotoxic CD95L trigger an c-IAP1/2-dependent signalling pathway that promotes the synthesis of pro-inflammatory mediators, such as IL-6, IL-8, CXCL1, MCP-1, and GMCSF [37]. Production of these cytokines not only promotes chemotaxis of phagocytes but also stimulates their ability to phagocyte and to clear apoptotic cells and subsequently mount an adaptive immune response. This study reveals that caspase-8 is instrumental in this c-IAP1/2–RIPK1–NFκb signalling pathway as a scaffold molecule, because inhibition of its activity does not alter this nonapoptotic signalling program. In accordance with these findings, caspase-8 is in fact a highly complex regulator of cell fate, protecting cells through inhibition of the necroptotic signal [121–123]; promoting cell migration [77, 124] and tissue inflammation independently of its proteolysis activity; and evoking apoptosis [13, 125, 126], via its enzymatic activity, in cells exposed to death ligands such as CD95L.

CD95 engagement is also able to affect the posttranslational modifications of inflammatory cytokines such as IL-1β and IL-18 [127]. Indeed, this process occurs in myeloid cells through caspase-8 activation [127]. In addition to mediating inflammation via the production and maturation of cytokines and chemokines, CD95 can also directly enhance cell migration of immune cells such as neutrophils [128]. CD95 also contributes to the recruitment of myeloid cell within inflammatory sites [65]. This chemoattractant action occurs through recruitment of the tyrosine kinase syk by CD95 and PI3K activation.

7.7.2 Dendritic Cells

Activation of CD95 in immature DCs induces their maturation, including the expression of MHC class II, B7, and DC-lysosome-associated membrane protein molecules and the secretion of proinflammatory cytokines, in particular interleukin IL-1β and TNF-α [129]. On the other hand, stimulation of pattern recognition receptors in DCs increases in the expression level of CD95 and, by doing so, promotes the elimination of APCs by CD95L-expressing activated T-lymphocytes [130]. In agreement with these data, selective knockout of CD95 in DCs in mice causes autoimmunity due to the resistance of these cells to the CD95L-mediated apoptotic signal and their consecutive accumulation in inflamed tissues [130]. A seminal paper from Karray's group showed that the genetic deletion of CD95L in T- and B-cells not only impairs elimination of autoimmune T-cells but also of APCs such as B-cells and DCs, and thereby causes autoimmunity in these mice [131]. The finely tuned regulation of activated $CD95^+$ APCs (i.e., B-cells and DCs) by CD95L-expressing T-cells [75, 132] is clearly demonstrated by the degree to which loss of the CD95-mediated apoptotic signal in these conditional tissue-selective knockout experiments contributes to the etiology of autoimmune pathologies. Viral infection induces elimination of DCs through a CD95-dependent mechanism leading to a sustained, chronic infection. Indeed, mice genetically engineered to express CD95-deficient DCs, or transfer of CD95-deficient DCs to normal mice, clear persistent viral infection more rapidly than mice carrying wild-type CD95-expressing DCs [133]. It seems that the main resistance of DCs to the CD95-mediated apoptotic signalling pathway relies on the overexpression of the anti-apoptotic factor BclxL [134].

In summary, CD95 participates in recruiting and activating APCs in inflamed organs and, later, eliminating mature DCs. By doing so, CD95 contributes to the mounting of an efficient and transient immune response essential to clear infections and to prevent autoimmunity. On the other hand, APCs with a deregulated CD95-mediated signalling pathway will contribute to autoimmunity.

7.7.3 CD95 and T- and B-Cells

7.7.3.1 T-Cells and Activation-Induced Cell Death (AICD)

Activated peripheral T-cells are eliminated by apoptosis to terminate the immune response, a cellular process designated immune contraction [135]. Indeed, most of activated T-cells (apart from memory T-cells) enter a deletion phase called activation-induced cell death (AICD). Initially, this AICD was reported to rely on CD95/CD95L [136, 137] but this is now known to be only true for T-cells recognizing self-Ags (see below).

CD95L is not found at the surface of naïve T-cells, but this ligand is rapidly expressed after TCR activation [136]. TCR activation is also associated with a rapid cleavage of caspase-8, which has been suggested as an essential step in T-cell activation. This caspase-8 activation apparently occurs via CD95 engagement [138], raising the hypothesis that, during the activation process, T-cells can only proliferate if their apoptotic machinery is functional. Caspase-8 activation is also instrumental in extinguishing the activation of the necroptotic signalling pathway induced by RIPK1 and RIPK3 [122, 123, 139]. Hence, it is difficult to decipher whether caspase-8 orchestrates T-cell activation by promoting cell proliferation, by abrogating its necrotic death or by doing both.

Although the pro-apoptotic Bcl2 member Bim does not participate in the CD95-mediated apoptotic signalling pathway [140], this apoptotic factor contributes to AICD by eliminating 80% of the activated T-lymphocytes in mice injected with the superantigen staphylococcal enterotoxin B (SEB). In agreement with these data, while CD95 is involved in the elimination of activated T-lymphocytes responding to weak auto-Ags and chronic infections [133], it fails to eliminate T-cells activated by strong Ags [141] generated by acute infections or cancer cells.

7.7.3.2 B-Cells

Despite the fact that the CD95–CD95L pair is dispensable in the elimination of autoreactive B-cells, this couple suppresses IgE antibody production in mice [142]. This observation is confirmed in human, because, although IgE accumulation was not described as a clinical symptom in ALPS patients, a recent analysis showed that 25% of ALPS patients exhibit high concentrations of IgE in their serum [142]. The study found that CD95 controls the emergence of a germinal center B-cell population the authors designate as germinal center rogue cells (GCrs), which do not follow the selection rules of normal B-cells, and undergo somatic mutations leading to the production of autoantibodies. The CD95L-expressing cells that kill GCrs remain yet to be identified, but this elimination does not occur through an autocrine process, Follicular B helper T-cells may contribute to this process.

7.7.3.3 Memory T-Cells

The role of CD95 in T-cell activation/maturation has been recently highlighted by elucidating the molecular mechanism involved in the deleterious effect of memory T-cells in the antitumor response mediated by adoptive cell transfer (ACT). In mixed T-cell populations, T memory cells accelerate the maturation of naïve T-cells exposed to Ags through the induction of a CD95-dependent PI3K signalling pathway [143]. This CD95 nonapoptotic response accelerates the differentiation/maturation process in naïve T-cells. Of note, inhibition of the CD95 signalling pathway improves the magnitude of the antitumor response exerted by ACT. This immune process has been designated "precocious differentiation" and occurs in both $CD4^+$ and $CD8^+$ naïve cells [143]. Primed naïve T-cells undergoing precocious differentiation do not generate T memory stem cells or T central memory populations, but instead produce T effector memory cells showing reduced proliferation and antitumor capacities. Of note and counter intuitively, high expression level of CD95 is considered a robust marker of these pluripotent T memory stem cells [144]. This collective decision induced by CD95L-expressing T memory cells may correspond to a cellular mechanism to synchronize the immune response and thereby may represent a way to extinguish it once the antitumor or anti-infectious response has been conducted.

7.7.3.4 Th17 Cells

Th17 cells orchestrate inflammation and the elimination of extracellular pathogens [145]. Among 22 "Th17-positive factors" involved in Th17 differentiation, Regev's group identified that the loss of CD95 leads to failure of Th17 differentiation of activated T-cells bathed in a medium complemented with TGFβ1 and IL-6 [146]. The authors showed that CD95, as a target of STAT3 and BATF transcription factors, is overexpressed early during Th17 differentiation and loss of CD95 promotes Th1 differentiation (IFNγ-R1) over that of Th17 cells.

7.7.4 T-Cell Activation

Soon after the cloning of CD95L, it was shown that simultaneous aggregation of CD95 with CD3 enhanced T-cell proliferation [25]. Moreover, CD95/TCR activation seems to be required to promote T-cell proliferation through the caspase-8-driven synthesis of IL2. In this cellular context, caspase-8 activation leads to the cleavage of a different subset of substrates from that processed in dying T-cells [138]. For instance, TCR/CD95-driven caspase-8 activation does not cause the cleavage of poly(ADP-ribose) polymerase (PARP) and caspase-3, both of which are processed in dying cells. Nonetheless, the exact role of CD95 in T-cell activation remains to be clarified. Indeed, unlike simultaneous stimulation of CD95 and TCR, the sequential activation of CD95 and TCR (CD95 aggregation performed 1 h prior to T-cell activation) prevents TCR activation [147]. This inhibitory process occurs through CD95-mediated ceramide/sphingosine production, which in turn inhibits the Ca^{2+} response and IL2 production [147].

Viruses also hijack the CD95/CD95L pathway to survive and spread. For instance, HIV infection of APCs induces CD95L expression, which prevents the initial steps of TCR activation in naïve T-cells such as the distribution of their receptor into lipid rafts [148]. These studies indicate that CD95 stimulation during or prior to TCR activation leads to the suppression of the immune response that may correspond to clonal anergy.

Although TCR engagement in T-cells induces de novo expression of CD95L [136, 149], activated T-cells fail to respond to the CD95-mediated apoptotic signalling pathway unless they undergo restimulation promoting the redistribution of CD95 into lipid rafts [150]. The redistribution of CD95 into these plasma membrane subdomains favors the implementation of the apoptotic signalling pathway [150, 151]. This restimulation induced cell death (RICD) ensures the clonotypic elimination of chronically stimulated T-cells that may have a pivotal role in killing T-cells specific for auto-Ags.

After cleavage by metalloprotease, soluble CD95L (that we call cl-CD95L to differentiate it from the soluble exosome-bound CD95L) is detected in serum. This naturally processed ligand activates through the implementation of PI3K and a Ca^{2+} signalling pathways the endothelial transmigration of activated T-cells, which accumulate in enflamed organs of systemic lupus erythematosus (SLE) patients [33]. This initial study raised the question of whether all T-cell subsets respond to cl-CD95L or whether only pro-inflammatory Th cells potentially involved in the SLE pathology progression, such as Th17 cells, respond to the accumulation of cl-CD95L associated with the aggressiveness of the pathology. IL-17-expressing cells such as Th17 cells are involved in kidney damage and in the pathology progression in SLE patients [152, 153]. A potential explanation for the accumulation of Th17 cells in damaged organs of SLE patients is that an abnormal level of Th17 trafficking occurs in these patients, promoting inflammation and tissue damage. Nonetheless, the mechanism of Th17 cell accumulation in damaged SLE organs remained unexplained. In cancer [32, 154] and lupus [8], endothelial cells covering blood vessels ectopically express membrane-bound CD95L [8, 33, 154]. Of note, we demonstrated that accumulation of cl-CD95L in lupus patients promotes a selective Th17/Th1-cell recruitment in inflamed organs, a cellular process conserved in both mouse and humans that causes organ damage in lupus patients. Another parameter appears to be involved; Th17 cells exposed to cl-CD95L upregulate expression of the adhesion molecule PSGL-1, which not only promotes tethering of lymphocytes to endothelial cells and subsequent rolling, but when highly expressed on T-cells also provokes the secretion of effector cytokines [155]. Therefore, cl-CD95L may also fuel the inflammatory process by altering the pattern of cytokine release in inflamed tissues. The sphingosine 1 phosphate (S1P) signalling pathway is a critical regulator of many normal and pathophysiological processes [156]. Unlike Treg cells, Th17 cells exposed to cl-CD95L upregulate S1P. Activation of the S1P signalling pathway in Th17 cells exposed to cl-CD95L provides a molecular mechanism to explain how Th17 cells migrate in the presence of this soluble ligand. The successful development of the S1P analogue FTY720, as a useful drug for treatment of multiple sclerosis [157] has proven that it is possible to specifically target S1P signalling in humans. These findings indicate that use of such S1P antagonists would be a potential therapeutic approach to prevent CD95-mediated Th17 transmigration in SLE patients.

Like many proteins, CD95 shows a "day job" and acts as a "night killer"; this schizophrenic attitude may be associated to the preservation of the collectivity and thereby molecules involved in the high pace of immune cell proliferation are also responsible for stopping the reaction and killing cells. The interplay between the apoptotic and nonapoptotic signalling pathways is still poorly understood and the characterization of the molecular mechanism controlling switch between these signals may provide pivotal data to resensitize tumor cell to death and also to prevent the lost control of the T-cells due to an increased cell proliferation and/or reduced cell death.

Acknowledgements This work was supported by grants from INCa PLBIO, Fondation ARC, La Ligue contre le Cancer (Comités d'Ille-et-Vilaine/du Morbihan/des Côtes d'Armor/du Finistère/du Maine et Loire), Cancéropole Grand Ouest, Région Bretagne and Rennes Métropole. AP is supported by La Ligue contre le Cancer and Région Bretagne.

References

1. Chtanova T, Tangye SG, Newton R, Frank N, Hodge MR, Rolph MS, Mackay CR (2004) T follicular helper cells express a distinctive transcriptional profile, reflecting their role as non-Th1/Th2 effector cells that provide help for B cells. J Immunol 173(1):68–78
2. Basu R, O'Quinn DB, Silberger DJ, Schoeb TR, Fouser L, Ouyang W, Hatton RD, Weaver CT (2012) Th22 cells are an important source of IL-22 for host protection against enteropathogenic bacteria. Immunity 37(6):1061–1075. doi:10.1016/j.immuni.2012.08.024
3. Gerlach K, Hwang Y, Nikolaev A, Atreya R, Dornhoff H, Steiner S, Lehr HA, Wirtz S, Vieth M, Waisman A, Rosenbauer F, McKenzie AN, Weigmann B, Neurath MF (2014) TH9 cells that express the transcription factor PU.1 drive T cell-mediated colitis via IL-9 receptor signaling in intestinal epithelial cells. Nat Immunol 15(7):676–686. doi:10.1038/ni.2920
4. Chu JL, Ramos P, Rosendorff A, Nikolic-Zugic J, Lacy E, Matsuzawa A, Elkon KB (1995) Massive upregulation of the Fas ligand in lpr and gld mice: implications for Fas regulation and the graft-versus-host disease-like wasting syndrome. J Exp Med 181(1):393–398
5. Nagata S, Golstein P (1995) The Fas death factor. Science 267(5203):1449–1456
6. Yang Y, Mercep M, Ware CF, Ashwell JD (1995) Fas and activation-induced Fas ligand mediate apoptosis of T cell hybridomas: inhibition of Fas ligand expression by retinoic acid and glucocorticoids. J Exp Med 181(5):1673–1682
7. Strasser A, Jost PJ, Nagata S (2009) The many roles of FAS receptor signaling in the immune system. Immunity 30(2):180–192. doi:10.1016/j.immuni.2009.01.001. S1074-7613(09)00069-7 [pii]
8. Poissonnier A, Sanseau D, Le Gallo M, Malleter M, Levoin N, Viel R, Morere L, Penna A, Blanco P, Dupuy A, Poizeau F, Fautrel A, Seneschal J, Jouan F, Ritz J, Forcade E, Rioux N, Contin-Bordes C, Ducret T, Vacher AM, Barrow PA, Flynn RJ, Vacher P, Legembre P (2016) CD95-mediated calcium signaling promotes T helper 17 trafficking to inflamed organs in lupus-prone mice. Immunity 45(1):209–223. doi:10.1016/j.immuni.2016.06.028
9. Alnemri ES, Livingston DJ, Nicholson DW, Salvesen G, Thornberry NA, Wong WW, Yuan J (1996) Human ICE/CED-3 protease nomenclature. Cell 87(2):171
10. Boldin MP, Varfolomeev EE, Pancer Z, Mett IL, Camonis JH, Wallach D (1995) A novel protein that interacts with the death domain of Fas/APO1 contains a sequence motif related to the death domain. J Biol Chem 270(14):7795–7798
11. Chinnaiyan AM, O'Rourke K, Tewari M, Dixit VM (1995) FADD, a novel death domain-containing protein, interacts with the death domain of Fas and initiates apoptosis. Cell 81(4):505–512. 0092-8674(95)90071-3 [pii]

12. Hsu H, Xiong J, Goeddel DV (1995) The TNF receptor 1-associated protein TRADD signals cell death and NF-kappa B activation. Cell 81(4):495–504. 0092-8674(95)90070-5 [pii]
13. Kischkel FC, Hellbardt S, Behrmann I, Germer M, Pawlita M, Krammer PH, Peter ME (1995) Cytotoxicity-dependent APO-1 (Fas/CD95)-associated proteins form a death-inducing signaling complex (DISC) with the receptor. EMBO J 14(22):5579–5588
14. Hengartner MO (2000) The biochemistry of apoptosis. Nature 407(6805):770–776
15. Li P, Nijhawan D, Budihardjo I, Srinivasula SM, Ahmad M, Alnemri ES, Wang X (1997) Cytochrome c and dATP-dependent formation of Apaf-1/caspase-9 complex initiates an apoptotic protease cascade. Cell 91(4):479–489
16. Itoh N, Yonehara S, Ishii A, Yonehara M, Mizushima S, Sameshima M, Hase A, Seto Y, Nagata S (1991) The polypeptide encoded by the cDNA for human cell surface antigen Fas can mediate apoptosis. Cell 66(2):233–243. 0092-8674(91)90614-5 [pii]
17. Loetscher H, Pan YC, Lahm HW, Gentz R, Brockhaus M, Tabuchi H, Lesslauer W (1990) Molecular cloning and expression of the human 55 kd tumor necrosis factor receptor. Cell 61(2):351–359
18. Pan G, O'Rourke K, Chinnaiyan AM, Gentz R, Ebner R, Ni J, Dixit VM (1997) The receptor for the cytotoxic ligand TRAIL. Science 276(5309):111–113
19. Walczak H, Degli-Esposti MA, Johnson RS, Smolak PJ, Waugh JY, Boiani N, Timour MS, Gerhart MJ, Schooley KA, Smith CA, Goodwin RG, Rauch CT (1997) TRAIL-R2: a novel apoptosis-mediating receptor for TRAIL. EMBO J 16(17):5386–5397. doi:10.1093/emboj/16.17.5386
20. Pan G, Bauer JH, Haridas V, Wang S, Liu D, Yu G, Vincenz C, Aggarwal BB, Ni J, Dixit VM (1998) Identification and functional characterization of DR6, a novel death domain-containing TNF receptor. FEBS Lett 431(3):351–356
21. Fouque A, Debure L, Legembre P (2014) The CD95/CD95L signaling pathway: a role in carcinogenesis. Biochim Biophys Acta. doi:10.1016/j.bbcan.2014.04.007
22. Hoogwater FJ, Steller EJ, Westendorp BF, Borel Rinkes IH, Kranenburg O (2012) CD95 signaling in colorectal cancer. Biochim Biophys Acta 1826(1):189–198. doi:10.1016/j.bbcan.2012.03.007
23. Martin-Villalba A, Llorens-Bobadilla E, Wollny D (2013) CD95 in cancer: tool or target? Trends Mol Med 19(6):329–335. doi:10.1016/j.molmed.2013.03.002
24. Peter ME, Hadji A, Murmann AE, Brockway S, Putzbach W, Pattanayak A, Ceppi P (2015) The role of CD95 and CD95 ligand in cancer. Cell Death Differ 22(5):885–886
25. Alderson MR, Armitage RJ, Maraskovsky E, Tough TW, Roux E, Schooley K, Ramsdell F, Lynch DH (1993) Fas transduces activation signals in normal human T lymphocytes. J Exp Med 178(6):2231–2235
26. Schulze-Osthoff K, Krammer PH, Droge W (1994) Divergent signalling via APO-1/Fas and the TNF receptor, two homologous molecules involved in physiological cell death. EMBO J 13(19):4587–4596
27. Eisele G, Roth P, Hasenbach K, Aulwurm S, Wolpert F, Tabatabai G, Wick W, Weller M (2011) APO010, a synthetic hexameric CD95 ligand, induces human glioma cell death in vitro and in vivo. Neuro-Oncology 13(2):155–164. doi:10.1093/neuonc/noq176
28. Verbrugge I, Wissink EH, Rooswinkel RW, Jongsma J, Beltraminelli N, Dupuis M, Borst J, Verheij M (2009) Combining radiotherapy with APO010 in cancer treatment. Clin Cancer Res 15(6):2031–2038. doi:10.1158/1078-0432.CCR-08-2125
29. Wick W, Fricke H, Junge K, Kobyakov G, Martens T, Heese O, Wiestler B, Schliesser MG, von Deimling A, Pichler J, Vetlova E, Harting I, Debus J, Hartmann C, Kunz C, Platten M, Bendszus M, Combs SE (2014) A phase II, randomized, study of weekly APG101+reirradiation versus reirradiation in progressive glioblastoma. Clin Cancer Res 20(24):6304–6313. doi:10.1158/1078-0432.CCR-14-0951-T
30. Trauth BC, Klas C, Peters AM, Matzku S, Moller P, Falk W, Debatin KM, Krammer PH (1989) Monoclonal antibody-mediated tumor regression by induction of apoptosis. Science 245(4915):301–305

31. Suda T, Takahashi T, Golstein P, Nagata S (1993) Molecular cloning and expression of the Fas ligand, a novel member of the tumor necrosis factor family. Cell 75(6):1169–1178
32. Malleter M, Tauzin S, Bessede A, Castellano R, Goubard A, Godey F, Leveque J, Jezequel P, Campion L, Campone M, Ducret T, MacGrogan G, Debure L, Collette Y, Vacher P, Legembre P (2013) CD95L cell surface cleavage triggers a prometastatic signaling pathway in triple-negative breast cancer. Cancer Res 73(22):6711–6721. doi:10.1158/0008-5472.CAN-13-1794
33. Tauzin S, Chaigne-Delalande B, Selva E, Khadra N, Daburon S, Contin-Bordes C, Blanco P, Le Seyec J, Ducret T, Counillon L, Moreau JF, Hofman P, Vacher P, Legembre P (2011) The naturally processed CD95L elicits a c-yes/calcium/PI3K-driven cell migration pathway. PLoS Biol 9(6):e1001090. doi:10.1371/journal.pbio.1001090
34. Schneider P, Holler N, Bodmer JL, Hahne M, Frei K, Fontana A, Tschopp J (1998) Conversion of membrane-bound Fas(CD95) ligand to its soluble form is associated with downregulation of its proapoptotic activity and loss of liver toxicity. J Exp Med 187(8):1205–1213
35. Soderstrom TS, Nyberg SD, Eriksson JE (2005) CD95 capping is ROCK-dependent and dispensable for apoptosis. J Cell Sci 118(Pt 10):2211–2223
36. Legembre P, Barnhart BC, Peter ME (2004) The relevance of NF-kappaB for CD95 signaling in tumor cells. Cell Cycle 3(10):1235–1239
37. Cullen SP, Henry CM, Kearney CJ, Logue SE, Feoktistova M, Tynan GA, Lavelle EC, Leverkus M, Martin SJ (2013) Fas/CD95-induced chemokines can serve as "find-me" signals for apoptotic cells. Mol Cell 49(6):1034–1048. doi:10.1016/j.molcel.2013.01.025
38. Smith CA, Farrah T, Goodwin RG (1994) The TNF receptor superfamily of cellular and viral proteins: activation, costimulation, and death. Cell 76(6):959–962
39. Locksley RM, Killeen N, Lenardo MJ (2001) The TNF and TNF receptor superfamilies: integrating mammalian biology. Cell 104(4):487–501
40. Bodmer JL, Schneider P, Tschopp J (2002) The molecular architecture of the TNF superfamily. Trends Biochem Sci 27(1):19–26
41. Edmond V, Ghali B, Penna A, Taupin JL, Daburon S, Moreau JF, Legembre P (2012) Precise mapping of the CD95 pre-ligand assembly domain. PLoS One 7(9):e46236. doi:10.1371/journal.pone.0046236
42. Papoff G, Hausler P, Eramo A, Pagano MG, Di Leve G, Signore A, Ruberti G (1999) Identification and characterization of a ligand-independent oligomerization domain in the extracellular region of the CD95 death receptor. J Biol Chem 274(53):38241–38250
43. Siegel RM, Frederiksen JK, Zacharias DA, Chan FK, Johnson M, Lynch D, Tsien RY, Lenardo MJ (2000) Fas preassociation required for apoptosis signaling and dominant inhibition by pathogenic mutations. Science 288(5475):2354–2357
44. Itoh N, Nagata S (1993) A novel protein domain required for apoptosis. Mutational analysis of human Fas antigen. J Biol Chem 268(15):10932–10937
45. Tartaglia LA, Ayres TM, Wong GH, Goeddel DV (1993) A novel domain within the 55 kd TNF receptor signals cell death. Cell 74(5):845–853. 0092-8674(93)90464-2 [pii]
46. Pennica D, Nedwin GE, Hayflick JS, Seeburg PH, Derynck R, Palladino MA, Kohr WJ, Aggarwal BB, Goeddel DV (1984) Human tumour necrosis factor: precursor structure, expression and homology to lymphotoxin. Nature 312(5996):724–729
47. Black RA, Rauch CT, Kozlosky CJ, Peschon JJ, Slack JL, Wolfson MF, Castner BJ, Stocking KL, Reddy P, Srinivasan S, Nelson N, Boiani N, Schooley KA, Gerhart M, Davis R, Fitzner JN, Johnson RS, Paxton RJ, March CJ, Cerretti DP (1997) A metalloproteinase disintegrin that releases tumour-necrosis factor-alpha from cells. Nature 385(6618):729–733. doi:10.1038/385729a0
48. Moss ML, Jin SL, Milla ME, Bickett DM, Burkhart W, Carter HL, Chen WJ, Clay WC, Didsbury JR, Hassler D, Hoffman CR, Kost TA, Lambert MH, Leesnitzer MA, McCauley P, McGeehan G, Mitchell J, Moyer M, Pahel G, Rocque W, Overton LK, Schoenen F, Seaton T, Su JL, Becherer JD et al (1997) Cloning of a disintegrin metalloproteinase that processes precursor tumour-necrosis factor-alpha. Nature 385(6618):733–736. doi:10.1038/385733a0

49. Grell M, Douni E, Wajant H, Lohden M, Clauss M, Maxeiner B, Georgopoulos S, Lesslauer W, Kollias G, Pfizenmaier K, Scheurich P (1995) The transmembrane form of tumor necrosis factor is the prime activating ligand of the 80 kDa tumor necrosis factor receptor. Cell 83(5):793–802
50. Cabal-Hierro L, Lazo PS (2012) Signal transduction by tumor necrosis factor receptors. Cell Signal 24(6):1297–1305. doi:10.1016/j.cellsig.2012.02.006
51. Takahashi T, Tanaka M, Brannan CI, Jenkins NA, Copeland NG, Suda T, Nagata S (1994) Generalized lymphoproliferative disease in mice, caused by a point mutation in the Fas ligand. Cell 76(6):969–976. 0092-8674(94)90375-1 [pii]
52. Montel AH, Bochan MR, Hobbs JA, Lynch DH, Brahmi Z (1995) Fas involvement in cytotoxicity mediated by human NK cells. Cell Immunol 166(2):236–246
53. Saas P, Walker PR, Hahne M, Quiquerez AL, Schnuriger V, Perrin G, French L, Van Meir EG, de Tribolet N, Tschopp J, Dietrich PY (1997) Fas ligand expression by astrocytoma in vivo: maintaining immune privilege in the brain? J Clin Invest 99(6):1173–1178. doi:10.1172/JCI119273
54. Griffith TS, Brunner T, Fletcher SM, Green DR, Ferguson TA (1995) Fas ligand-induced apoptosis as a mechanism of immune privilege. Science 270(5239):1189–1192
55. Stuart PM, Griffith TS, Usui N, Pepose J, Yu X, Ferguson TA (1997) CD95 ligand (FasL)-induced apoptosis is necessary for corneal allograft survival. J Clin Invest 99(3):396–402. doi:10.1172/JCI119173
56. Bellgrau D, Gold D, Selawry H, Moore J, Franzusoff A, Duke RC (1995) A role for CD95 ligand in preventing graft rejection. Nature 377(6550):630–632
57. Chen JJ, Sun Y, Nabel GJ (1998) Regulation of the proinflammatory effects of Fas ligand (CD95L). Science 282(5394):1714–1717
58. Hahne M, Rimoldi D, Schroter M, Romero P, Schreier M, French LE, Schneider P, Bornand T, Fontana A, Lienard D, Cerottini J, Tschopp J (1996) Melanoma cell expression of Fas(Apo-1/CD95) ligand: implications for tumor immune escape. Science 274(5291):1363–1366
59. O'Connell J, O'Sullivan GC, Collins JK, Shanahan F (1996) The Fas counterattack: Fas-mediated T cell killing by colon cancer cells expressing Fas ligand. J Exp Med 184(3):1075–1082
60. Allison J, Georgiou HM, Strasser A, Vaux DL (1997) Transgenic expression of CD95 ligand on islet beta cells induces a granulocytic infiltration but does not confer immune privilege upon islet allografts. Proc Natl Acad Sci U S A 94(8):3943–3947
61. Kang SM, Schneider DB, Lin Z, Hanahan D, Dichek DA, Stock PG, Baekkeskov S (1997) Fas ligand expression in islets of Langerhans does not confer immune privilege and instead targets them for rapid destruction. Nat Med 3(7):738–743
62. Restifo NP (2001) Countering the 'counterattack' hypothesis. Nat Med 7(3):259. doi:10.1038/85357. 85357 [pii]
63. Park SM, Schickel R, Peter ME (2005) Nonapoptotic functions of FADD-binding death receptors and their signaling molecules. Curr Opin Cell Biol 17(6):610–616. doi:10.1016/j.ceb.2005.09.010
64. Chervonsky AV, Wang Y, Wong FS, Visintin I, Flavell RA, Janeway CA Jr, Matis LA (1997) The role of Fas in autoimmune diabetes. Cell 89(1):17–24
65. Letellier E, Kumar S, Sancho-Martinez I, Krauth S, Funke-Kaiser A, Laudenklos S, Konecki K, Klussmann S, Corsini NS, Kleber S, Drost N, Neumann A, Levi-Strauss M, Brors B, Gretz N, Edler L, Fischer C, Hill O, Thiemann M, Biglari B, Karray S, Martin-Villalba A (2010) CD95-ligand on peripheral myeloid cells activates Syk kinase to trigger their recruitment to the inflammatory site. Immunity 32(2):240–252. doi:10.1016/j.immuni.2010.01.011. S1074-7613(10)00041-5 [pii]
66. Barnhart BC, Legembre P, Pietras E, Bubici C, Franzoso G, Peter ME (2004) CD95 ligand induces motility and invasiveness of apoptosis-resistant tumor cells. EMBO J 23(15):3175–3185. doi:10.1038/sj.emboj.7600325

67. Kleber S, Sancho-Martinez I, Wiestler B, Beisel A, Gieffers C, Hill O, Thiemann M, Mueller W, Sykora J, Kuhn A, Schreglmann N, Letellier E, Zuliani C, Klussmann S, Teodorczyk M, Grone HJ, Ganten TM, Sultmann H, Tuttenberg J, von Deimling A, Regnier-Vigouroux A, Herold-Mende C, Martin-Villalba A (2008) Yes and PI3K bind CD95 to signal invasion of glioblastoma. Cancer Cell 13(3):235–248. doi:10.1016/j.ccr.2008.02.003. S1535-6108(08)00043-3 [pii]
68. Matsuno H, Yudoh K, Watanabe Y, Nakazawa F, Aono H, Kimura T (2001) Stromelysin-1 (MMP-3) in synovial fluid of patients with rheumatoid arthritis has potential to cleave membrane bound Fas ligand. J Rheumatol 28(1):22–28
69. Vargo-Gogola T, Crawford HC, Fingleton B, Matrisian LM (2002) Identification of novel matrix metalloproteinase-7 (matrilysin) cleavage sites in murine and human Fas ligand. Arch Biochem Biophys 408(2):155–161
70. Kiaei M, Kipiani K, Calingasan NY, Wille E, Chen J, Heissig B, Rafii S, Lorenzl S, Beal MF (2007) Matrix metalloproteinase-9 regulates TNF-alpha and FasL expression in neuronal, glial cells and its absence extends life in a transgenic mouse model of amyotrophic lateral sclerosis. Exp Neurol 205(1):74–81. doi:10.1016/j.expneurol.2007.01.036. S0014-4886(07)00039-8 [pii]
71. Kirkin V, Cahuzac N, Guardiola-Serrano F, Huault S, Luckerath K, Friedmann E, Novac N, Wels WS, Martoglio B, Hueber AO, Zornig M (2007) The Fas ligand intracellular domain is released by ADAM10 and SPPL2a cleavage in T-cells. Cell Death Differ 14(9):1678–1687. doi:10.1038/sj.cdd.4402175. 4402175 [pii]
72. Schulte M, Reiss K, Lettau M, Maretzky T, Ludwig A, Hartmann D, de Strooper B, Janssen O, Saftig P (2007) ADAM10 regulates FasL cell surface expression and modulates FasL-induced cytotoxicity and activation-induced cell death. Cell Death Differ 14(5):1040–1049. doi:10.1038/sj.cdd.4402101. 4402101 [pii]
73. Holler N, Tardivel A, Kovacsovics-Bankowski M, Hertig S, Gaide O, Martinon F, Tinel A, Deperthes D, Calderara S, Schulthess T, Engel J, Schneider P, Tschopp J (2003) Two adjacent trimeric Fas ligands are required for Fas signaling and formation of a death-inducing signaling complex. Mol Cell Biol 23(4):1428–1440
74. Suda T, Hashimoto H, Tanaka M, Ochi T, Nagata S (1997) Membrane Fas ligand kills human peripheral blood T lymphocytes, and soluble Fas ligand blocks the killing. J Exp Med 186(12):2045–2050
75. O'Reilly LA, Tai L, Lee L, Kruse EA, Grabow S, Fairlie WD, Haynes NM, Tarlinton DM, Zhang JG, Belz GT, Smyth MJ, Bouillet P, Robb L, Strasser A (2009) Membrane-bound Fas ligand only is essential for Fas-induced apoptosis. Nature 461(7264):659–663. doi:10.1038/nature08402. nature08402 [pii]
76. Cursi S, Rufini A, Stagni V, Condo I, Matafora V, Bachi A, Bonifazi AP, Coppola L, Superti-Furga G, Testi R, Barila D (2006) Src kinase phosphorylates caspase-8 on Tyr380: a novel mechanism of apoptosis suppression. EMBO J 25(9):1895–1905. doi:10.1038/sj.emboj.7601085
77. Senft J, Helfer B, Frisch SM (2007) Caspase-8 interacts with the p85 subunit of phosphatidylinositol 3-kinase to regulate cell adhesion and motility. Cancer Res 67(24):11505–11509. doi:10.1158/0008-5472.CAN-07-5755
78. Steller EJ, Borel Rinkes IH, Kranenburg O (2011) How CD95 stimulates invasion. Cell Cycle 10(22):3857–3862. doi:10.4161/cc.10.22.18290
79. Steller EJ, Ritsma L, Raats DA, Hoogwater FJ, Emmink BL, Govaert KM, Laoukili J, Rinkes IH, van Rheenen J, Kranenburg O (2011) The death receptor CD95 activates the cofilin pathway to stimulate tumour cell invasion. EMBO Rep 12(9):931–937. doi:10.1038/embor.2011.129
80. Herrero R, Kajikawa O, Matute-Bello G, Wang Y, Hagimoto N, Mongovin S, Wong V, Park DR, Brot N, Heinecke JW, Rosen H, Goodman RB, Fu X, Martin TR (2011) The biological activity of FasL in human and mouse lungs is determined by the structure of its stalk region. J Clin Invest 121(3):1174–1190. doi:10.1172/JCI43004
81. Alonso R, Mazzeo C, Rodriguez MC, Marsh M, Fraile-Ramos A, Calvo V, Avila-Flores A, Merida I, Izquierdo M (2011) Diacylglycerol kinase alpha regulates the formation and polarisation of mature multivesicular bodies involved in the secretion of Fas ligand-containing exosomes in T lymphocytes. Cell Death Differ 18(7):1161–1173. doi:10.1038/cdd.2010.184

82. Bianco NR, Kim SH, Morelli AE, Robbins PD (2007) Modulation of the immune response using dendritic cell-derived exosomes. Methods Mol Biol 380:443–455
83. Abusamra AJ, Zhong Z, Zheng X, Li M, Ichim TE, Chin JL, Min WP (2005) Tumor exosomes expressing Fas ligand mediate CD8+ T-cell apoptosis. Blood Cells Mol Dis 35(2):169–173. doi:10.1016/j.bcmd.2005.07.001
84. Bui JD, Schreiber RD (2007) Cancer immunosurveillance, immunoediting and inflammation: independent or interdependent processes? Curr Opin Immunol 19(2):203–208. doi:10.1016/j.coi.2007.02.001. S0952-7915(07)00009-X [pii]
85. Peter ME, Legembre P, Barnhart BC (2005) Does CD95 have tumor promoting activities? Biochim Biophys Acta 1755(1):25–36. doi:10.1016/j.bbcan.2005.01.001
86. Fisher GH, Rosenberg FJ, Straus SE, Dale JK, Middleton LA, Lin AY, Strober W, Lenardo MJ, Puck JM (1995) Dominant interfering Fas gene mutations impair apoptosis in a human autoimmune lymphoproliferative syndrome. Cell 81(6):935–946
87. Rieux-Laucat F, Le Deist F, Hivroz C, Roberts IA, Debatin KM, Fischer A, de Villartay JP (1995) Mutations in Fas associated with human lymphoproliferative syndrome and autoimmunity. Science 268(5215):1347–1349
88. Drappa J, Vaishnaw AK, Sullivan KE, Chu JL, Elkon KB (1996) Fas gene mutations in the Canale-Smith syndrome, an inherited lymphoproliferative disorder associated with autoimmunity. N Engl J Med 335(22):1643–1649
89. Straus SE, Jaffe ES, Puck JM, Dale JK, Elkon KB, Rosen-Wolff A, Peters AM, Sneller MC, Hallahan CW, Wang J, Fischer RE, Jackson CM, Lin AY, Baumler C, Siegert E, Marx A, Vaishnaw AK, Grodzicky T, Fleisher TA, Lenardo MJ (2001) The development of lymphomas in families with autoimmune lymphoproliferative syndrome with germline Fas mutations and defective lymphocyte apoptosis. Blood 98(1):194–200
90. Legembre P, Barnhart BC, Zheng L, Vijayan S, Straus SE, Puck J, Dale JK, Lenardo M, Peter ME (2004) Induction of apoptosis and activation of NF-kappaB by CD95 require different signalling thresholds. EMBO Rep 5(11):1084–1089. doi:10.1038/sj.embor.7400280
91. Bivona TG, Hieronymus H, Parker J, Chang K, Taron M, Rosell R, Moonsamy P, Dahlman K, Miller VA, Costa C, Hannon G, Sawyers CL (2011) FAS and NF-kappaB signalling modulate dependence of lung cancers on mutant EGFR. Nature 471(7339):523–526. doi:10.1038/nature09870. nature09870 [pii]
92. Chen L, Park SM, Tumanov AV, Hau A, Sawada K, Feig C, Turner JR, Fu YX, Romero IL, Lengyel E, Peter ME (2010) CD95 promotes tumour growth. Nature 465(7297):492–496. doi:10.1038/nature09075
93. Bellone G, Smirne C, Carbone A, Mareschi K, Dughera L, Farina EC, Alabiso O, Valente G, Emanuelli G, Rodeck U (2000) Production and pro-apoptotic activity of soluble CD95 ligand in pancreatic carcinoma. Clin Cancer Res 6(6):2448–2455
94. Malleter M, Tauzin S, Bessede A, Castellano R, Goubard A, Godey F, Leveque J, Jezequel P, Campion L, Campone M, Ducret T, Macgrogan G, Debure L, Collette Y, Vacher P, Legembre P (2013) CD95L cell surface cleavage triggers a pro-metastatic signaling pathway in triple negative breast cancer. Cancer Res. doi:10.1158/0008-5472.CAN-13-1794
95. Tanaka M, Suda T, Haze K, Nakamura N, Sato K, Kimura F, Motoyoshi K, Mizuki M, Tagawa S, Ohga S, Hatake K, Drummond AH, Nagata S (1996) Fas ligand in human serum. Nat Med 2(3):317–322
96. Hashimoto H, Tanaka M, Suda T, Tomita T, Hayashida K, Takeuchi E, Kaneko M, Takano H, Nagata S, Ochi T (1998) Soluble Fas ligand in the joints of patients with rheumatoid arthritis and osteoarthritis. Arthritis Rheum 41(4):657–662. doi:10.1002/1529-0131(199804)41:4<657::AID-ART12>3.0.CO;2-N
97. Das H, Imoto S, Murayama T, Kajimoto K, Sugimoto T, Isobe T, Nakagawa T, Nishimura R, Koizumi T (1999) Levels of soluble FasL and FasL gene expression during the development of graft-versus-host disease in DLT-treated patients. Br J Haematol 104(4):795–800
98. Kanda Y, Tanaka Y, Shirakawa K, Yatomi T, Nakamura N, Kami M, Saito T, Izutsu K, Asai T, Yuji K, Ogawa S, Honda H, Mitani K, Chiba S, Yazaki Y, Hirai H (1998) Increased soluble Fas-ligand in sera of bone marrow transplant recipients with acute graft-versus-host disease. Bone Marrow Transplant 22(8):751–754. doi:10.1038/sj.bmt.1701427

99. Tomokuni A, Otsuki T, Isozaki Y, Kita S, Ueki H, Kusaka M, Kishimoto T, Ueki A (1999) Serum levels of soluble Fas ligand in patients with silicosis. Clin Exp Immunol 118(3):441–444
100. Chan FK, Chun HJ, Zheng L, Siegel RM, Bui KL, Lenardo MJ (2000) A domain in TNF receptors that mediates ligand-independent receptor assembly and signaling. Science 288(5475):2351–2354
101. Lang I, Fick A, Schafer V, Giner T, Siegmund D, Wajant H (2012) Signaling active CD95 receptor molecules trigger co-translocation of inactive CD95 molecules into lipid rafts. J Biol Chem 287(28):24026–24042. doi:10.1074/jbc.M111.328211
102. Huang B, Eberstadt M, Olejniczak ET, Meadows RP, Fesik SW (1996) NMR structure and mutagenesis of the Fas (APO-1/CD95) death domain. Nature 384(6610):638–641. doi:10.1038/384638a0
103. Scott FL, Stec B, Pop C, Dobaczewska MK, Lee JJ, Monosov E, Robinson H, Salvesen GS, Schwarzenbacher R, Riedl SJ (2009) The Fas-FADD death domain complex structure unravels signalling by receptor clustering. Nature 457(7232):1019–1022. doi:10.1038/nature07606. nature07606 [pii]
104. Esposito D, Sankar A, Morgner N, Robinson CV, Rittinger K, Driscoll PC (2010) Solution NMR investigation of the CD95/FADD homotypic death domain complex suggests lack of engagement of the CD95 C terminus. Structure 18(10):1378–1390. doi:10.1016/j.str.2010.08.006. S0969-2126(10)00301-1 [pii]
105. Wang L, Yang JK, Kabaleeswaran V, Rice AJ, Cruz AC, Park AY, Yin Q, Damko E, Jang SB, Raunser S, Robinson CV, Siegel RM, Walz T, Wu H (2010) The Fas-FADD death domain complex structure reveals the basis of DISC assembly and disease mutations. Nat Struct Mol Biol 17(11):1324–1329. doi:10.1038/nsmb.1920
106. Monet M, Poet M, Tauzin S, Fouque A, Cophignon A, Lagadic-Gossmann D, Vacher P, Legembre P, Counillon L (2016) The cleaved FAS ligand activates the Na(+)/H(+) exchanger NHE1 through Akt/ROCK1 to stimulate cell motility. Sci Rep 6:28008. doi:10.1038/srep28008
107. Muppidi JR, Lobito AA, Ramaswamy M, Yang JK, Wang L, Wu H, Siegel RM (2006) Homotypic FADD interactions through a conserved RXDLL motif are required for death receptor-induced apoptosis. Cell Death Differ 13(10):1641–1650. doi:10.1038/sj.cdd.4401855
108. Irmler M, Thome M, Hahne M, Schneider P, Hofmann K, Steiner V, Bodmer JL, Schroter M, Burns K, Mattmann C, Rimoldi D, French LE, Tschopp J (1997) Inhibition of death receptor signals by cellular FLIP. Nature 388(6638):190–195
109. Thome M, Schneider P, Hofmann K, Fickenscher H, Meinl E, Neipel F, Mattmann C, Burns K, Bodmer JL, Schroter M, Scaffidi C, Krammer PH, Peter ME, Tschopp J (1997) Viral FLICE-inhibitory proteins (FLIPs) prevent apoptosis induced by death receptors. Nature 386(6624):517–521
110. Condorelli G, Vigliotta G, Cafieri A, Trencia A, Andalo P, Oriente F, Miele C, Caruso M, Formisano P, Beguinot F (1999) PED/PEA-15: an anti-apoptotic molecule that regulates FAS/TNFR1-induced apoptosis. Oncogene 18(31):4409–4415. doi:10.1038/sj.onc.1202831
111. Kimura M, Matsuzawa A (1994) Autoimmunity in mice bearing lprcg: a novel mutant gene. Int Rev Immunol 11(3):193–210
112. Watanabe-Fukunaga R, Brannan CI, Copeland NG, Jenkins NA, Nagata S (1992) Lymphoproliferation disorder in mice explained by defects in Fas antigen that mediates apoptosis. Nature 356(6367):314–317. doi:10.1038/356314a0
113. Adachi M, Watanabe-Fukunaga R, Nagata S (1993) Aberrant transcription caused by the insertion of an early transposable element in an intron of the Fas antigen gene of lpr mice. Proc Natl Acad Sci U S A 90(5):1756–1760
114. Chu JL, Drappa J, Parnassa A, Elkon KB (1993) The defect in Fas mRNA expression in MRL/lpr mice is associated with insertion of the retrotransposon, ETn. J Exp Med 178(2):723–730
115. Matsuzawa A, Moriyama T, Kaneko T, Tanaka M, Kimura M, Ikeda H, Katagiri T (1990) A new allele of the lpr locus, lprcg, that complements the gld gene in induction of lymphadenopathy in the mouse. J Exp Med 171(2):519–531

116. Heinzelmann F, Jendrossek V, Lauber K, Nowak K, Eldh T, Boras R, Handrick R, Henkel M, Martin C, Uhlig S, Kohler D, Eltzschig HK, Wehrmann M, Budach W, Belka C (2006) Irradiation-induced pneumonitis mediated by the CD95/CD95-ligand system. J Natl Cancer Inst 98(17):1248–1251. doi:10.1093/jnci/djj335
117. Martin DA, Zheng L, Siegel RM, Huang B, Fisher GH, Wang J, Jackson CE, Puck JM, Dale J, Straus SE, Peter ME, Krammer PH, Fesik S, Lenardo MJ (1999) Defective CD95/APO-1/Fas signal complex formation in the human autoimmune lymphoproliferative syndrome, type Ia. Proc Natl Acad Sci U S A 96(8):4552–4557
118. Orlinick JR, Elkon KB, Chao MV (1997) Separate domains of the human fas ligand dictate self-association and receptor binding. J Biol Chem 272(51):32221–32229
119. Hadji A, Ceppi P, Murmann AE, Brockway S, Pattanayak A, Bhinder B, Hau A, De Chant S, Parimi V, Kolesza P, Richards J, Chandel N, Djaballah H, Peter ME (2014) Death induced by CD95 or CD95 ligand elimination. Cell Rep. doi:10.1016/j.celrep.2014.02.035
120. Buonocore S, Flamand V, Claessen N, Heeringa P, Goldman M, Florquin S (2004) Dendritic cells overexpressing Fas-ligand induce pulmonary vasculitis in mice. Clin Exp Immunol 137(1):74–80. doi:10.1111/j.1365-2249.2004.02514.x
121. Green DR, Oberst A, Dillon CP, Weinlich R, Salvesen GS (2011) RIPK-dependent necrosis and its regulation by caspases: a mystery in five acts. Mol Cell 44(1):9–16. doi:10.1016/j.molcel.2011.09.003
122. Kaiser WJ, Upton JW, Long AB, Livingston-Rosanoff D, Daley-Bauer LP, Hakem R, Caspary T, Mocarski ES (2011) RIP3 mediates the embryonic lethality of caspase-8-deficient mice. Nature 471(7338):368–372. doi:10.1038/nature09857
123. Oberst A, Dillon CP, Weinlich R, McCormick LL, Fitzgerald P, Pop C, Hakem R, Salvesen GS, Green DR (2011) Catalytic activity of the caspase-8-FLIP(L) complex inhibits RIPK3-dependent necrosis. Nature 471(7338):363–367. doi:10.1038/nature09852
124. Finlay D, Howes A, Vuori K (2009) Critical role for caspase-8 in epidermal growth factor signaling. Cancer Res 69(12):5023–5029. doi:10.1158/0008-5472.CAN-08-3731
125. Fernandes-Alnemri T, Armstrong RC, Krebs J, Srinivasula SM, Wang L, Bullrich F, Fritz LC, Trapani JA, Tomaselli KJ, Litwack G, Alnemri ES (1996) In vitro activation of CPP32 and Mch3 by Mch4, a novel human apoptotic cysteine protease containing two FADD-like domains. Proc Natl Acad Sci U S A 93(15):7464–7469
126. Muzio M, Chinnaiyan AM, Kischkel FC, O'Rourke K, Shevchenko A, Ni J, Scaffidi C, Bretz JD, Zhang M, Gentz R, Mann M, Krammer PH, Peter ME, Dixit VM (1996) FLICE, a novel FADD-homologous ICE/CED-3-like protease, is recruited to the CD95 (Fas/APO-1) death--inducing signaling complex. Cell 85(6):817–827
127. Bossaller L, Chiang PI, Schmidt-Lauber C, Ganesan S, Kaiser WJ, Rathinam VA, Mocarski ES, Subramanian D, Green DR, Silverman N, Fitzgerald KA, Marshak-Rothstein A, Latz E (2012) Cutting edge: FAS (CD95) mediates noncanonical IL-1beta and IL-18 maturation via caspase-8 in an RIP3-independent manner. J Immunol 189(12):5508–5512. doi:10.4049/jimmunol.1202121
128. Dupont PJ, Warrens AN (2007) Fas ligand exerts its pro-inflammatory effects via neutrophil recruitment but not activation. Immunology 120(1):133–139. doi:10.1111/j.1365-2567.2006.02504.x
129. Rescigno M, Piguet V, Valzasina B, Lens S, Zubler R, French L, Kindler V, Tschopp J, Ricciardi-Castagnoli P (2000) Fas engagement induces the maturation of dendritic cells (DCs), the release of interleukin (IL)-1beta, and the production of interferon gamma in the absence of IL-12 during DC-T cell cognate interaction: a new role for Fas ligand in inflammatory responses. J Exp Med 192(11):1661–1668
130. Stranges PB, Watson J, Cooper CJ, Choisy-Rossi CM, Stonebraker AC, Beighton RA, Hartig H, Sundberg JP, Servick S, Kaufmann G, Fink PJ, Chervonsky AV (2007) Elimination of antigen-presenting cells and autoreactive T cells by Fas contributes to prevention of autoimmunity. Immunity 26(5):629–641. doi:10.1016/j.immuni.2007.03.016
131. Mabrouk I, Buart S, Hasmim M, Michiels C, Connault E, Opolon P, Chiocchia G, Levi-Strauss M, Chouaib S, Karray S (2008) Prevention of autoimmunity and control of recall response to exogenous antigen by Fas death receptor ligand expression on T cells. Immunity 29(6):922–933. doi:10.1016/j.immuni.2008.10.007

132. Sàb T, Chaigne-Delalande B, Selva E, Khadra N, Daburon S, Càc C-B, Blanco P, Le Seyec J, Ducret T, Counillon L, J-Fàü M, Hofman P, Vacher P, Legembre P (2011) The naturally processed CD95L elicits a c-yes/calcium/PI3K-driven cell migration pathway. PLoS Biol 9(6):e1001090
133. Varanasi V, Khan AA, Chervonsky AV (2014) Loss of the death receptor CD95 (Fas) expression by dendritic cells protects from a chronic viral infection. Proc Natl Acad Sci U S A 111(23):8559–8564. doi:10.1073/pnas.1401750111
134. Lundqvist A, Nagata T, Kiessling R, Pisa P (2002) Mature dendritic cells are protected from Fas/CD95-mediated apoptosis by upregulation of Bcl-X(L). Cancer Immunol Immunother 51(3):139–144. doi:10.1007/s00262-002-0265-7
135. Krueger A, Fas SC, Baumann S, Krammer PH (2003) The role of CD95 in the regulation of peripheral T-cell apoptosis. Immunol Rev 193:58–69
136. Ju ST, Panka DJ, Cui H, Ettinger R, el-Khatib M, Sherr DH, Stanger BZ, Marshak-Rothstein A (1995) Fas(CD95)/FasL interactions required for programmed cell death after T-cell activation. Nature 373(6513):444–448. doi:10.1038/373444a0
137. Krammer PH (2000) CD95's deadly mission in the immune system. Nature 407(6805):789–795. doi:10.1038/35037728
138. Kennedy NJ, Kataoka T, Tschopp J, Budd RC (1999) Caspase activation is required for T cell proliferation. J Exp Med 190(12):1891–1896
139. Peter ME (2011) Programmed cell death: apoptosis meets necrosis. Nature 471(7338):310–312. doi:10.1038/471310a
140. Bouillet P, Metcalf D, Huang DC, Tarlinton DM, Kay TW, Kontgen F, Adams JM, Strasser A (1999) Proapoptotic Bcl-2 relative Bim required for certain apoptotic responses, leukocyte homeostasis, and to preclude autoimmunity. Science 286(5445):1735–1738
141. Hildeman DA, Zhu Y, Mitchell TC, Bouillet P, Strasser A, Kappler J, Marrack P (2002) Activated T cell death in vivo mediated by proapoptotic bcl-2 family member bim. Immunity 16(6):759–767
142. Butt D, Chan TD, Bourne K, Hermes JR, Nguyen A, Statham A, O'Reilly LA, Strasser A, Price S, Schofield P, Christ D, Basten A, Ma CS, Tangye SG, Phan TG, Rao VK, Brink R (2015) FAS inactivation releases unconventional germinal center B cells that escape antigen control and drive IgE and autoantibody production. Immunity 42(5):890–902. doi:10.1016/j.immuni.2015.04.010
143. Klebanoff CA, Scott CD, Leonardi AJ, Yamamoto TN, Cruz AC, Ouyang C, Ramaswamy M, Roychoudhuri R, Ji Y, Eil RL, Sukumar M, Crompton JG, Palmer DC, Borman ZA, Clever D, Thomas SK, Patel S, Yu Z, Muranski P, Liu H, Wang E, Marincola FM, Gros A, Gattinoni L, Rosenberg SA, Siegel RM, Restifo NP (2016) Memory T cell-driven differentiation of naive cells impairs adoptive immunotherapy. J Clin Invest 126(1):318–334. doi:10.1172/JCI81217
144. Gattinoni L, Lugli E, Ji Y, Pos Z, Paulos CM, Quigley MF, Almeida JR, Gostick E, Yu Z, Carpenito C, Wang E, Douek DC, Price DA, June CH, Marincola FM, Roederer M, Restifo NP (2011) A human memory T cell subset with stem cell-like properties. Nat Med 17(10):1290–1297. doi:10.1038/nm.2446
145. Bettelli E, Korn T, Kuchroo VK (2007) Th17: the third member of the effector T cell trilogy. Curr Opin Immunol 19(6):652–657. doi:10.1016/j.coi.2007.07.020
146. Yosef N, Shalek AK, Gaublomme JT, Jin H, Lee Y, Awasthi A, Wu C, Karwacz K, Xiao S, Jorgolli M, Gennert D, Satija R, Shakya A, Lu DY, Trombetta JJ, Pillai MR, Ratcliffe PJ, Coleman ML, Bix M, Tantin D, Park H, Kuchroo VK, Regev A (2013) Dynamic regulatory network controlling TH17 cell differentiation. Nature 496(7446):461–468. doi:10.1038/nature11981
147. Lepple-Wienhues A, Belka C, Laun T, Jekle A, Walter B, Wieland U, Welz M, Heil L, Kun J, Busch G, Weller M, Bamberg M, Gulbins E, Lang F (1999) Stimulation of CD95 (Fas) blocks T lymphocyte calcium channels through sphingomyelinase and sphingolipids. Proc Natl Acad Sci U S A 96(24):13795–13800

148. Strauss G, Lindquist JA, Arhel N, Felder E, Karl S, Haas TL, Fulda S, Walczak H, Kirchhoff F, Debatin KM (2009) CD95 co-stimulation blocks activation of naive T cells by inhibiting T cell receptor signaling. J Exp Med 206(6):1379–1393. doi:10.1084/jem.20082363. jem.20082363 [pii]
149. Dhein J, Walczak H, Baumler C, Debatin KM, Krammer PH (1995) Autocrine T-cell suicide mediated by APO-1/(Fas/CD95). Nature 373(6513):438–441
150. Muppidi JR, Siegel RM (2004) Ligand-independent redistribution of Fas (CD95) into lipid rafts mediates clonotypic T cell death. Nat Immunol 5(2):182–189
151. Legembre P, Daburon S, Moreau P, Ichas F, de Giorgi F, Moreau JF, Taupin JL (2005) Amplification of Fas-mediated apoptosis in type II cells via microdomain recruitment. Mol Cell Biol 25(15):6811–6820. doi:10.1128/MCB.25.15.6811-6820.2005
152. Steinmetz OM, Turner JE, Paust HJ, Lindner M, Peters A, Heiss K, Velden J, Hopfer H, Fehr S, Krieger T, Meyer-Schwesinger C, Meyer TN, Helmchen U, Mittrucker HW, Stahl RA, Panzer U (2009) CXCR3 mediates renal Th1 and Th17 immune response in murine lupus nephritis. J Immunol 183(7):4693–4704. doi:10.4049/jimmunol.0802626
153. Yang J, Chu Y, Yang X, Gao D, Zhu L, Yang X, Wan L, Li M (2009) Th17 and natural Treg cell population dynamics in systemic lupus erythematosus. Arthritis Rheum 60(5):1472–1483. doi:10.1002/art.24499
154. Motz GT, Santoro SP, Wang LP, Garrabrant T, Lastra RR, Hagemann IS, Lal P, Feldman MD, Benencia F, Coukos G (2014) Tumor endothelium FasL establishes a selective immune barrier promoting tolerance in tumors. Nat Med. doi:10.1038/nm.3541
155. Baaten BJ, Cooper AM, Swain SL, Bradley LM (2013) Location, location, location: the impact of migratory heterogeneity on T cell function. Front Immunol 4:311. doi:10.3389/fimmu.2013.00311
156. Maceyka M, Harikumar KB, Milstien S, Spiegel S (2012) Sphingosine-1-phosphate signaling and its role in disease. Trends Cell Biol 22(1):50–60. doi:10.1016/j.tcb.2011.09.003
157. Brinkmann V, Billich A, Baumruker T, Heining P, Schmouder R, Francis G, Aradhye S, Burtin P (2010) Fingolimod (FTY720): discovery and development of an oral drug to treat multiple sclerosis. Nat Rev Drug Discov 9(11):883–897. doi:10.1038/nrd3248

Chapter 8
TLR3 Is a Death Receptor Target in Cancer Therapy

Yann Estornes, Toufic Renno, and Serge Lebecque

Abstract TLR3 is a pattern-recognition receptor specialized in detecting extracellular double-stranded RNAs (dsRNAs) that sign the presence of virus. Accordingly, TLR3 triggers a Type I-IFN dominated inflammatory response in immune and non-immune normal cells. Remarkably, TLR3 behaves also as a death receptor activating the extrinsic pathway of apoptosis in a broad variety of human epithelial cancer cells. In addition, TLR3 is highly expressed by myeloid dendritic cells that undergo maturation in the presence of Poly(I:C), a synthetic dsRNA that mimics viral dsRNA. In particular, the $BDCA3^{+}$ subset of human dendritic cells that is specialized in antigen cross-presentation express the highest level of TLR3. Therefore, the double activity of TLR3 ligand to trigger apoptosis and inflammation of epithelial cancer cells and to initiate dendritic cells maturation suggests that TLR3 ligand may provide simultaneously the two components required for tumor autovaccination: the tumor-associated antigens released in immunogenic apoptotic bodies and the adjuvant to enhance their cross-presentation by dendritic cells to T cells. Here, we review the rationale for targeting TLR3 in cancer and for its combination with immune-checkpoint inhibitors.

Keywords TLR3 • Caspase-8 • Apoptosis • dsRNA

Y. Estornes • T. Renno
Centre de Recherche en Cancérologie de Lyon, UMR INSERM 1052–CNRS 5286, Centre Léon Bérard Batiment Cheney D, 6ème étage, 28, rue Laënnec, Lyon, France

S. Lebecque (✉)
Centre de Recherche en Cancérologie de Lyon, UMR INSERM 1052–CNRS 5286, Centre Léon Bérard Batiment Cheney D, 6ème étage, 28, rue Laënnec, Lyon, France

Université Claude Bernard Lyon 1, Lyon, France

Hospices Civils de Lyon, Centre Hospitalier Lyon Sud, Pierre Bénite, France
e-mail: serge.lebecque@univ-lyon1.fr

O. Micheau (ed.), *TRAIL, Fas Ligand, TNF and TLR3 in Cancer*, Resistance to Targeted Anti-Cancer Therapeutics, DOI 10.1007/978-3-319-56805-8_8

8.1 Introduction

Toll-like Receptor 3 (TLR3) is one of the ten human members of the TLR family of Pattern Recognition Receptor (PRR) that participates to the innate immune response against viral infection through recognition of dsRNA. However, beside triggering inflammation, TLR3 can also behave as a Death Receptor (DR) and cause the demise of cells through direct activation of the extrinsic pathway of apoptosis. DRs are a subset of the Tumor Necrosis Factor (TNF) Receptor superfamily of plasma membrane receptors characterized by a cytoplasmic sequence of ~80 amino acids known as the death domain (DD) [1] In human, 8 DRs have been identified: TNFR1, CD95/Apo1/Fas, Apo2/TRAIL receptors DR4 (TNFSF10A) and DR5 (TNFRSF10B), Apo3/LARD/TNFRSF25, DR6/TNFRSF, ectodysplasin A receptor (EDAR), and p75 neurotrophin receptor (NGFR). Triggering of DR leads to the activation of three main signal transduction pathways: NF-kB-mediated inflammation, mitogen-associated protein kinase-mediated stress response and caspase 8/10-mediated apoptosis. Selective triggering of DR-mediated apoptosis in cancer cells, in particular through TRAIL receptors is a novel approach in cancer therapy that has shown impressive preclinical results, but clinical trials with TRAIL receptor agonists have been disappointing [2]. Here we review the features of apoptosis, cell activation, and inflammation triggered by TLR3 that make this receptor a promising target for cancer therapy.

8.2 TLR3 is a PRR that Recognizes dsRNA

8.2.1 The TLR3 Gene and Protein

Human TLR3 is a type 1 transmembrane receptor of 906 aa consisting of an extracellular domain (ECD) made of 23 leucine-rich repeat (LRR) motifs, a transmembrane (TM) domain, and an intracellular Toll and IL-1R (TIR) domain. The ECD of TLR3 forms a horseshoe-shaped fold with one face devoid of glycosylation and belongs to the single-domain fold because, as shown in the X-ray structure [3, 4], its LRR domain has uniform β-sheet angles and a continuous asparagine network [5]. Three distinctive features put TLR3 somehow apart from the nine other members of the human Toll-like receptor family of PRR: first, the TLR3 gene located on chromosome 4q35.1 is composed of 5 exons, in contrast to the other TLRs that contain only one exon; second, a comparison of the TLRs from 96 species revealed that the LRR domains of TLR3 and TLR7 are the most highly conserved [6] and one of the four intracellular human TLRs (TLR3, TLR7, TLR8, and TLR9) that have evolved under the strongest purifying selection throughout human history [7]. TLR3 recognizes dsRNA [8], and it was therefore thought that TLR3 acted as a sentinel against viruses. It has been speculated that the extreme conservation of TLR3 ECD may result from the concurrent constraints imposed by the protection against viruses and the danger of autoimmune disease potentially triggered by self RNA [7]; third, in contrast with the nine other human TLRs that all use MYD88, TLR3 signaling pathway is mediated exclusively by the TIR domain-containing adapter inducing IFN-β (TRIF) also called Toll-interleukin 1 receptor domain (TIR)-containing adaptor molecule (TICAM-1) which is recruited to TLR3 by interaction with the TIR domains of TLR3 dimers [9, 10]. Crystallization studies have shown that TLR3 binds to dsRNA of at least 45 bp in length through two sites located at the N- and C-terminal ends of the ECD, and intermolecular contacts between the C-terminal domains of two TLR3-ECDs coordinate and stabilize the TLR3 dimer [4, 11, 12]. However, shorter dsRNA appear to bind TLR3 ECD, especially at low pH (<5.0) [13]. Thus, the binding of dsRNA to the TLR3-ECD with an affinity that increases with buffer acidity and, to some extent, with ligand size, represents the first key step in TLR3 signaling, and the minimal signaling unit appears to be one TLR3 dimer [14, 15].

8.2.2 *Expression of TLR3 in Normal Tissues and Their Response to TLR3 Activation*

The strongest expression of TLR3 is observed in myeloid and epithelial cells. At the mRNA level, monocyte-derived DC (mDC) were initially reported to be the resting human leukocytes to express the largest amount of TLR3 mRNA, and maturation of mDC by inflammatory signal such as TNF-α, LPS, or IL-1 was associated with the downregulation of TLR3 mRNA level [16, 17]. In mice however, macrophages display the strongest expression of TLR3 mRNA [8, 18]. In both species, TLR3 expression was further increased after viral infection or treatment with IFN-I [19, 20]. Among DC subpopulations, the $CD8\alpha^{+}$ [20] and $BDCA3^{+}$ subsets that represent the most effective cross-presenting DC in mouse and human, respectively, were found to express the highest level of TLR3. Moreover, in situ hybridization confirmed the expression of the receptor by DC present in the T cell-dependent areas of human lymph nodes while Langerhans cells were negative [16] or weakly positive [21]. In addition, both human and mouse mast cells express a functional TLR3 [22].

The expression of TLR3 has been reliably demonstrated in many types of primary human epithelial cells including keratinocytes [23], trophoblasts [24, 25], bronchial epithelial cells [19, 26], pancreatic islet cells [27], kidney glomerular mesangial and tubular cells [28], uterine epithelial cells [29, 30], endothelial cells [31], human retinal pigment epithelial cells [32], hepatocytes [33], ileal and colonic epithelial cells [34], nasal epithelial cells [35], cervical epithelial cells [36], corneal epithelial cells [37], smooth muscle cells of mid-sized arteries [38], synovial lining fibroblasts [39], and skin fibroblasts [40]. In CNS, TLR3 mRNA is expressed by primary cultures of both human microglia cells and astrocytes [41, 42] and detected in neurons by immunohistochemistry [43]. Noticeably, the expression of TLR3 can be upregulated in several cell types so as that they become responsive to Poly(I:C) after either viral infection or pretreatment with type I IFN [31]. Regarding the control of TLR3 expression, IRF3 and p53 were shown to enhance *TLR3* transcription

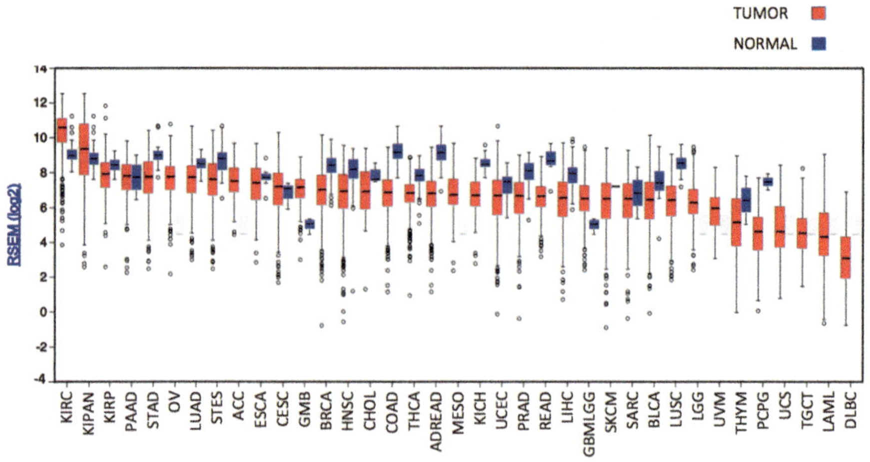

ACC	Adrenocortical carcinoma	KICH	Kidney Chromophobe	PAAD	Pancreatic adenocarcinoma
BLCA	Bladder Urothelial Carcinoma	KIPAN	Pan-kidney cohort (KICH+KIRC+KIRP)	PCPG	Pheochromocytoma and Paraganglioma
BRCA	Breast invasive carcinoma	KIRC	Kidney renal clear cell carcinoma	PRAD	Prostate adenocarcinoma
CESC	Cervical squamous cell carcinoma and endocervical adenocarcinoma	KIRP	Kidney renal papillary cell carcinoma	READ	Rectum adenocarcinoma
CHOL	Cholangiocarcinoma	LAML	Acute Myeloid Leukemia	SARC	Sarcoma
COAD	Colon adenocarcinoma	LGG	Brain Lower Grade Glioma	SKCM	Skin Cutaneous Melanoma
COADREA	Colorectal adenocarcinoma	LIHC	Liver hepatocellular carcinoma	STAD	Stomach adenocarcinoma
DLBC	Lymphoid Neoplasm Diffuse Large B-cell Lymphoma	LUAD	Lung adenocarcinoma	STES	Stomach and Esophageal carcinoma
ESCA	Esophageal carcinoma	LUSC	Lung squamous cell carcinoma	TGCT	Testicular Germ Cell Tumors
GBM	Glioblastoma multiforme	MESO	Mesothelioma	THCA	Thyroid carcinoma
GBMLGG	Glioma	OV	Ovarian serous cystadenocarcinoma	THYM	Thymoma
HNSC	Head and Neck squamous cell carcinoma			UCEC	Uterine Corpus Endometrial Carcinoma
				UCS	Uterine Carcinosarcoma
				UVM	Uveal Melanoma

Fig. 8.1 Relative expression of TLR3mRNA in cancer vs. normal human tissues. The results shown here are based on data generated by the TCGA Research Network: http://cancergenome.nih.gov/. The figure and information regarding the cohorts of cancers can be directly retrieved from the TCGA website at http://firebrowse.org/viewGene.html?gene=TLR3#

[44], while E2F1 has an inhibitory activity [45]. TLR3 is found exclusively in the intracellular endocytic compartment and/or in the Golgi apparatus, except in lung fibroblasts where TLR3 expression on the cell surface has been reported [40]. Figure 8.1 compares the TLR3 mRNA expression in normal vs. cancer tissues.

The common activities of TLR3 in normal cells reflect the signaling pathways that appear to concur to trigger an antiviral immune response through activation of IRF3, NF-kB, and AP1 transcription factors. Like other nucleotide-sensing TLRs (TLR7, TLR9), TLR3 is recruited from the endoplasmic reticulum to endosomes by the transmembrane protein UNC93B1 [46]. However, in contrast with TLR7 or 9, the constitutive cleavage by cathepsins of the majority of TLR3 in resting cells suggests that its trafficking to endolysosome is independent of ligand binding [47, 48]. Unlike other TLRs, phosphorylation of Tyr759 and Tyr858 in the cytoplasmic domain of TLR3 is required to activate downstream signaling. The recruitment of the epidermal growth factor receptor (EGFR) by dsRNA-bound TLR3 leading to

Tyr858 phosphorylation is an early event of the signaling process [49], which is followed by Src recruitment and Tyr759 phosphorylation [50]. In addition, phosphoinositide 3-kinase [51] and Bruton's tyrosine kinase [52] have been implicated in TLR3 phosphorylation, which is a prerequisite for TRIF recruitment. An alanine that replaces the conserved proline residue present in the BB-loop of most TLRs' TIR domains appears to be responsible for the direct recruitment of TRIF rather than MyD88 to initiate signaling [53]. The N-terminal domain of TRIF mediates the formation of a signalosome complex containing key molecules, such as NAP1 [54] and TRAF3 [55]. The signalosome drives the recruitment and activation of the kinases IKKε and TBK-1, which in turn phosphorylates IRF3 [56, 57], enabling its dimerization, nuclear translocation and transcription of *IFN-β*. Full activation of IRF3 appears to require its additional PI3K-dependent phosphorylation [51]. Autocrine IFN-β activates the transcription factors signal transducer and activator of transcription (STAT) 1 and 2, resulting in the transcription of type-1 IFN target genes and subsequent antiviral responses [58]. IRF3 signaling is under the negative feedback control of the TLR3-induced and NF-kB-dependent deubiquitinase A20 [59]. The same N-terminal region of TRIF also recruits the K63-linked ubiquitin E3 ligase TRAF6, thereby activating TAK1, a member of the MAPKKK family that activates canonical IKKs (IKKα and IKKβ), allowing NF-kB to translocate to the nucleus [60]. TAK1 simultaneously activates the MAPK (JNK, p38, and ERK) pathway, leading to activation of members of the AP-1 family of transcription factors. The C-terminal region of TRIF contains a receptor-interacting protein (RIP) homotypic interaction motif (RHIM), which associates with the receptor-interacting protein kinases RIPK1 and RIPK3. cIAP1/2 mediated K63-linked polyubiquitination triggers the recruitment of TRAF6 and transforming growth factor-beta activated kinase 1 (TAK1), which enhance both NF-kB and MAPK activation [61]. As a result of activating the IRF3, NF-kB, and AP1 transcription factors, TLR3 triggers a strong inflammatory response in non-transformed human epithelial cells with no apparent cytotoxicity [59, 62–64]. Type I IFN, RANTES, IP-10, IL-6, IL-8, TNF-α, GM-CSF, Mip-3a, and serum amyloid A represent the secreted proteins most frequently reported in response to TLR3 activation. Importantly, a large number of negative and positive regulators of TLR3 signaling that target TRIF, TRAF3, RIPK1, and TRAF6 have been described (reviewed in [65]). Beside eliciting an inflammatory response, whether TLR3 can trigger the death of non-transformed cells remains unclear. Overexpression of exogenous TRIF leads to the RHIM domain-dependent recruitment of RIPK1 and RIPK3, FADD and caspase-8, resulting in cell apoptosis. However, normal human cells of different origins were found to be resistant to the cytotoxicity of Poly(I:C). In contrast, mouse peritoneal macrophages underwent TRIF-dependent apoptosis when exposed to Poly(I:C) together with the proteasome inhibitor MG132 [66], but the autocrine role of TNF-α had not been ruled out. Likewise, primary mouse β-pancreatic cells exposed to IFN-I or II [67, 68] and primary porcine retinal pigment epithelium cells [69] were shown to undergo apoptosis following Poly(I:C) treatment, but again the role of TLR3 was not directly established. The same is true for the ability of dsRNA isolated from rotavirus to kill mouse primary intestinal epithelial cells [70]. In vivo, small intestinal injury, which represent the limiting toxicity of Poly(I:C) in mice, has been attributed to a direct apoptotic effect of TLR3 on normal intestinal epithelial cells (IECs). However, TLR3 signaling was found to induce IECs to express Rae1, which mediates epithelial destruction and mucosal injury by interacting with the activating receptor NKG2D expressed on intestinal intraepithelial NK cells [71]. Lastly, mouse neuronal precursor cells undergo TLR3-dependent apoptosis when exposed to Poly(I:C), but the death of the cells might be triggered indirectly via Fas [72]. In summary, TLR3 is expressed by a large variety of non-transformed immune and epithelial cells where it triggers inflammation without clear evidence of direct cytotoxicity. However, it remains possible that normal cells infected by some viruses might become sensitive to TLR3-triggered apoptosis.

8.3 TLR3 Activation by Pathogen-Derived and Self dsRNAs

All the natural TLR3 ligands identified up to now are dsRNAs coming from pathogens or from endogenous sources. TLR3 has the theoretical ability to play a key role of sentinel against viral infection, as dsRNA may represent either the genome of some viruses or the intermediates of their replication generated during most viral infections [73]. The exact nature of dsRNA produced during viral infection that stimulates TLR3 is generally missing, except for poliovirus-derived single-stranded RNA segments harboring stem structures with bulge/internal loops [74]. Epstein–Barr virus (EBV)-encoded small RNA (EBER) released from human EBV-infected cells represent a second example of well-defined viral ligand that activates signaling from TLR3 [75].

Studies of experimental viral infection with TLR3 KO mice have revealed the role of the receptor in defense against many RNA viruses. However, several parameters such as the strain of the TLR3 KO mice, the dose and mode of inoculation of the virus and the readouts must be considered to interpret the published data. TLR3 KO mice are more susceptible to death following challenge with encephalomyocarditis virus, coxsackievirus group B3 (CVB3), CVB4, and poliovirus, and they show impaired control of infection by respiratory syncytial virus, but also of infection of the CNS by herpes simplex virus 2 (HSV-2), a DNA virus (reviewed in [76]). In human, the importance of TLR3 in viral protection has been strikingly demonstrated by the discovery that mutations affecting not only TLR3 but also UNC93B1, TRIF, TRAF3, or TBK1 can all be associated with life-threatening childhood HSV-1 encephalitis while remaining normally resistant to other common viruses [77–81]. Incidentally, it has been reported that dsRNA from helminth schistosoma activates TLR3 in DC [82].

Regarding self-RNAs that are tenfold more abundant than DNA in cells, they represent a potential source of natural ligands for TLR3. Indirect evidence for endogenous ligand comes from the observation that TLR3 is a negative regulator of embryonic neural progenitor cell proliferation during mouse development, even though the trigger was not identified [83]. It was first described that endogenous mRNA, which is single-stranded but contains double-stranded regions and is released from necrotic cells, can activate TLR3 [84]. However, in contrast to in vitro-transcribed mRNA that activates TLR3, the poly-A tail and nucleoside modifications present on in vivo transcribed mammalian mRNA suppress this activation [84–86]. RNA released by necrotic cells in rheumatoid arthritis synovial fluid was the first description of an endogenous TLR3 ligand potentially involved in pathologic inflammation [39]. Similarly, RNA liberated by necrotic neurons [87], necrotic neutrophils [88] necrotic keratinocytes [89], and dying retinal cells [90] appears to be involved in TLR3-triggered inflammation. It was later reported that U1-snRNA is liberated by ultraviolet-damaged cells and drives skin inflammation through TLR3 activation [91]. Composed of 164 nucleotides and characterized by stretches of double-stranded RNA U1-snRNA (the defining part of U1-RNP) is the most abundant small nuclear RNA in eukaryotic cells and has been shown to activate TLR3 [92]. In cells undergoing apoptosis, U1-snRNA is concentrated in apoptotic bodies, and thus can activate TLR3 found in the endosomes of phagocytes during efferocytosis [93]. Recently, tumor exosomal snRNA has been shown to promote lung premetastatic niche formation by activating alveolar epithelial TLR3 in mouse tumor models [94].

8.4 Synthetic Ligands for TLR3

All TLR3 agonist that have been described are dsRNA, and while their sequences do not appear to play a dominant role, their length and structure are important for TLR3 binding and activation. In particular long dsRNAs are more potent inducers of TLR3 signaling than short ones. Synthetic poly(I:C) is the most often used ligand, although it is a nonspecific agonist of TLR3 [8]. Indeed, Poly(I:C) has an undefined chemical structure and very poor homogeneity, being composed of a mix of single-stranded and double-stranded RNA molecules ranging from about 1.5 to 8 kb [95] that are imperfectly annealed. As a consequence Poly(I:C) can also activate the cytosolic dsRNA receptors MDA5 and RIG-I [95–97]. Poly-ICLC (Hiltonol® from Oncovir), a form of Poly(I:C) stabilized with polylysine and carboxymethylcellulose activates TLR3 and is a potent inducer of serum type I IFN [98]. However, the capacity of polylysine to enhance cell transfection suggests that Poly-ICLC could activate not only TLR3 but also cytosolic sensors such as MDA5, the 2′-5′-oligoadenylate synthetase (OAS) and the p68 protein kinase PKR. Nevertheless, Phase I/II clinical trials with local administration of Hiltonol as adjuvant indicate that low doses of Hiltonol are not particularly toxic. PolyI:polyC12U (Ampligene® from Hemispherix) is another modification of Poly(I:C) where uracil replaces every 12th cytosine in order to decrease the toxicity (and the potency) of Poly(I:C) and to insure the TLR3 specificity [99]. Poly(A:U) is also a synthetic ligand which appears to be more specific for TLR3, at least in human, but which has substantially lower potency than poly(I:C) [100] possibly due to decreased ligand uptake and/or stability. Nevertheless, Poly(A:U) has been shown to have beneficial effect when injected in gastric and breast cancer patients [101, 102]. Recent publications have reported the activation of TLR3 by the short (23-bp) dsRNA BM06, but experimental evidence of TLR3 specificity is still missing [103, 104]. Seya et al. have developed an original and TLR3-specific chimeric ligand (ssODN-dsRNA) named ARNAX.

It consists of a viral ssRNA spontaneously folding into dsRNA stretches covalently linked to a short phosphorothioate ODN required for recognition by scavenger receptors at the cell surface and internalization [105, 106]. Lastly, RGC100 produced by Riboxx is a new ligand specific for TLR3 with a defined chemical structure, homogenous length (100 bp) and high resistance to RNAses [107]. Of note, the requirement for receptor multimerization through cross-linking of mAb directed to recombinant TLR3 expressed at the cell membrane [15, 100] and the acidic condition in endosomes/lysosomes where the endogenous receptor resides can explain the failure so far to generate agonistic anti-TLR3 mAb. In contrast, blocking anti-TLR3 mAbs have been generated and found to be active in vitro [40, 108].

8.5 Sides Effects of TLR3 Ligand

Intravenous injection of Poly(A:U) elicits only mild side effects. However, the manifestations of acute toxicity following systemic administration of different formulations of Poly(I:C) that activates non only TLR3, but also RIG-I and MDA5, included fever, hypotension, myalgia, and arthralgia [109] that likely resulted from massive cytokines release [110, 111]. In contrast to Poly(I:C), a selective TLR3 ligand does not trigger systemic cytokinemia following i.p. injection in mice [105]. Activation by TLR3 ligands of mDC, macrophages and epithelial cells suggests that they should be able to induce and/or exacerbate some autoimmune diseases. Indeed, viral infections can trigger disease activity in autoimmunity in general, and elevated IFN-I levels promote the progression of autoimmune tissue injury in systemic lupus erythematous. Thus, when short (34-bp) viral dsRNA was injected i.v. in lupus-prone $MRL^{lpr/lpr}$ mice, it was found to accumulate in glomerular mesangial cells which responded to Poly(I:C) by secreting IFN-β, IL-6, and CCL2 in vitro. Furthermore, repeated i.p. injections of Poly(I:C) in $MRL^{lpr/lpr}$ mice increased the secretion of CCL2 and CCL5 which both recruit leukocytes in the kidney, and markedly aggravated the glomerulonephritis associated with severe tubulo-interstitial injuries [28]. In conclusion, while acute toxicity appears to be significantly reduced for TLR3-specific ligands compared with Poly(I:C), long term exacerbation of autoimmune manifestations is intrinsically associated with the potent adjuvant activity of dsRNA.

8.6 Expression of TLR3 by Cancer Cells and Their Response to TLR3 Activation

Tumor data available online from the Broad institute (Fig. 8.1) show that TLR3 mRNA is highly expressed in a high proportion of epithelial tumors, in particular kidney, pancreas and ovarian cancers. The expression of TLR3 by tumor cells themselves has been confirmed by IHC in nasopharyngeal adenocarcinoma cells [112], oesophageal squamous cell carcinomas, cervical squamous cell carcinomas [113],

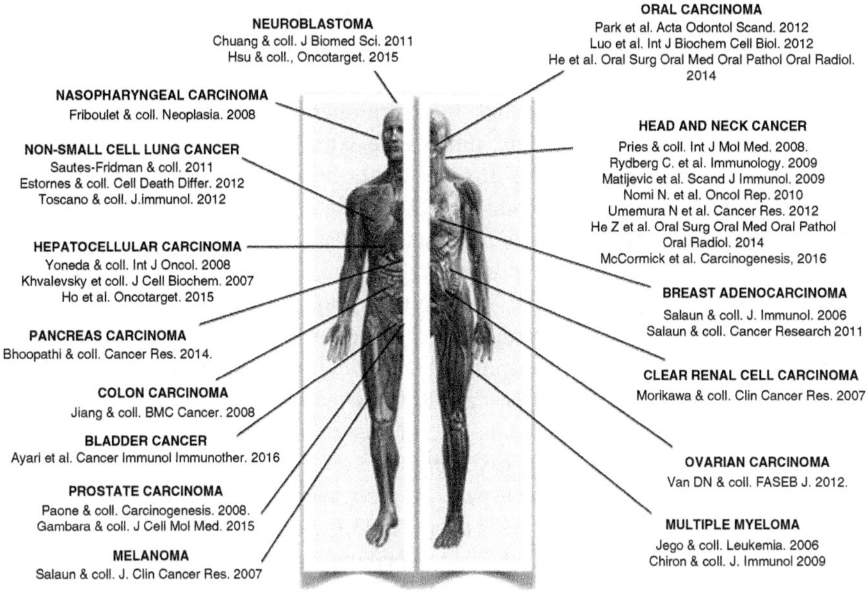

Fig. 8.2 The human epithelial cancer types for which a pro-apoptotic activity of TLR3 ligand in vitro has been reported are listed

oral squamous cancer cells [114–116], colon carcinoma [117], hepatocellular carcinoma [118, 119], papillary thyroid cancer cells [120], prostate cancer [121], ovarian cancer [122], esophageal cancer [123], breast cancer [102], mesothelioma cells [124], cervical cancer [113], endometrial carcinoma [125], and lung small cells and non-small cell cancers and adenocarcinomas (our submitted data). Data from the Human Protein Atlas available online (http://www.proteinatlas.org/ENSG00000164342-TLR3/cancer) confirm those observations and illustrate the expression of TLR3 in pancreatic, endometrial, melanoma, and urothelial cancer cells. Those analyses have revealed the heterogeneity of TLR3 staining in tumors, and it would be interesting to determine whether this might reflect, at least in part, different status of cancer cells (i.e., cancer cells' stemness, epithelial–mesenchymal transition, or senescence). The therapeutic importance of targeting TLR3 expressed by tumor cells themselves was suggested by a retrospective analysis of a clinical trial wherein breast cancer patients had been treated with Poly(A:U) injections. It was indeed shown that the clinical benefit was strictly limited to patients whose tumor cells expressed TLR3 [102].

TLR3 ligands have been found to decrease the proliferation of cancer cells through the autocrine effect of type I IFN signaling and blockade of cell cycle through combined downregulation of cyclin D1 and upregulation of cyclin-dependent kinase inhibitor p27 [126]. In addition, the first direct pro-apoptotic activity of TLR3 ligand has been demonstrated in cancer cells wherein TLR3 behaves like a death receptor [127]. Figure 8.2 summarizes the data from the literature showing that many types of human epithelial cancer cells undergo apoptosis upon TLR3 activation. Occasional reports have implicated PKC-alpha-dependent mechanism [128], or survivin [129], but the generality of these observations remains to be confirmed.

TLR3 mediates apoptosis through the recruitment and activation of caspase-8 into an atypical death complex, and initiates the extrinsic pathway of apoptosis in a similar way as the DRs of the TNF-R superfamily. dsRNA triggers the formation of a multiprotein death complex containing TLR3, the adapter TRIF, RIPK1, cellular FLICE-Like Inhibitory Protein (cFLIP), and procaspase-8/procaspase-10. Hence, TLR3-mediated death complex resembles the Death-Inducing Signaling Complex (DISC) initiated by the TRAIL-R, Fas, TNF-R1, and CD40. The DISC formation mediated by DRs relies on a homotypic interaction between the Death Domain (DD) within the DR and the adaptor FADD which then recruits Death Effector Domain (DED)-containing procaspase-8/procaspase-10. Activation of procaspase-8/procaspase-10 within TRAIL-R- and Fas-associated DISC relies on DED-mediated chain formation to drive procaspase dimerization, and activation [130–133]. Activated caspase-8/caspase-10 then initiate the extrinsic pathway of apoptosis and caspases cascade. However, TLR3 is devoid of a cytosolic DD, and the current model proposes that TLR3 engagement by dsRNA triggers the recruitment of the adapter TRIF via a homotypic interaction between the RHIM domain within the receptor and TRIF. TRIF then recruits RIPK1 which contains a RHIM domain, but also a DD allowing the recruitment of FADD, and subsequently procaspase-8/procaspase-10 [134–137]. Due to its dependence on RIPK1, this death platform associated to TLR3/TRIF is also called Ripoptosome [135, 138]. Several negative regulators of the stability and/or activity of TLR3-death complex have been reported. Cellular Inhibitor of APoptosis (cIAP) 1 and 2 ubiquitin ligases limit the formation/stabilization of the TLR3 death complex probably via RIPK1 polyubiquitylation [134, 135, 139, 140], as reported for TNF-R1 signaling [141, 142]. Consistent with this hypothesis, TRAF2 and TRADD are also detected within TLR3 death complex to form the ubiquitin ligase complex TRAF2-TRADD-cIAPs [134]. c-FLIP, a well-known regulator of caspase-8, is also detected within TLR3 death complex [134, 135]. cFLIP potently inhibits the pro-apoptotic activity of this atypical DISC, potentially in a similar way as described downstream the DRs. The preferential formation of c-FLIP$_L$/caspase-8 heterodimer [143] has a limited but selective catalytic activity toward proximal substrate like RIPK1, which leads to the liberation of caspase-8 pro-apoptotic p10-p20 fragments [130, 144]. Hence, c-FLIP$_L$, when expressed above a certain threshold, prevents caspase-8 pro-apoptotic activity, and can also destabilize the ripoptosome [135].

In humans, apoptosis induction via TLR3 is limited to tumor cells, suggesting that sensitivity to apoptosis is somehow acquired during transformation. However, the molecular determinants of this differential sensitivity remain unclear. Although the expression of the receptor and the existence of a functional signaling pathway to caspase-8-dependent apoptosis are clearly required for cancer cells to die following TLR3 activation, the level of TLR3 expression does not appear to dictate the cell fate in the presence of dsRNA, at least in vitro. In addition, one study reported that TLR3 overexpression by tumor cells in prostate carcinoma was associated with poor clinical outcome, but another publication showed no evidence for correlation between TLR3 expression and either clinical grade or prognosis in oesophageal cancer [123]. As observed with TNF, inhibition of protein synthesis with cycloheximide sensitizes cancer cells to TLR3-triggered apoptosis [145, 146]. The role of c-IAP2 in the resistance to TLR3-triggered apoptosis was first demonstrated in EBV-associated nasopharyngeal carcinomas [119]. We recently observed that c-FLIP, a protein with a short half-life whose expression is critically dependent on NF-kB-driven transcription, represents the major regulator of TLR3-driven apoptosis in human lung and head-and-neck cancer cells (manuscript submitted). Recently, the linear ubiquitin chain assembly complex (LUBAC) has been shown to participate in the NF-kB and MAPK signaling pathway downstream of TLR3 and to be required to prevent TLR3-triggered apoptosis of the human transformed keratinocyte cell line (HaCaT) [147]. Consistent with this, the increased sensitivity of metastatic vs. primary Head and Neck Squamous Cell Carcinoma (HNSCC) cells has been ascribed to the inability of the former to activate NF-kB activation in response to TLR3 ligand [63]. Altogether, these data suggest that differences in TLR3 signaling complexes that remain to be identified but lead to differential activation of NF-kB and MAPK could explain why human tumors epithelial cells frequently succumb to TLR3 ligand while normal cells are resistant. One study has suggested that reduced RIPK1 expression sensitizes HNSCC cells to TLR3-triggered apoptosis, but simultaneously promotes several other pro-tumorigenic properties of the cells [148].

In the presence of chemical or viral caspase inhibitor, or following caspase-8 genetic ablation, DRs have also been shown to induce another form of regulated cell death, with features of necrosis, called necroptosis. Mechanistically, necroptosis depends on the formation of a cytosolic signaling platform called necrosome which contains the key components RIPK1, RIPK3, and mixed lineage kinase domain-like (MLKL) ([149–151], and see for review [152]). MLKL then undergoes a conformational change that relies on RIPK3-dependent phosphorylation, and translocates to the plasma membrane, leading to its permeabilization [153–156]. It has also been reported that TLR3 mediates necroptosis in transformed and non-transformed cells. Mouse Macrophages [157, 158], rat and mouse microglia [159], mouse fibroblasts [158, 160, 161], but also mouse colon cancer CT26 cells [161] massively die by necroptosis upon treatment with Poly(I:C) in condition of caspases inhibition by Z-VAD. Although the requirement of RIPK3 and MLKL for TLR3-mediated necroptosis has been well demonstrated by chemical and genetic approaches [157–160], the role of RIPK1 remains to be clarified. TRIF can bind RIPK1 and/or RIPK3 via homotypic interaction between their respective RHIM domains [157, 162]. However, while RIPK1 allosteric inhibitor necrostatin-1 [163] blocks TLR3-mediated necroptosis in murine cells [158, 159, 161], it has no effect, together with RIPK1 knockdown, in mouse fibroblasts [158]. Like for apoptosis induction, necroptosis induced by Poly(I:C) is fully dependent on TLR3/TRIF, and independent of the TNFR pathway [158, 161]. It is important to notice that RIPK3 is frequently downregulated in human transformed cells, at least in part through the methylation of *RIPK3* genomic DNA, hence limiting the possibility of inducing necroptosis through TLR3 targeting in human cancers [164, 165].

In contrast, the possibility that TLR3 activation in cancer cells might favor tumor progression is suggested by some reports. Indeed, TLR3 ligand was found to reduce, although modestly, the spontaneous apoptosis of two human breast cancer cell lines and to induce c-Myc-dependent cell proliferation in human head-and-neck cancer cell lines in vitro [166, 167]. TLR3 triggering was also found to enhance the proliferation of 1 out of 7 human multiple myeloma cell lines analyzed [168]. In addition, it has been suggested that activation of TLR3 in tumor cells may enhance metastasis of pharyngeal and papillary thyroid cancer [120, 169] and facilitate evasion of immune surveillance through the secretion of chemokines with immunosuppressive effects [170]. Altogether, the published data suggest that TLR3 activation mostly inhibits the growth of many types of epithelial cancer cells, mostly through the induction of apoptosis accompanied by inflammation, although a role of necroptosis cannot be excluded.

8.7 Combotherapy with TLR3 Ligands

Several approaches have been explored to increase the ability of TLR3 to inhibit cell tumor growth. Upregulation of TLR3 expression with IFN-I sensitizes resistant melanoma cell lines to the apoptosis triggered by dsRNA [145]. Similarly, the DNA-damaging reagent 5-fluorouracil was found to upregulate in a p53-dependent manner the expression of TLR3, thereby increasing the apoptosis triggered by Poly(I:C) in human colon carcinoma HCT116 cells [171]. Similar p53-dependent synergy between doxorubicin and Poly(I:C) has been reported in HCT116 cells [172]. The synergy with doxorubicin was confirmed in breast cancer cell lines [173], and extended to paclitaxel [174], 5-FU and methotrexate [175], gemcitabine [176], and carboplatin [177]. Regarding the mechanisms of synergy with chemotherapeutic agents, we found that the suppression of c-FLIP expression by paclitaxel is required for enhancing the apoptosis of cancer cells triggered by TLR3 (manuscript submitted). A similar mechanism has been reported to explain the synergy between IL-24 and influenza A virus for inducing TLR3-dependent apoptosis of human cancer cells [137]. DR-dependent apoptosis is highly sensitive to NF-kB blocking agents, which downregulate the expression of three anti-apoptotic proteins, cIAP1/2 and cFLIP. Thus, cIAPs have been successfully targeted with Smac mimetics to enhance the apoptosis triggered by TNF and TRAIL [178], and FasL [179]. The possibility to sensitize tumor cells to TLR3 ligand by Smac-mimetics was supported by the observation that cIAP overexpression protects EBV-related nasopharyngeal carcinoma cells from death triggered following activation of TLR3 by EBER. Indeed, suppression of cIAP2 with a smac mimetic strongly synergized with Poly(I:C) to kill nasopharyngeal carcinoma cells [180], while normal nasopharyngeal cells remained resistant to the combination [112]. Bernardo et al. have reported yet another mechanism of synergy between retinoic acid and TLR3 ligand to kill human cancer cells through the upregulation and apoptotic signaling of TRAIL [181]. Obviously, the synergy of anticancer drugs may also involve other anticancer activities of TLR3 ligand. For example, the adjuvant activity of poly-ICLC and the indirect activation of NK cells potentiate the antitumor effects of the anti-EGFR cetuximab against head-and-neck cancer cells [182]. Likewise, combination of the multi-kinase inhibitor sorafenib with a synthetic dsRNA was shown to reduce hepatocellular carcinoma tumor growth through direct induction of tumor cell death, activation of host T cells, NK cells, macrophages and DC, and restoration of tumor cells' immunogenicity in the local microenvironment [183, 184]. Changes in the microenvironment were also invoked to explain how Poly(I:C) potentiates Bacillus Calmette-Guérin immunotherapy for bladder cancer [185]. The immunogenic activity of TLR3 likely contributes to the synergy reported into tumor-bearing mice between Poly(I:C) and localized irradiation [186] or anti-PD-L1 mAb [187]. In conclusion, several chemotherapeutic agents as well as ionizing radiations appear to synergize with TLR3 ligand to kill cancer cells directly and/or through an indirect effect mediated by the immune cells.

8.8 TLR3 and Tumor Autovaccination

The superior efficacy of Poly(I:C) in combination with peptide as an adjuvant for tumor vaccination in mice has been amply demonstrated, and result from the combined direct effects on different types of immune and nonimmune cells, including tumor cells themselves, and indirect effects through the production of IFN-I and other cytokines and chemokines [188]. Regarding the adaptive immune response, a subset of human DCs that highly express TLR3 exhibits a better capacity for cross-presenting apoptotic and necrotic cells-derived antigens to CD8 T cells after TLR3 stimulation. In fact, the use of TLR3 ligands as adjuvants in vaccine therapy is based in part on the selective high expression of TLR3 in human BDCA3$^+$ CD141$^+$ DCs and mouse CD8a$^+$ DC subsets [189]. Importantly, IFN-α initiates a positive feedback on DC by enhancing their expression of TLR3, TRIF, and IRF3, thereby augmenting their secretion of IFN-I and IFN-λ (IL-28 and IL-29) in response to TLR3 agonist [190]. In mice, Poly(I:C) acts on splenic CD8α$^+$ DC to cross-prime T cells and on intratumoral DC and macrophages to secrete chemokines (including CCL5, CXCL9, and CXCL10) that attract CTLs [191]. Moreover, after i.v. injection of B16-F10 cells, activation of DCs with Poly(I:C) led to the production of IFN type I and generated an effective CTL response against metastatic lung cancer progression [192]. Indeed, the CTLs activated by TLR3-stimulated DC show increased IFN-γ and TNF-α production and they are relatively protected against apoptosis during the contraction phase of the primary response [193]. Moreover, when used as vaccine adjuvant, Poly(I:C) stimulates the production of IL-12 by mDC (and macrophages), thereby favoring a TH1-biased CD4 T cell-mediated protective response [194]. Lastly, ligation of TLR on DC was shown to block the suppressor activity of regulatory T cells via the secretion of IL-6. Considering the innate immune response, two populations of myeloid cells present at the tumor site do express TLR3 as well: the Myeloid Derived Suppressor Cells (MDSCs), whose frequency and immunosuppressive function are decreased in tumor-bearing mice treated with Poly(I:C) [195] and the Tumor Associated Macrophages (TAMs) that Poly(I:C) converts from M2 tumor-supportive to tumoricidal M1 cells [196]. In addition, dsRNA activates DC and macrophages but also TLR3$^+$ tumor and normal epithelial cells, as well as endothelial cells to secrete type I IFNs that directly suppress tumor cell replication and reduce tumor growth via antiangiogenic properties. Moreover, type I IFNs stimulate DC to cross-present tumor-associated antigen [197], support the clonal expansion and effector differentiation of CD8$^+$ T cells [198], augment NK cell-mediated tumor lysis and enhance the tumoricidal effects of macrophages and pDC (reviewed in [199]).

Beside the powerful adjuvant activity of TLR3 ligand described above, the discovery that activation of TLR3 directly triggers simultaneously the apoptosis and an inflammatory response in human epithelial cancer cells expressing the receptor opens the promising possibility to reach tumor autovaccination without the need for identifying and injecting patient-individualized Tumor-Associated Antigens (TAAs). While dying, TLR3-targeted cancer cells release apoptotic bodies containing an optimized form of TAA for autovaccination: TAAs have been shown to accumulate in apoptotic bodies, and apoptotic bodies-associated dsRNA may represent an even more powerful ligand than free dsRNA for TLR3$^+$ CD8α^+/BDCA3$^+$ mDC that will engulf them [200]. As a result, in cell-associated form of poly(I:C), very low levels of antigen were sufficient to induce robust cross-priming responses in naive mice, further supporting the proposal made a decade ago that "Tumour cells loaded with dsRNA could therefore constitute potent vaccines for cancer immunotherapy" [200]. Importantly, tumor autovaccination based on TLR3-dependent apoptosis has not been addressed properly in mice yet, as, in contrast to human cancer cells, mouse cancer cell lines are resistant to cell death when exposed to TLR3 ligand (our unpublished data). However, when CT26 tumor-bearing mice were treated with Poly(I:C) and the caspase inhibitor zVAD, the necroptotic death of cancer cells contributed to their elimination by CTLs [161]. Of note, in the absence of decription of human cancer cells undergoing necroptosis, it remains uncertain whether such type of cell death could participate in the inflammatory demise of human cancer cells in response to TLR3 ligand, as can occur in mouse tumor [161].

Tumor autovaccination generated by TLR3 ligand would represent useful priming before administration of immune checkpoint inhibitors directed against CTLA-4, PD-1/PD-L1, LAG3, IDO and the additional ones to be confirmed (Fig. 8.3). Indeed, despite the striking efficacy of immune checkpoint inhibitors in an ever-extending variety of cancers, <25% of patients show a prolonged survival. Several factors that have been demonstrated to limit their therapeutic activity, including a low level of expression of the targeted molecules (PD1, PD-L1, CTLA4), a low load of somatic mutations in tumor cells, and the accumulation of MDSC at the site of the tumor. However, the first reason for failure of T cell-targeted immune checkpoint inhibitors currently in the clinic appears to be the absence of tumor-specific CD8$^+$ T cells within the tumor, a situation referred to as "immunological desert" at the tumor site. Therefore, it has become urgent to design innovative vaccine strate-

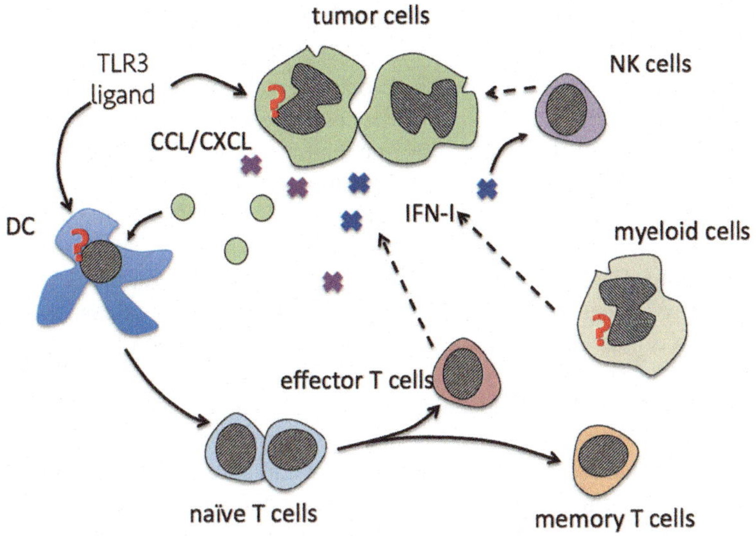

Fig. 8.3 Schematic model of tumor autovaccination by targeting TLR3 in cancer. At the tumor site, TLR3 (represented by red question marks) is mainly expressed by DC, by epithelial cancer cells and by myeloid cells (TAM and MDSC). TLR3 ligand will trigger the "inflammatory apoptosis" of cancer cells and the secretion of chemokines (*blue crosses*) and cytokines (*pink crosses*), and apoptotic bodies will be taken up by tumor-infliltrating DC which, following their activation, will cross-present the full repertoire of TAAs to naïve CD8$^+$ T cells. Effector CTLs will be generated and attracted to the tumor site by the chemokines released by TLR3-activated tumor cells while memory T cells will be generated that could fight back in case of cancer relapse. Through the direct activation by TLR3 ligand, tumor-supportive myeloid cells will be converted into tumor-suppressive cells, while activated DC will indirectly enhance the cytotoxicity of NK cells. Type-I IFNs will assist many aspects of the antitumor activity (see details in the text)

gies for generating a broad repertoire of tumor-specific CD8$^+$ T cells and for driving them in the tumor, two benefits that can be expected from treatment with TLR3 ligand. The rationale for combining TLR3 targeting with immune checkpoint inhibitors is further supported by the observation that TLR3 triggering regulates PD-L1 (CD274) expression in human neuroblastoma cells [201]. Interestingly, the correlation between the inflammatory signature resulting from endogenous retrovirus transcription and immune checkpoint inhibitors response in cancer patients provides indirect evidence for the importance of TLR3 activation in the context of tumor immunotherapy [202]. Several clinical trials using either local injection of Hiltonol® as adjuvant for peptide-based cancer vaccine, or i.p./i.v. administration of Ampligen® in cancer patients in combination with DC-based vaccination are presently underway [203]. However, little attention has been paid so far to the expression and the sensitivity of cancer cells to TLR3-triggered apoptosis that will be required for triggering tumor autovaccination.

8.9 Conclusions

TLR3 ligands have long been considered as attractive adjuvants for cancer vaccine, but the finding that they trigger directly the death of various types of epithelial cancer cells and the recent characterization of potent, specific, and well-defined dsRNA agonists has renewed interest in their clinical potential. Indeed, accumulated evidences suggest that, through the simultaneous provision of TAAs for presentation by DC and activation of various immune cells, TLR3 ligands could trigger tumor autovaccination. The benefit that TLR3 ligands would bring to tumor therapy can be the result of several activities: (1) the "inflammatory apoptosis" of cancer cells that express the receptor; (2) the intratumoral production and action of Type I IFNs on immune cells, most particularly on TAA cross-presenting DC and on NK cells, and on nonimmune cells, while avoiding the side effects associated with systemic administration of these cytokines; (3) the local secretion of cytokines and chemokines that boost and recruit effector and memory tumor-specific CTLs and TH17 to the tumor site; (4) the inhibition of Tregs; and (5) the enhancement of the innate antitumor response and the repolarization of tumor infiltrating myeloid cells, including the activation of their cytotoxicity [204]. At a time when immune checkpoint inhibitors are changing the way we envision cancer treatment, TLR3 appears as a promising target for generating tumor-specific CTLs, for driving them to the tumor site and eventually for enhancing the frequency of patients that could benefit from tumor immunotherapy.

References

1. Nagata S (1997) Apoptosis by death factor. Cell 88(3):355–365
2. Ashkenazi A (2015) Targeting the extrinsic apoptotic pathway in cancer: lessons learned and future directions. J Clin Invest 125(2):487–489
3. Bell JK, Botos I, Hall PR, Askins J, Shiloach J, Segal DM et al (2005) The molecular structure of the Toll-like receptor 3 ligand-binding domain. Proc Natl Acad Sci U S A 102(31):10976–10980
4. Liu L, Botos I, Wang Y, Leonard JN, Shiloach J, Segal DM et al (2008) Structural basis of toll-like receptor 3 signaling with double-stranded RNA. Science 320(5874):379–381
5. Kang JY, Lee J-O (2011) Structural biology of the Toll-like receptor family. Annu Rev Biochem 80:917–941
6. Mikami T, Miyashita H, Takatsuka S, Kuroki Y, Matsushima N (2012) Molecular evolution of vertebrate Toll-like receptors: evolutionary rate difference between their leucine-rich repeats and their TIR domains. Gene 503(2):235–243
7. Barreiro LB, Ben-Ali M, Quach H, Laval G, Patin E, Pickrell JK et al (2009) Evolutionary dynamics of human Toll-like receptors and their different contributions to host defense. PLoS Genet 5(7):e1000562
8. Alexopoulou L, Holt AC, Medzhitov R, Flavell RA (2001) Recognition of double-stranded RNA and activation of NF-kappaB by Toll-like receptor 3. Nature 413(6857):732–738
9. Yamamoto M, Sato S, Mori K, Hoshino K, Takeuchi O, Takeda K et al (2002) Cutting edge: a novel Toll/IL-1 receptor domain-containing adapter that preferentially activates the IFN-beta promoter in the Toll-like receptor signaling. J Immunol 169(12):6668–6672

10. Oshiumi H, Matsumoto M, Funami K, Akazawa T, Seya T (2003) TICAM-1, an adaptor molecule that participates in Toll-like receptor 3-mediated interferon-beta induction. Nat Immunol 4(2):161–167
11. Botos I, Liu L, Wang Y, Segal DM, Davies DR (2009) The toll-like receptor 3:dsRNA signaling complex. Biochim Biophys Acta 1789(9–10):667–674
12. Wang Y, Liu L, Davies DR, Segal DM (2010) Dimerization of Toll-like receptor 3 (TLR3) is required for ligand binding. J Biol Chem 285(47):36836–36841
13. Fukuda K, Tsujita T, Matsumoto M, Seya T, Sakiyama H, Nishikawa F et al (2006) Analysis of the interaction between human TLR3 ectodomain and nucleic acids. Nucleic Acids Symp Ser 50(1):249–250
14. Leonard JN, Ghirlando R, Askins J, Bell JK, Margulies DH, Davies DR et al (2008) The TLR3 signaling complex forms by cooperative receptor dimerization. Proc Natl Acad Sci U S A 105(1):258–263
15. de Bouteiller O, Merck E, Hasan UA, Hubac S, Benguigui B, Trinchieri G et al (2005) Recognition of double-stranded RNA by human toll-like receptor 3 and downstream receptor signaling requires multimerization and an acidic pH. J Biol Chem 280(46):38133–38145
16. Muzio M, Bosisio D, Polentarutti N, D'amico G, Stoppacciaro A, Mancinelli R et al (2000) Differential expression and regulation of toll-like receptors (TLR) in human leukocytes: selective expression of TLR3 in dendritic cells. J Immunol 164(11):5998–6004
17. Visintin A, Mazzoni A, Spitzer JH, Wyllie DH, Dower SK, Segal DM (2001) Regulation of Toll-like receptors in human monocytes and dendritic cells. J Immunol 166(1):249–255
18. Heinz S, Haehnel V, Karaghiosoff M, Schwarzfischer L, Müller M, Krause SW et al (2003) Species-specific regulation of Toll-like receptor 3 genes in men and mice. J Biol Chem 278(24):21502–21509
19. Miettinen M, Sareneva T, Julkunen I, Matikainen S (2001) IFNs activate toll-like receptor gene expression in viral infections. Genes Immun 2(6):349–355
20. Edwards AD, Diebold SS, Slack EMC, Tomizawa H, Hemmi H, Kaisho T et al (2003) Toll-like receptor expression in murine DC subsets: lack of TLR7 expression by CD8 alpha+ DC correlates with unresponsiveness to imidazoquinolines. Eur J Immunol 33(4):827–833
21. Fujita H, Asahina A, Mitsui H, Tamaki K (2004) Langerhans cells exhibit low responsiveness to double-stranded RNA. Biochem Biophys Res Commun 319(3):832–839
22. Kulka M, Alexopoulou L, Flavell RA, Metcalfe DD (2004) Activation of mast cells by double-stranded RNA: evidence for activation through Toll-like receptor 3. J Allergy Clin Immunol 114(1):174–182
23. Tohyama M, Dai X, Sayama K, Yamasaki K, Shirakata Y, Hanakawa Y et al (2005) dsRNA-mediated innate immunity of epidermal keratinocytes. Biochem Biophys Res Commun 335(2):505–511
24. Abrahams VM, Visintin I, Aldo PB, Guller S, Romero R, Mor G (2005) A role for TLRs in the regulation of immune cell migration by first trimester trophoblast cells. J Immunol 175(12):8096–8104
25. Pineda A, Verdin-Terán SL, Camacho A, Moreno-Fierros L (2011) Expression of toll-like receptor TLR-2, TLR-3, TLR-4 and TLR-9 is increased in placentas from patients with preeclampsia. Arch Med Res 42(5):382–391
26. Tanabe M, Kurita-Taniguchi M, Takeuchi K, Takeda M, Ayata M, Ogura H et al (2003) Mechanism of up-regulation of human Toll-like receptor 3 secondary to infection of measles virus-attenuated strains. Biochem Biophys Res Commun 311(1):39–48
27. Wen L, Peng J, Li Z, Wong FS (2004) The effect of innate immunity on autoimmune diabetes and the expression of Toll-like receptors on pancreatic islets. J Immunol 172(5):3173–3180
28. Patole PS, Gröne H-J, Segerer S, Ciubar R, Belemezova E, Henger A et al (2005) Viral double-stranded RNA aggravates lupus nephritis through Toll-like receptor 3 on glomerular mesangial cells and antigen-presenting cells. J Am Soc Nephrol 16(5):1326–1338
29. Young SL, Lyddon TD, Jorgenson RL, Misfeldt ML (2004) Expression of Toll-like receptors in human endometrial epithelial cells and cell lines. Am J Reprod Immunol 52(1):67–73

30. Schaefer TM, Fahey JV, Wright JA, Wira CR (2005) Innate immunity in the human female reproductive tract: antiviral response of uterine epithelial cells to the TLR3 agonist poly(I:C). J Immunol 174(2):992–1002
31. Tissari J, Sirén J, Meri S, Julkunen I, Matikainen S (2005) IFN-alpha enhances TLR3-mediated antiviral cytokine expression in human endothelial and epithelial cells by up-regulating TLR3 expression. J Immunol 174(7):4289–4294
32. Kumar MV, Nagineni CN, Chin MS, Hooks JJ, Detrick B (2004) Innate immunity in the retina: Toll-like receptor (TLR) signaling in human retinal pigment epithelial cells. J Neuroimmunol 153(1–2):7–15
33. Takii Y, Nakamura M, Ito M, Yokoyama T, Komori A, Shimizu-Yoshida Y et al (2005) Enhanced expression of type I interferon and toll-like receptor-3 in primary biliary cirrhosis. Lab Invest 85(7):908–920
34. Cario E, Podolsky DK (2000) Differential alteration in intestinal epithelial cell expression of toll-like receptor 3 (TLR3) and TLR4 in inflammatory bowel disease. Infect Immun 68(12):7010–7017
35. Fransson M, Adner M, Erjefält J, Jansson L, Uddman R, Cardell L-O (2005) Up-regulation of Toll-like receptors 2, 3 and 4 in allergic rhinitis. Respir Res 6:100
36. Andersen JM, Al-Khairy D, Ingalls RR (2006) Innate immunity at the mucosal surface: role of toll-like receptor 3 and toll-like receptor 9 in cervical epithelial cell responses to microbial pathogens. Biol Reprod 74(5):824–831
37. Kumar A, Zhang J, Yu F-SX (2006) Toll-like receptor 3 agonist poly(I:C)-induced antiviral response in human corneal epithelial cells. Immunology 117(1):11–21
38. Wörnle M, Schmid H, Banas B, Merkle M, Henger A, Roeder M et al (2006) Novel role of toll-like receptor 3 in hepatitis C-associated glomerulonephritis. Am J Pathol 168(2):370–385
39. Brentano F, Schorr O, Gay RE, Gay S, Kyburz D (2005) RNA released from necrotic synovial fluid cells activates rheumatoid arthritis synovial fibroblasts via Toll-like receptor 3. Arthritis Rheum 52(9):2656–2665
40. Matsumoto M, Kikkawa S, Kohase M, Miyake K, Seya T (2002) Establishment of a monoclonal antibody against human Toll-like receptor 3 that blocks double-stranded RNA-mediated signaling. Biochem Biophys Res Commun 293(5):1364–1369
41. Bsibsi M, Ravid R, Gveric D, van Noort JM (2002) Broad expression of Toll-like receptors in the human central nervous system. J Neuropathol Exp Neurol 61(11):1013–1021
42. Farina C, Krumbholz M, Giese T, Hartmann G, Aloisi F, Meinl E (2005) Preferential expression and function of Toll-like receptor 3 in human astrocytes. J Neuroimmunol 159(1–2):12–19
43. Jackson AC, Rossiter JP, Lafon M (2006) Expression of Toll-like receptor 3 in the human cerebellar cortex in rabies, herpes simplex encephalitis, and other neurological diseases. J Neurovirol 12(3):229–234
44. Taura M, Eguma A, Suico MA, Shuto T, Koga T, Komatsu K et al (2008) p53 regulates Toll-like receptor 3 expression and function in human epithelial cell lines. Mol Cell Biol 28(21):6557–6567
45. Taura M, Suico MA, Koyama K, Komatsu K, Miyakita R, Matsumoto C et al (2012) Rb/E2F1 regulates the innate immune receptor Toll-like receptor 3 in epithelial cells. Mol Cell Biol 32(8):1581–1590
46. Kim Y-M, Brinkmann MM, Paquet M-E, Ploegh HL (2008) UNC93B1 delivers nucleotide-sensing toll-like receptors to endolysosomes. Nature 452(7184):234–238
47. Toscano F, Estornes Y, Virard F, Garcia-Cattaneo A, Pierrot A, Vanbervliet B et al (2013) Cleaved/associated TLR3 represents the primary form of the signaling receptor. J Immunol 190(2):764–773
48. Ewald SE, Engel A, Lee J, Wang M, Bogyo M, Barton GM (2011) Nucleic acid recognition by Toll-like receptors is coupled to stepwise processing by cathepsins and asparagine endopeptidase. J Exp Med 208(4):643–651
49. Yamashita M, Chattopadhyay S, Fensterl V, Saikia P, Wetzel JL, Sen GC (2012) Epidermal growth factor receptor is essential for Toll-like receptor 3 signaling. Sci Signal 5(233):ra50

50. Johnsen IB, Nguyen TT, Ringdal M, Tryggestad AM, Bakke O, Lien E et al (2006) Toll-like receptor 3 associates with c-Src tyrosine kinase on endosomes to initiate antiviral signaling. EMBO J 25(14):3335–3346
51. Sarkar SN, Peters KL, Elco CP, Sakamoto S, Pal S, Sen GC (2004) Novel roles of TLR3 tyrosine phosphorylation and PI3 kinase in double-stranded RNA signaling. Nat Struct Mol Biol 11(11):1060–1067
52. Lee K-G, Xu S, Kang Z-H, Huo J, Huang M, Liu D et al (2012) Bruton's tyrosine kinase phosphorylates Toll-like receptor 3 to initiate antiviral response. Proc Natl Acad Sci U S A 109(15):5791–5796
53. Verstak B, Arnot CJ, Gay NJ (2013) An alanine-to-proline mutation in the BB-loop of TLR3 Toll/IL-1R domain switches signalling adaptor specificity from TRIF to MyD88. J Immunol 191(12):6101–6109
54. Sasai M, Oshiumi H, Matsumoto M, Inoue N, Fujita F, Nakanishi M et al (2005) Cutting edge: NF-kappaB-activating kinase-associated protein 1 participates in TLR3/Toll-IL-1 homology domain-containing adapter molecule-1-mediated IFN regulatory factor 3 activation. J Immunol 174(1):27–30
55. Oganesyan G, Saha SK, Guo B, He JQ, Shahangian A, Zarnegar B et al (2006) Critical role of TRAF3 in the Toll-like receptor-dependent and -independent antiviral response. Nature 439(7073):208–211
56. Sharma S, tenOever BR, Grandvaux N, Zhou G-P, Lin R, Hiscott J (2003) Triggering the interferon antiviral response through an IKK-related pathway. Science 300(5622):1148–1151
57. Fitzgerald KA, McWhirter SM, Faia KL, Rowe DC, Latz E, Golenbock DT et al (2003) IKKepsilon and TBK1 are essential components of the IRF3 signaling pathway. Nat Immunol 4(5):491–496
58. Ng CT, Mendoza JL, Garcia KC, Oldstone MBA (2016) Alpha and Beta type 1 interferon signaling: passage for diverse biologic outcomes. Cell 164(3):349–352
59. Ritter M, Mennerich D, Weith A, Seither P (2005) Characterization of Toll-like receptors in primary lung epithelial cells: strong impact of the TLR3 ligand poly(I:C) on the regulation of Toll-like receptors, adaptor proteins and inflammatory response. J Inflamm (Lond) 2:16
60. Saitoh T, Yamamoto M, Miyagishi M, Taira K, Nakanishi M, Fujita T et al (2005) A20 is a negative regulator of IFN regulatory factor 3 signaling. J Immunol 174(3):1507–1512
61. Jiang Z, Mak TW, Sen G, Li X (2004) Toll-like receptor 3-mediated activation of NF-kappaB and IRF3 diverges at Toll-IL-1 receptor domain-containing adapter inducing IFN-beta. Proc Natl Acad Sci U S A 101(10):3533–3538
62. Rydberg C, Månsson A, Uddman R, Riesbeck K, Cardell L-O (2009) Toll-like receptor agonists induce inflammation and cell death in a model of head and neck squamous cell carcinomas. Immunology 128(1 Suppl):e600–e611
63. Umemura N, Zhu J, Mburu YK, Forero A, Hsieh PN, Muthuswamy R et al (2012) Defective NF-κB signaling in metastatic head and neck cancer cells leads to enhanced apoptosis by dsRNA. Cancer Res 72(1):45–55
64. Sha Q, Truong-Tran AQ, Plitt JR, Beck LA, Schleimer RP (2004) Activation of airway epithelial cells by toll-like receptor agonists. Am J Respir Cell Mol Biol 31(3):358–364
65. Perales-Linares R, Navas-Martin S (2013) Toll-like receptor 3 in viral pathogenesis: friend or foe? Immunology 140(2):153–167
66. Ruckdeschel K, Pfaffinger G, Haase R, Sing A, Weighardt H, Häcker G et al (2004) Signaling of apoptosis through TLRs critically involves toll/IL-1 receptor domain-containing adapter inducing IFN-beta, but not MyD88, in bacteria-infected murine macrophages. J Immunol 173(5):3320–3328
67. Rasschaert J, Ladrière L, Urbain M, Dogusan Z, Katabua B, Sato S et al (2005) Toll-like receptor 3 and STAT-1 contribute to double-stranded RNA+ interferon-gamma-induced apoptosis in primary pancreatic beta-cells. J Biol Chem 280(40):33984–33991
68. Dogusan Z, García M, Flamez D, Alexopoulou L, Goldman M, Gysemans C et al (2008) Double-stranded RNA induces pancreatic beta-cell apoptosis by activation of the toll-like receptor 3 and interferon regulatory factor 3 pathways. Diabetes 57(5):1236–1245

69. Klettner A, Koinzer S, Meyer T, Roider J (2013) Toll-like receptor 3 activation in retinal pigment epithelium cells – mitogen-activated protein kinase pathways of cell death and vascular endothelial growth factor secretion. Acta Ophthalmol 91(3):e211–e218
70. Sato A, Iizuka M, Nakagomi O, Suzuki M, Horie Y, Konno S et al (2006) Rotavirus double-stranded RNA induces apoptosis and diminishes wound repair in rat intestinal epithelial cells. J Gastroenterol Hepatol 21(3):521–530
71. Zhou R, Wei H, Sun R, Zhang J, Tian Z (2007) NKG2D recognition mediates Toll-like receptor 3 signaling-induced breakdown of epithelial homeostasis in the small intestines of mice. Proc Natl Acad Sci U S A 104(18):7512–7515
72. Yaddanapudi K, De Miranda J, Hornig M, Lipkin WI (2011) Toll-like receptor 3 regulates neural stem cell proliferation by modulating the Sonic Hedgehog pathway. PLoS One 6(10):e26766
73. Jacobs BL, Langland JO (1996) When two strands are better than one: the mediators and modulators of the cellular responses to double-stranded RNA. Virology 219(2):339–349
74. Tatematsu M, Nishikawa F, Seya T, Matsumoto M (2013) Toll-like receptor 3 recognizes incomplete stem structures in single-stranded viral RNA. Nat Commun 4:1833
75. Iwakiri D, Zhou L, Samanta M, Matsumoto M, Ebihara T, Seya T et al (2009) Epstein-Barr virus (EBV)–encoded small RNA is released from EBV-infected cells and activates signaling from toll-like receptor 3. J Exp Med 206(10):2091
76. Zhang S-Y, Herman M, Ciancanelli MJ, Pérez de Diego R, Sancho-Shimizu V, Abel L et al (2013) TLR3 immunity to infection in mice and humans. Curr Opin Immunol 25(1):19–33
77. Zhang S-Y, Jouanguy E, Ugolini S, Smahi A, Elain G, Romero P et al (2007) TLR3 deficiency in patients with herpes simplex encephalitis. Science 317(5844):1522–1527
78. Casrouge A, Zhang S-Y, Eidenschenk C, Jouanguy E, Puel A, Yang K et al (2006) Herpes simplex virus encephalitis in human UNC-93B deficiency. Science 314(5797):308–312
79. Sancho-Shimizu V, Pérez de Diego R, Lorenzo L, Halwani R, Alangari A, Israelsson E et al (2011) Herpes simplex encephalitis in children with autosomal recessive and dominant TRIF deficiency. J Clin Invest 121(12):4889–4902
80. Pérez de Diego R, Sancho-Shimizu V, Lorenzo L, Puel A, Plancoulaine S, Picard C et al (2010) Human TRAF3 adaptor molecule deficiency leads to impaired Toll-like receptor 3 response and susceptibility to herpes simplex encephalitis. Immunity 33(3):400–411
81. Herman M, Ciancanelli M, Ou Y-H, Lorenzo L, Klaudel-Dreszler M, Pauwels E et al (2012) Heterozygous TBK1 mutations impair TLR3 immunity and underlie herpes simplex encephalitis of childhood. J Exp Med 209(9):1567–1582
82. Aksoy E, Zouain CS, Vanhoutte F, Fontaine J, Pavelka N, Thieblemont N et al (2005) Double-stranded RNAs from the helminth parasite Schistosoma activate TLR3 in dendritic cells. J Biol Chem 280(1):277–283
83. Lathia JD, Okun E, Tang S-C, Griffioen K, Cheng A, Mughal MR et al (2008) Toll-like receptor 3 is a negative regulator of embryonic neural progenitor cell proliferation. J Neurosci 28(51):13978–13984
84. Karikó K, Ni H, Capodici J, Lamphier M, Weissman D (2004) mRNA is an endogenous ligand for Toll-like receptor 3. J Biol Chem 279(13):12542–12550
85. Koski GK, Karikó K, Xu S, Weissman D, Cohen PA, Czerniecki BJ (2004) Cutting edge: innate immune system discriminates between RNA containing bacterial versus eukaryotic structural features that prime for high-level IL-12 secretion by dendritic cells. J Immunol 172(7):3989–3993
86. Karikó K, Buckstein M, Ni H, Weissman D (2005) Suppression of RNA recognition by Toll-like receptors: the impact of nucleoside modification and the evolutionary origin of RNA. Immunity 23(2):165–175
87. Lee H, Jo E-K, Choi S-Y, Oh SB, Park K, Kim JS et al (2006) Necrotic neuronal cells induce inflammatory Schwann cell activation via TLR2 and TLR3: implication in Wallerian degeneration. Biochem Biophys Res Commun 350(3):742–747
88. Cavassani KA, Ishii M, Wen H, Schaller MA, Lincoln PM, Lukacs NW et al (2008) TLR3 is an endogenous sensor of tissue necrosis during acute inflammatory events. J Exp Med 205(11):2609–2621

89. Lin Q, Fang D, Fang J, Ren X, Yang X, Wen F et al (2011) Impaired wound healing with defective expression of chemokines and recruitment of myeloid cells in TLR3-deficient mice. J Immunol 186(6):3710–3717
90. Shiose S, Chen Y, Okano K, Roy S, Kohno H, Tang J et al (2011) Toll-like receptor 3 is required for development of retinopathy caused by impaired all-trans-retinal clearance in mice. J Biol Chem 286(17):15543–15555
91. Bernard JJ, Cowing-Zitron C, Nakatsuji T, Muehleisen B, Muto J, Borkowski AW et al (2012) Ultraviolet radiation damages self noncoding RNA and is detected by TLR3. Nat Med 18(8):1286–1290
92. Hoffman RW, Gazitt T, Foecking MF, Ortmann RA, Misfeldt M, Jorgenson R et al (2004) U1 RNA induces innate immunity signaling. Arthritis Rheum 50(9):2891–2896
93. Malmegrim KCR, Pruijn GJM, van Venrooij WJ (2002) The fate of the U1 snRNP autoantigen during apoptosis: implications for systemic autoimmunity. Isr Med Assoc J 4(9):706–712
94. Liu Y, Gu Y, Han Y, Zhang Q, Jiang Z, Zhang X et al (2016) Tumor Exosomal RNAs promote lung pre-metastatic niche formation by activating alveolar epithelial TLR3 to recruit neutrophils. Cancer Cell 30(2):243–256
95. Kato H, Takeuchi O, Mikamo-Satoh E, Hirai R, Kawai T, Matsushita K et al (2008) Length-dependent recognition of double-stranded ribonucleic acids by retinoic acid-inducible gene-I and melanoma differentiation-associated gene 5. J Exp Med 205(7):1601–1610
96. Kato H, Takeuchi O, Sato S, Yoneyama M, Yamamoto M, Matsui K et al (2006) Differential roles of MDA5 and RIG-I helicases in the recognition of RNA viruses. Nature 441(7089):101–105
97. Gitlin L, Barchet W, Gilfillan S, Cella M, Beutler B, Flavell RA et al (2006) Essential role of mda-5 in type I IFN responses to polyriboinosinic:polyribocytidylic acid and encephalomyocarditis picornavirus. Proc Natl Acad Sci U S A 103(22):8459–8464
98. Levy HB, Baer G, Baron S, Buckler CE, Gibbs CJ, Iadarola MJ et al (1975) A modified polyriboinosinic-polyribocytidylic acid complex that induces interferon in primates. J Infect Dis 132(4):434–439
99. Gowen BB, Wong M-H, Jung K-H, Sanders AB, Mitchell WM, Alexopoulou L et al (2007) TLR3 is essential for the induction of protective immunity against Punta Toro virus infection by the double-stranded RNA (dsRNA), poly(I:C12U), but not poly(I:C): differential recognition of synthetic dsRNA molecules. J Immunol 178(8):5200–5208
100. Okahira S, Nishikawa F, Nishikawa S, Akazawa T, Seya T, Matsumoto M (2005) Interferon-beta induction through toll-like receptor 3 depends on double-stranded RNA structure. DNA Cell Biol 24(10):614–623
101. Jeung H-C, Moon YW, Rha SY, Yoo NC, Roh JK, Noh SH et al (2008) Phase III trial of adjuvant 5-fluorouracil and adriamycin versus 5-fluorouracil, adriamycin, and polyadenylic-polyuridylic acid (poly A:U) for locally advanced gastric cancer after curative surgery: final results of 15-year follow-up. Ann Oncol 19(3):520–526
102. Salaun B, Zitvogel L, Asselin-Paturel C, Morel Y, Chemin K, Dubois C et al (2011) TLR3 as a biomarker for the therapeutic efficacy of double-stranded RNA in breast cancer. Cancer Res 71(5):1607–1614
103. Chen L, Xu Y-Y, Zhou J-M, Wu Y-Y, E Q, Zhu Y-Y (2012) TLR3 dsRNA agonist inhibits growth and invasion of HepG2.2.15 HCC cells. Oncol Rep 28(1):200–206
104. Xu Y-Y, Chen L, Zhou J-M, Wu Y-Y, Zhu Y-Y (2013) Inhibitory effect of dsRNA TLR3 agonist in a rat hepatocellular carcinoma model. Mol Med Rep 8(4):1037–1042
105. Matsumoto M, Tatematsu M, Nishikawa F, Azuma M, Ishii N, Morii-Sakai A et al (2015) Defined TLR3-specific adjuvant that induces NK and CTL activation without significant cytokine production in vivo. Nat Commun 6:6280
106. Seya T, Takeda Y, Matsumoto M (2016) Tumor vaccines with dsRNA adjuvant ARNAX induces antigen-specific tumor shrinkage without cytokinemia. Oncoimmunology 5(2): e1043506
107. Naumann K, Wehner R, Schwarze A, Petzold C, Schmitz M, Rohayem J (2013) Activation of dendritic cells by the novel Toll-like receptor 3 agonist RGC100. Clin Dev Immunol 2013:283649

108. Duffy KE, Lamb RJ, San Mateo LR, Jordan JL, Canziani G, Brigham-Burke M et al (2007) Down modulation of human TLR3 function by a monoclonal antibody. Cell Immunol 248(2):103–114
109. Levine AS, Levy HB (1978) Phase I-II trials of poly IC stabilized with poly-L-lysine. Cancer Treat Rep 62(11):1907–1912
110. Lampkin BC, Levine AS, Levy H, Krivit W, Hammond D (1985) Phase II trial of a complex polyriboinosinic-polyribocytidylic acid with poly-L-lysine and carboxymethyl cellulose in the treatment of children with acute leukemia and neuroblastoma: a report from the Children's Cancer Study Group. Cancer Res 45(11 Pt 2):5904–5909
111. Seya T, Azuma M, Matsumoto M (2013) Targeting TLR3 with no RIG-I/MDA5 activation is effective in immunotherapy for cancer. Expert Opin Ther Targets 17(5):533–544
112. Vérillaud B, Gressette M, Morel Y, Paturel C, Herman P, Lo KW et al (2012) Toll-like receptor 3 in Epstein-Barr virus-associated nasopharyngeal carcinomas: consistent expression and cytotoxic effects of its synthetic ligand poly(A:U) combined to a Smac-mimetic. Infect Agent Cancer 7(1):36
113. Hasimu A, Ge L, Li Q-Z, Zhang R-P, Guo X (2011) Expressions of Toll-like receptors 3, 4, 7, and 9 in cervical lesions and their correlation with HPV16 infection in Uighur women. Chin J Cancer 30(5):344–350
114. Luo Q, Hu S, Yan M, Sun Z, Chen W, Chen F (2012) Activation of Toll-like receptor 3 induces apoptosis of oral squamous carcinoma cells in vitro and in vivo. Int J Biochem Cell Biol 44(8):1266–1275
115. He Z, Huang X, Ni Y, Shi P, Wang Z, Han W et al (2014) Functional toll-like receptor 3 expressed by oral squamous cell carcinoma induced cell apoptosis and decreased migration. Oral Surg Oral Med Oral Pathol Oral Radiol 118(1):92–100
116. Chuang H-C, Huang C-C, Chien C-Y, Chuang J-H (2012) Toll-like receptor 3-mediated tumor invasion in head and neck cancer. Oral Oncol 48(3):226–232
117. Nojiri K, Sugimoto K, Shiraki K, Tameda M, Inagaki Y, Kusagawa S et al (2013) The expression and function of Toll-like receptors 3 and 9 in human colon carcinoma. Oncol Rep 29(5):1737–1743
118. Chew V, Tow C, Huang C, Bard-Chapeau E, Copeland NG, Jenkins NA et al (2012) Toll-like receptor 3 expressing tumor parenchyma and infiltrating natural killer cells in hepatocellular carcinoma patients. J Natl Cancer Inst 104(23):1796–1807
119. Yuan M-M, Xu Y-Y, Chen L, Li X-Y, Qin J, Shen Y (2015) TLR3 expression correlates with apoptosis, proliferation and angiogenesis in hepatocellular carcinoma and predicts prognosis. BMC Cancer 15:245
120. Li D, Gu R, Yang X, Hu C, Li Y, Gao M et al (2014) TLR3 correlated with cervical lymph node metastasis in patients with papillary thyroid cancer. Int J Clin Exp Med 7(12):5111
121. Gambara G, Desideri M, Stoppacciaro A, Padula F, Cesaris PD, Starace D et al (2015) TLR3 engagement induces IRF-3-dependent apoptosis in androgen-sensitive prostate cancer cells and inhibits tumour growth in vivo. J Cell Mol Med 19(2):327
122. Zhou M, McFarland-Mancini MM, Funk HM, Husseinzadeh N, Mounajjed T, Drew AF (2009) Toll-like receptor expression in normal ovary and ovarian tumors. Cancer Immunol Immunother 58(9):1375–1385
123. Helminen O, Huhta H, Lehenkari PP, Saarnio J, Karttunen TJ, Kauppila JH (2016) Nucleic acid-sensing toll-like receptors 3, 7 and 8 in esophageal epithelium, barrett's esophagus, dysplasia and adenocarcinoma. Oncoimmunology 5(5):e1127495
124. Combaz-Lair C, Galateau-Sallé F, McLeer-Florin A, Le Stang N, David-Boudet L, Duruisseaux M et al (2016) Immune biomarkers PD-1/PD-L1 and TLR3 in malignant pleural mesotheliomas. Hum Pathol 52:9–18
125. Allhorn S, Böing C, Koch AA, Kimmig R, Gashaw I (2008) TLR3 and TLR4 expression in healthy and diseased human endometrium. Reprod Biol Endocrinol 6:40
126. Hasan UA, Caux C, Perrot I, Doffin AC, Menetrier-Caux C, Trinchieri G, Tommasino M, Vlach J (2007) Cell proliferation and survival induced by Toll-like receptors is antagonized by type I IFNs. Proc Natl Acad Sci U S A 104(19):8047–8052

127. Salaun B, Coste I, Rissoan M-C, Lebecque SJ, Renno T (2006) TLR3 can directly trigger apoptosis in human cancer cells. J Immunol 176(8):4894–4901
128. Paone A, Starace D, Galli R, Padula F, De Cesaris P, Filippini A et al (2008) Toll-like receptor 3 triggers apoptosis of human prostate cancer cells through a PKC-alpha-dependent mechanism. Carcinogenesis 29(7):1334–1342
129. Nomi N, Kodama S, Suzuki M (2010) Toll-like receptor 3 signaling induces apoptosis in human head and neck cancer via survivin associated pathway. Oncol Rep 24(1):225–231
130. Hughes MA, Harper N, Butterworth M, Cain K, Cohen GM, MacFarlane M (2009) Reconstitution of the death-inducing signaling complex reveals a substrate switch that determines CD95-mediated death or survival. Mol Cell 35(3):265–279
131. Oberst A, Pop C, Tremblay AG, Blais V, Denault J-B, Salvesen GS et al (2010) Inducible dimerization and inducible cleavage reveal a requirement for both processes in caspase-8 activation. J Biol Chem 285(22):16632–16642
132. Dickens LS, Boyd RS, Jukes-Jones R, Hughes MA, Robinson GL, Fairall L et al (2012) A death effector domain chain DISC model reveals a crucial role for caspase-8 chain assembly in mediating apoptotic cell death. Mol Cell 47(2):291–305
133. Schleich K, Warnken U, Fricker N, Oztürk S, Richter P, Kammerer K et al (2012) Stoichiometry of the CD95 death-inducing signaling complex: experimental and modeling evidence for a death effector domain chain model. Mol Cell 47(2):306–319
134. Estornes Y, Toscano F, Virard F, Jacquemin G, Pierrot A, Vanbervliet B et al (2012) dsRNA induces apoptosis through an atypical death complex associating TLR3 to caspase-8. Cell Death Differ 19(9):1482–1494
135. Feoktistova M, Geserick P, Kellert B, Dimitrova DP, Langlais C, Hupe M et al (2011) cIAPs block Ripoptosome formation, a RIP1/caspase-8 containing intracellular cell death complex differentially regulated by cFLIP isoforms. Mol Cell 43(3):449–463
136. Kaiser WJ, Offermann MK (2005) Apoptosis induced by the toll-like receptor adaptor TRIF is dependent on its receptor interacting protein homotypic interaction motif. J Immunol 174(8):4942–4952
137. Weiss R, Sachet M, Zinngrebe J, Aschacher T, Krainer M, Hegedus B et al (2013) IL-24 sensitizes tumor cells to TLR3-mediated apoptosis. Cell Death Differ 20(6):823–833
138. Tenev T, Bianchi K, Darding M, Broemer M, Langlais C, Wallberg F et al (2011) The Ripoptosome, a signaling platform that assembles in response to genotoxic stress and loss of IAPs. Mol Cell 43(3):432–448
139. Friboulet L, Pioche-Durieu C, Rodriguez S, Valent A, Souquère S, Ripoche H et al (2008) Recurrent overexpression of c-IAP2 in EBV-associated nasopharyngeal carcinomas: critical role in resistance to Toll-like receptor 3-mediated apoptosis. Neoplasia 10(11):1183–1194
140. Weber A, Kirejczyk Z, Besch R, Potthoff S, Leverkus M, Häcker G (2010) Proapoptotic signalling through Toll-like receptor-3 involves TRIF-dependent activation of caspase-8 and is under the control of inhibitor of apoptosis proteins in melanoma cells. Cell Death Differ 17(6):942–951
141. O'Donnell MA, Legarda-Addison D, Skountzos P, Yeh WC, Ting AT (2007) Ubiquitination of RIP1 regulates an NF-kappaB-independent cell-death switch in TNF signaling. Curr Biol 17(5):418–424
142. Varfolomeev E, Goncharov T, Fedorova AV, Dynek JN, Zobel K, Deshayes K et al (2008) c-IAP1 and c-IAP2 are critical mediators of tumor necrosis factor alpha (TNFalpha)-induced NF-kappaB activation. J Biol Chem 283(36):24295–24299
143. Boatright KM, Deis C, Denault J-B, Sutherlin DP, Salvesen GS (2004) Activation of caspases-8 and -10 by FLIP(L). Biochem J 382(Pt 2):651–657
144. Pop C, Oberst A, Drag M, Van Raam BJ, Riedl SJ, Green DR et al (2011) FLIP(L) induces caspase 8 activity in the absence of interdomain caspase 8 cleavage and alters substrate specificity. Biochem J 433(3):447–457
145. Salaun B, Lebecque S, Matikainen S, Rimoldi D, Romero P (2007) Toll-like receptor 3 expressed by melanoma cells as a target for therapy? Clin Cancer Res 13(15 Pt 1):4565–4574

146. Jiang Q, Wei H, Tian Z (2008) Poly I:C enhances cycloheximide-induced apoptosis of tumor cells through TLR3 pathway. BMC Cancer 8:12
147. Zinngrebe J, Rieser E, Taraborrelli L, Peltzer N, Hartwig T, Ren H et al (2016) LUBAC deficiency perturbs TLR3 signaling to cause immunodeficiency and autoinflammation. J Exp Med 213(12):2671–2689
148. McCormick KD, Ghosh A, Trivedi S, Wang L, Coyne CB, Ferris RL et al (2016) Innate immune signaling through differential RIPK1 expression promote tumor progression in head and neck squamous cell carcinoma. Carcinogenesis 37(5):522–529
149. Cho YS, Challa S, Moquin D, Genga R, Ray TD, Guildford M et al (2009) Phosphorylation-driven assembly of the RIP1-RIP3 complex regulates programmed necrosis and virus-induced inflammation. Cell 137(6):1112–1123
150. He S, Wang L, Miao L, Wang T, Du F, Zhao L et al (2009) Receptor interacting protein kinase-3 determines cellular necrotic response to TNF-alpha. Cell 137(6):1100–1111
151. Zhang D-W, Shao J, Lin J, Zhang N, Lu B-J, Lin S-C et al (2009) RIP3, an energy metabolism regulator that switches TNF-induced cell death from apoptosis to necrosis. Science 325(5938):332–336
152. Vanden Berghe T, Linkermann A, Jouan-Lanhouet S, Walczak H, Vandenabeele P (2014) Regulated necrosis: the expanding network of non-apoptotic cell death pathways. Nat Rev Mol Cell Biol 15(2):135–147
153. Chen W, Zhou Z, Li L, Zhong C-Q, Zheng X, Wu X et al (2013) Diverse sequence determinants control human and mouse receptor interacting protein 3 (RIP3) and mixed lineage kinase domain-like (MLKL) interaction in necroptotic signaling. J Biol Chem 288(23):16247–16261
154. Cai Z, Jitkaew S, Zhao J, Chiang H-C, Choksi S, Liu J et al (2014) Plasma membrane translocation of trimerized MLKL protein is required for TNF-induced necroptosis. Nat Cell Biol 16(1):55–65
155. Dondelinger Y, Declercq W, Montessuit S, Roelandt R, Goncalves A, Bruggeman I et al (2014) MLKL compromises plasma membrane integrity by binding to phosphatidylinositol phosphates. Cell Rep 7(4):971–981
156. Hildebrand JM, Tanzer MC, Lucet IS, Young SN, Spall SK, Sharma P et al (2014) Activation of the pseudokinase MLKL unleashes the four-helix bundle domain to induce membrane localization and necroptotic cell death. Proc Natl Acad Sci U S A 111(42):15072–15077
157. He S, Liang Y, Shao F, Wang X (2011) Toll-like receptors activate programmed necrosis in macrophages through a receptor-interacting kinase-3-mediated pathway. Proc Natl Acad Sci U S A 108(50):20054–20059
158. Kaiser WJ, Sridharan H, Huang C, Mandal P, Upton JW, Gough PJ et al (2013) Toll-like receptor 3-mediated necrosis via TRIF, RIP3, and MLKL. J Biol Chem 288(43):31268–31279
159. Kim SJ, Li J (2013) Caspase blockade induces RIP3-mediated programmed necrosis in Toll-like receptor-activated microglia. Cell Death Dis 4:e716
160. Mandal P, Berger SB, Pillay S, Moriwaki K, Huang C, Guo H et al (2014) RIP3 induces apoptosis independent of pronecrotic kinase activity. Mol Cell 56(4):481–495
161. Takemura R, Takaki H, Okada S, Shime H, Akazawa T, Oshiumi H et al (2015) PolyI:C-induced, TLR3/RIP3-dependent Necroptosis backs up immune effector-mediated tumor elimination in vivo. Cancer Immunol Res 3(8):902–914
162. Meylan E, Burns K, Hofmann K, Blancheteau V, Martinon F, Kelliher M et al (2004) RIP1 is an essential mediator of Toll-like receptor 3-induced NF-kappa B activation. Nat Immunol 5(5):503–507
163. Degterev A, Hitomi J, Germscheid M, Ch'en IL, Korkina O, Teng X et al (2008) Identification of RIP1 kinase as a specific cellular target of necrostatins. Nat Chem Biol 4(5):313–321
164. Koo G-B, Morgan MJ, Lee D-G, Kim W-J, Yoon J-H, Koo JS et al (2015) Methylation-dependent loss of RIP3 expression in cancer represses programmed necrosis in response to chemotherapeutics. Cell Res 25(6):707–725
165. Geserick P, Wang J, Schilling R, Horn S, Harris PA, Bertin J et al (2015) Absence of RIPK3 predicts necroptosis resistance in malignant melanoma. Cell Death Dis 6:e1884

166. Bondhopadhyay B, Moirangthem A, Basu A (2015) Innate adjuvant receptor Toll-like receptor 3 can promote breast cancer through cell surface. Tumour Biol 36(2):1261–1271
167. Pries R, Hogrefe L, Xie L, Frenzel H, Brocks C, Ditz C et al (2008) Induction of c-Myc-dependent cell proliferation through toll-like receptor 3 in head and neck cancer. Int J Mol Med 21(2):209–215
168. Chiron D, Pellat-Deceunynck C, Amiot M, Bataille R, Jego G (2009) TLR3 ligand induces NF-{kappa}B activation and various fates of multiple myeloma cells depending on IFN-{alpha} production. J Immunol 182(7):4471–4478
169. Matijevic T, Pavelic J (2011) The dual role of TLR3 in metastatic cell line. Clin Exp Metastasis 28(7):701–712
170. Conforti R, Ma Y, Morel Y, Paturel C, Terme M, Viaud S et al (2010) Opposing effects of toll-like receptor (TLR3) signaling in tumors can be therapeutically uncoupled to optimize the anticancer efficacy of TLR3 ligands. Cancer Res 70(2):490–500
171. Taura M, Fukuda R, Suico MA, Eguma A, Koga T, Shuto T et al (2010) TLR3 induction by anticancer drugs potentiates poly I:C-induced tumor cell apoptosis. Cancer Sci 101(7):1610–1617
172. Menendez D, Lowe JM, Snipe J, Resnick MA (2016) Ligand dependent restoration of human TLR3 signaling and death in p53 mutant cells. Oncotarget 7(38):61630–61642
173. Ultimo A, Giménez C, Bartovsky P, Aznar E, Sancenón F, Marcos MD et al (2016) Targeting innate immunity with dsRNA-conjugated Mesoporous silica nanoparticles promotes antitumor effects on breast cancer cells. Chemistry 22(5):1582–1586
174. Park J-H, Jeon D-I, Yoon H-E, Kwon S-M, Kim S-A, Ahn S-G et al (2012) Poly I:C inhibits cell proliferation and enhances the growth inhibitory effect of paclitaxel in oral sqaumous cell carcinoma. Acta Odontol Scand 70(3):241–245
175. Matijević T, Kirinec G, Pavelić J (2011) Antitumor activity from the combined application of poly(I:C) and chemotherapeutics in human metastatic pharyngeal cell lines. Chemotherapy 57(6):460–467
176. Le UM, Yanasarn N, Löhr CV, Fischer KA, Cui Z (2008) Tumor chemo-immunotherapy using gemcitabine and a synthetic dsRNA. Cancer Biol Ther 7(3):440–447
177. Van DN, Roberts CF, Marion JD, Lépine S, Harikumar KB, Schreiter J et al (2012) Innate immune agonist, dsRNA, induces apoptosis in ovarian cancer cells and enhances the potency of cytotoxic chemotherapeutics. FASEB J 26(8):3188–3198
178. Li L, Thomas RM, Suzuki H, De Brabander JK, Wang X, Harran PG (2004) A small molecule Smac mimic potentiates TRAIL- and TNFalpha-mediated cell death. Science 305(5689):1471–1474
179. Brands RC, Herbst F, Hartmann S, Seher A, Linz C, Kübler AC et al (2016) Cytotoxic effects of SMAC-mimetic compound LCL161 in head and neck cancer cell lines. Clin Oral Investig 20(9):2325–2332
180. Friboulet L, Gourzones C, Tsao SW, Morel Y, Paturel C, Témam S et al (2010) Poly(I:C) induces intense expression of c-IAP2 and cooperates with an IAP inhibitor in induction of apoptosis in cancer cells. BMC Cancer 10:327
181. Bernardo AR, Cosgaya JM, Aranda A, Jiménez-Lara AM (2013) Synergy between RA and TLR3 promotes type I IFN-dependent apoptosis through upregulation of TRAIL pathway in breast cancer cells. Cell Death Dis 4:e479
182. Ming Lim C, Stephenson R, Salazar AM, Ferris RL (2013) TLR3 agonists improve the immunostimulatory potential of cetuximab against EGFR(+) head and neck cancer cells. Oncoimmunology. 2(6):e24677
183. Xu Y-Y, Chen L, Wang G-L, Zhou J-M, Zhang Y-X, Wei Y-Z et al (2013) A synthetic dsRNA, as a TLR3 pathwaysynergist, combined with sorafenib suppresses HCC in vitro and in vivo. BMC Cancer 13:527
184. Ho V, Lim TS, Lee J, Steinberg J, Szmyd R, Tham M et al (2015) TLR3 agonist and Sorafenib combinatorial therapy promotes immune activation and controls hepatocellular carcinoma progression. Oncotarget 6(29):27252–27266

185. Ayari C, Besançon M, Bergeron A, LaRue H, Bussières V, Fradet Y (2016) Poly(I:C) potentiates Bacillus Calmette-Guérin immunotherapy for bladder cancer. Cancer Immunol Immunother 65(2):223–234
186. Le UM, Kaurin DGL, Sloat BR, Yanasarn N, Cui Z (2009) Localized irradiation of tumors prior to synthetic dsRNA therapy enhanced the resultant anti-tumor activity. Radiother Oncol 90(2):273–279
187. Nagato T, Lee Y-R, Harabuchi Y, Celis E (2014) Combinatorial immunotherapy of polyinosinic-polycytidylic acid and blockade of programmed death-ligand 1 induce effective CD8 T-cell responses against established tumors. Clin Cancer Res 20(5):1223–1234
188. Trumpfheller C, Longhi MP, Caskey M, Idoyaga J, Bozzacco L, Keler T et al (2012) Dendritic cell-targeted protein vaccines: a novel approach to induce T-cell immunity. J Intern Med 271(2):183–192
189. Jongbloed SL, Kassianos AJ, McDonald KJ, Clark GJ, Ju X, Angel CE et al (2010) Human CD141+ (BDCA-3)+ dendritic cells (DCs) represent a unique myeloid DC subset that cross-presents necrotic cell antigens. J Exp Med 207(6):1247–1260
190. Lauterbach H, Bathke B, Gilles S, Traidl-Hoffmann C, Luber CA, Fejer G et al (2010) Mouse CD8alpha+ DCs and human BDCA3+ DCs are major producers of IFN-lambda in response to poly IC. J Exp Med 207(12):2703–2717
191. Azuma M, Takeda Y, Nakajima H, Sugiyama H, Ebihara T, Oshiumi H et al (2016) Biphasic function of TLR3 adjuvant on tumor and spleen dendritic cells promotes tumor T cell infiltration and regression in a vaccine therapy. Oncoimmunology. 5(8):e1188244
192. Forte G, Rega A, Morello S, Luciano A, Arra C, Pinto A et al (2012) Polyinosinic-polycytidylic acid limits tumor outgrowth in a mouse model of metastatic lung cancer. J Immunol 188(11):5357–5364
193. Salem ML, Kadima AN, Cole DJ, Gillanders WE (2005) Defining the antigen-specific T-cell response to vaccination and poly(I:C)/TLR3 signaling: evidence of enhanced primary and memory CD8 T-cell responses and antitumor immunity. J Immunother 28(3):220–228
194. Trumpfheller C, Caskey M, Nchinda G, Longhi MP, Mizenina O, Huang Y et al (2008) The microbial mimic poly IC induces durable and protective CD4+ T cell immunity together with a dendritic cell targeted vaccine. Proc Natl Acad Sci U S A 105(7):2574–2579
195. Forghani P, Waller EK (2015) Poly (I: C) modulates the immunosuppressive activity of myeloid-derived suppressor cells in a murine model of breast cancer. Breast Cancer Res Treat 153(1):21–30
196. Shime H, Matsumoto M, Oshiumi H, Tanaka S, Nakane A, Iwakura Y et al (2012) Toll-like receptor 3 signaling converts tumor-supporting myeloid cells to tumoricidal effectors. Proc Natl Acad Sci U S A 109(6):2066–2071
197. Diamond MS, Kinder M, Matsushita H, Mashayekhi M, Dunn GP, Archambault JM et al (2011) Type I interferon is selectively required by dendritic cells for immune rejection of tumors. J Exp Med 208(10):1989–2003
198. Curtsinger JM, Valenzuela JO, Agarwal P, Lins D, Mescher MF (2005) Type I IFNs provide a third signal to CD8 T cells to stimulate clonal expansion and differentiation. J Immunol 174(8):4465–4469
199. Zitvogel L, Galluzzi L, Kepp O, Smyth MJ, Kroemer G (2015) Type I interferons in anticancer immunity. Nat Rev Immunol 15(7):405–414
200. Schulz O, Diebold SS, Chen M, Näslund TI, Nolte MA, Alexopoulou L et al (2005) Toll-like receptor 3 promotes cross-priming to virus-infected cells. Nature 433(7028):887–892
201. Boes M, Meyer-Wentrup F (2015) TLR3 triggering regulates PD-L1 (CD274) expression in human neuroblastoma cells. Cancer Lett 361(1):49–56
202. Chiappinelli KB, Strissel PL, Desrichard A, Li H, Henke C, Akman B et al (2015) Inhibiting DNA methylation causes an interferon response in cancer via dsRNA including endogenous retroviruses. Cell 162(5):974–986

203. Iribarren K, Bloy N, Buqué A, Cremer I, Eggermont A, Fridman WH et al (2016) Trial watch: Immunostimulation with Toll-like receptor agonists in cancer therapy. Oncoimmunology. 5(3):e1088631
204. Shime H, Matsumoto M, Seya T (2016) Double-stranded RNA promotes CTL-independent tumor cytolysis mediated by CD11b(+)Ly6G(+) intratumor myeloid cells through the TICAM-1 signaling pathway. Cell Death Differ 24(3):385–396

Chapter 9
Fas/CD95, Lipid Rafts, and Cancer

Faustino Mollinedo and Consuelo Gajate

Abstract Cholesterol/sphingolipid-rich membrane domains, known as lipid rafts, are critical for the compartmentalization of signalling processes. Initially, lipid rafts were found to host signalling pathways related to cell survival and the immune system, but with the advent of the new millennium, lipid rafts were also found to host Fas/CD95 death receptor and to be involved in cell death signalling. In the last 15 years it has become clear that lipid rafts are crucial for the triggering of apoptosis mediated by Fas/CD95. Accumulating evidence has led to the notion that lipid rafts serve as scaffolds for the recruitment and clustering of Fas/CD95 death receptor and downstream signalling molecules, thus leading to the formation of the so-called clusters of apoptotic signalling molecule-enriched rafts (CASMERs) that could be pharmacologically modulated. Despite the molecular mechanisms that regulate the recruitment of Fas/CD95 in lipid rafts remain to be unraveled, a number of protein modifications, together with additional proteins and signalling pathways have been suggested to play a role in both Fas/CD95-mediated apoptosis as well as death receptor association with lipid rafts. In this chapter, we discuss the involvement of lipid rafts in the regulation of Fas/CD95-induced apoptosis and its implications as a promising avenue for cancer therapy.

Keywords Fas • CD95 • Apoptotic molecules • Apoptotic signalling • Non-apoptotic signalling • Lipid rafts • Cancer • Anticancer drugs • Chemotherapy • CASMER

9.1 Introduction

Fas (CD95/APO-1) is the prototype of "death receptors" in the tumor necrosis factor (TNF) receptor superfamily [1, 2]. Studies on Fas/CD95 have focused primarily on its role in apoptosis, which were greatly supported by the fact that specific mutations in Fas/CD95 and FasL/CD95L led to the lack of apoptosis in lymphocytes

F. Mollinedo (✉) • C. Gajate (✉)
Laboratory of Cell Death and Cancer Therapy, Department of Cellular and Molecular Medicine, Centro de Investigaciones Biológicas, Consejo Superior de Investigaciones Científicas (CSIC), C/ Ramiro de Maeztu 9, E-28040 Madrid, Spain
e-mail: fmollin@cib.csic.es; cgajate@cib.csic.es

O. Micheau (ed.), *TRAIL, Fas Ligand, TNF and TLR3 in Cancer*, Resistance to Targeted Anti-Cancer Therapeutics, DOI 10.1007/978-3-319-56805-8_9

leading to massive lymphadenopathy and autoimmune lymphoproliferative syndrome in *lpr* (lymphoproliferation), and *gld* (generalized lymphoproliferative disease) mice, respectively, causing autoantibody formation with autoimmune manifestations, and the accumulation of abnormal double negative T cells [3–5]. The equivalent human disorder is known as autoimmune lymphoproliferative syndrome (ALPS), which is characterized by immune dysregulation mainly due to defective Fas/CD95-mediated apoptosis that leads to a defect in lymphocyte apoptosis, and patients develop lymphadenopathy, splenomegaly, increased risk of lymphoma, and autoimmune disease with an abnormal accumulation of double negative T cells [6–12]. However, despite Fas/CD95 have long viewed as a death receptor mediating apoptosis induction in a wide range of apoptosis-based physiologic processes (e.g., T-cell-dependent cytotoxicity, deletion of autoreactive T and B cells, activation-induced cell death, tumor surveillance, immune privilege) and pathologic degenerative diseases (e.g., autoimmunity, fulminant hepatitis, and neurodegeneration) [13–15], Fas/CD95 has also been shown to have multiple non-apoptotic and tumor-promoting activities [16–20], making difficult to discern the role of Fas/CD95 death receptor as a friend or a foe in cancer.

Since the first demonstration of the clustering of Fas/CD95 in lipid rafts in 2001 [21], a wide number of studies have been focused on the association of Fas/CD95 with lipid rafts and its functional relevance in apoptotic cell death [12, 22–25]. Lipid rafts have been defined as "small (10–200 nm) heterogenous, highly dynamic, sterol- and sphingolipid-enriched domains that compartmentalize cellular processes" [26]. Because the lipid and protein composition of membrane rafts differs from that of the surrounding membrane, rafts provide an additional level of compartmentalization, serving as sorting platforms and hubs for signal transduction proteins. Accumulating evidence indicates that a high local concentration of Fas/CD95 can be achieved in lipid rafts, the latter serving as platforms for coupling adaptor and effector proteins required for Fas/CD95 downstream signalling, thus facilitating and amplifying signalling processes by transient local assembly of various cross-interacting molecules [12, 22, 23, 25, 27]. This is of particular importance in Fas/CD95-mediated signal transduction because death receptors lack enzymatic activity and the subsequent apoptotic signalling pathway is triggered and transmitted by protein–protein interactions [12, 23, 25, 28].

9.2 Fas/CD95 Death Receptor and Apoptosis

Human mature CD95 (aka as Fas or APO-1) is a 45–48 kDa (319 amino acids) single spanning transmembrane receptor, and a prototypical death receptor of the TNF receptor (TNFR), that contains: a 157-amino acid N-terminal extracellular region, comprising three cysteine-rich domains (CRDs), which binds to its cognate ligand FasL/CD95L; a 17-amino acid transmembrane domain, and a C-terminal cytoplasmic domain of 145 amino acids that harbors a "death domain" (DD) required to transmit apoptotic signals (Fig. 9.1) [25, 29–32]. This DD contains

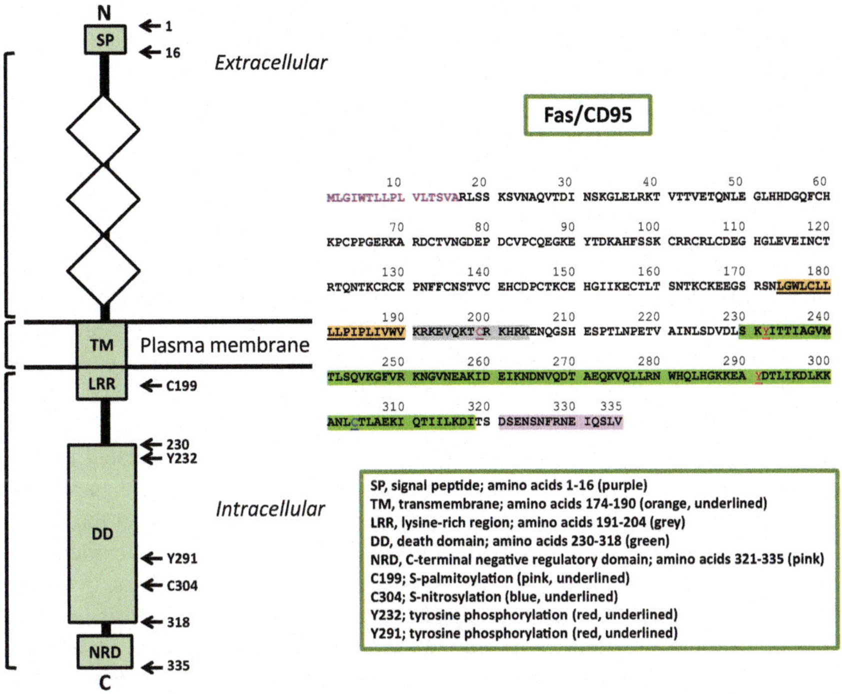

Fig. 9.1 Primary sequence and schematic diagram of human CD95 death receptor, highlighting the amino acid residues and signatures involved in raft localization and posttranslational protein modification. Human CD95 contains a signal peptide (SP; amino acid residues 1–16), and thus the mature CD95 protein consists of 319 amino acids (aas) with a N-terminal extracellular domain of 157 aas, a short (17 aas) transmembrane region (TM) and a C-terminal cytoplasmic domain of 145 aas. Relevant domains and amino acid residues for CD95 binding to lipid rafts (lysine-rich region, LRR, C199 and C304), tyrosine phosphorylation (Y232 and Y291), and apoptotic activity (death domain, DD, and C-terminal negative regulatory domain, NRD) are indicated. See text for further details

about 88 amino acids (Fig. 9.1), is homologous to other DDs present in additional death receptors, and plays a critical role in transmitting death signalling from the cell surface to the interior of the cell [25, 32–34]. Fas/CD95 does not possess enzymatic activity, but acts by binding to other proteins through its DD, which is a protein–protein interaction domain that enables Fas/CD95 and other DD-containing death receptors to interact by homotypic binding with the bipartite DD adapter protein Fas-associated death domain protein (FADD) [35, 36]. Following physiological Fas/CD95 activation by its cognate ligand FasL/CD95L, the death receptor undergoes a conformational change in the intracellular domain of the receptor that results in receptor aggregation at the cell membrane and the recruitment of FADD through interaction between the DDs of FADD and the clustered Fas/CD95 receptors [35, 37–39]. FADD also contains a "death effector domain" (DED) that binds to an analogous DED domain repeated in tandem within the zymogen form of procaspase-8 [40], leading to its recruitment and self-activation, which in turn activates downstream effector caspases and signalling processes that eventually lead to apoptosis [41]. Thus, Fas/CD95-mediated apoptosis involves the formation of the so-called "death inducing signalling complex" (DISC) [42], composed of Fas/CD95, FADD and procaspase-8.

In addition to the apoptotic response, Fas/CD95 has been also shown to promote necroptotic cell death through the DD-containing kinase receptor interacting protein (RIP1) [43, 44], as well as autophagy in cells with low levels of caspase-8 [45] or following the participation of distinct kinases [46, 47]. Nevertheless, CD95/Fas behaves mainly as an apoptosis-inducing receptor expressed on many tissues and tumor cells. During tumor progression CD95 is frequently downregulated, and tumor cells lose apoptosis sensitivity. Dysregulation and mutations have been reported in Fas/CD95 in several malignant cells of various histological origins, with most of the mutations distributed within the DD domain, thus leading to resistance to Fas/CD95-mediated apoptosis [48–51]. Reduced Fas/CD95-mediated apoptosis is a well-established factor in tumor cell survival, and expression of Fas/CD95 is decreased in several different tumor types [52–59]. However, the fact that the Fas/CD95 mutation rate is not usually high in cancer, and the increasing evidence for a Fas/CD95 engagement in transmitting non-apoptotic signals, thus leading to tumor-promoting activities [19, 60, 61], suggests that other additional factors apart from primary structure are going to play a critical role in the final outcome regarding cell death triggering. Interestingly, accumulating evidence has shown that Fas/CD95 signalling cascades are often disrupted in tumor cells, leading to the triggering of Fas/CD95-mediated pro-survival, rather than apoptotic pathways [50, 62–65]. These non-apoptotic functions of Fas/CD95 contribute to tumor-promoting phenotypes [19, 66–70], and Fas/CD95 knockout in tumor cell xenografts was found to prevent tumor growth, thus suggesting that Fas/CD95 has a growth-promoting role during tumorigenesis [17]. The regulatory factors that switch the role of Fas/CD95 towards either cell death or cell survival remain to be elucidated, but it could be envisaged that these regulatory factors might include the particular location of the death receptor in certain membrane domains where it could interact with distinct proteins, generating altogether a molecular microenvironment predisposed to launch either an apoptotic or non-apoptotic signalling.

9.3 Fas/CD95 Non-apoptotic Signalling

Despite Fas/CD95 is a major molecule in triggering and modulating receptor-mediated cell death, it is now well accepted that CD95 is a receptor with pleiotropic functions, including apoptotic and non-apoptotic signals. Recent studies have shown an increasing number of non-apoptotic responses emanating from Fas/CD95. The Fas/CD95-FasL/CD95L system has now been involved in a wide variety of functional non-apoptotic responses, including migration and invasion, particularly in apoptosis-resistant malignant cells [16, 18, 71–73], inflammation [66, 74, 75–78,

79–82], neurite sprouting and outgrowth [14, 83–85], as well as cell proliferation [64, 86–88]. Fas/CD95 can trigger the three main mitogen-activated protein kinase (MAPK) pathways p38, JNK1/2, and ERK1/2 [83, 88–90], tyrosine protein kinase signalling [16, 91, 92], as well as the transcription factor NF-κB [93], leading to the abovementioned Fas/CD95-mediated non-apoptotic responses [20, 64, 94].

However, a major unresolved question is to identify how the Fas/CD95 system switches between apoptotic and non-apoptotic responses. This switch seems to occur at different levels of signalling transduction, ranging from how the death receptor is located in specific membrane domains, thus allowing different interactions with signalling molecules, to cross-talk with other signalling pathways, which could lead to distinct and even opposite cellular outcomes [2, 20].

Interestingly, Fas/CD95 stimulation has been shown to lead to the activation of the phosphatydilinositol-3-kinase (PI3K) pathway in glioblastoma multiforme [16], as well as to tyrosine phosphorylation through Src family kinases in different cell types [95, 96], which are recruited to Fas/CD95 [91, 97]. Stimulation of Fas/CD95 has also been shown to result in tyrosine phosphorylation of the receptor [98, 99], which contains a tyrosine-containing motif YXXL within the DD of Fas/CD95, similar to the canonical immunoreceptor tyrosine activation motifs (ITAMs) or immunoreceptor tyrosine inhibitory motifs (ITIMs). This link between the Fas/CD95 system and the PI3K pathway or tyrosine phosphorylation could explain, at least in part, the involvement of Fas/CD95 in survival signalling. In this context, It has been recently demonstrated that phosphorylation of Y232 and Y291, within the DD, is critical to FasL/CD95L-induced non-apoptotic signalling of Fas/CD95 and is regulated by Src family kinases and the protein tyrosine phosphatase SHP-1 [100]. On these grounds, it could be envisaged that Fas/CD95 signalling outcome might be determined by the tyrosine phosphorylation status of its DD.

9.4 Proteins Affecting Fas/CD95-Mediated Apoptotic Signalling with Implications in Fas/CD95-Mediated Chemotherapeutic Regimens

A number of proteins affecting the Fas/CD95 apoptotic activity through their interaction with the death receptor (Daxx, FAF1, FAIM, FAP-1, FIST/HIPK3, Lifeguard, Sentrin/SUMO-1, Ubc9) or with DISC constituents (FLASH, FLIP, TOSO) have been previously reviewed [33]. The cellular FADD-like interleukin-1β-converting enzyme (FLICE)-inhibitory protein (c-FLIP) negatively regulates apoptotic signalling downstream of death receptors, being a key inhibitor of procaspase-8 activation in the Fas/CD95-DISC apoptotic signalling. c-FLIP plays a major role as a master switch in determining life/death cell fate decisions, behaves as a guardian of the threshold of extrinsic apoptosis, and the amount of c-FLIP in the cell at the moment of death receptor stimulation defines the timing of cell death; its function having been largely discussed in previous reviews [101–104]. c-FLIP expression has been

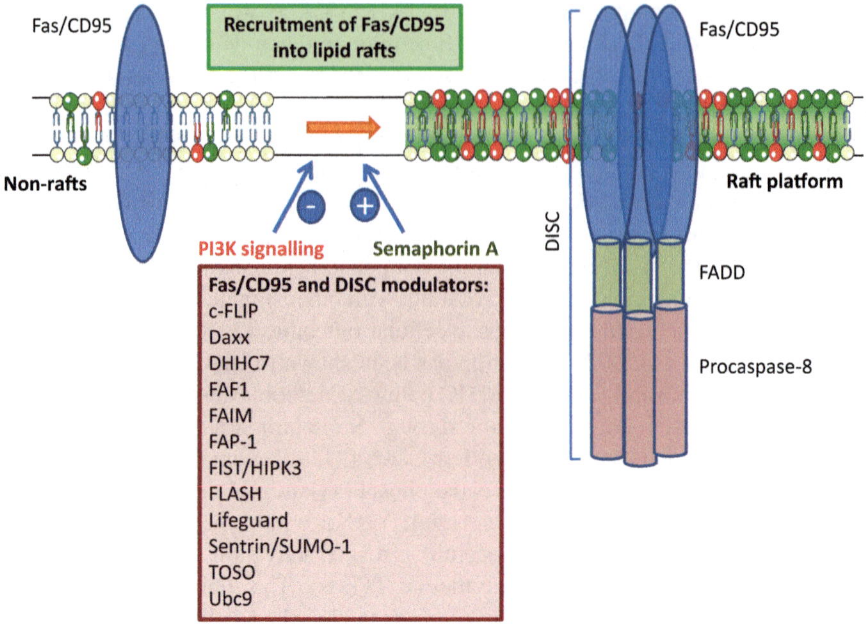

Fig. 9.2 Proteins and signalling pathways affecting Fas/CD95-mediated apoptosis and recruitment of Fas/CD95 into lipid rafts. See text for further details

detected to be increased in certain tumors, and c-FLIP overexpression results in tumor cell escape from T-cell immunity [105]. In addition to the role of c-FLIP in the pathogenesis of hematologic cancers [105–108], further proteins (Fig. 9.2) have been reported to influence the Fas/CD95 apoptotic signalling pathway by affecting its cell surface expression and pro-apoptotic activity. Several of these proteins are suggested to play a role in cancer development and progression [33], and other proteins affecting Fas/CD95-mediated apoptosis, which are not so frequently reviewed in their relation to cancer, are discussed below. Moreover, the human intracellular serine protease inhibitor (serpin), protease inhibitor 9 (PI9), has been shown to inhibit FasL/CD95L-mediated apoptosis in some cell lines in a cell type-specific manner by binding to the intermediate active forms of caspase-8 (p43/41) and caspase-10 (p47/43), thereby preventing further activation of the downstream target caspase-3 and execution of apoptosis [109].

9.4.1 FAP-1

The protein-tyrosine phosphatase **F**as-**a**ssociated **p**hosphatase-1 (FAP-1), aka PTPL1, PTPN13, PTP1E, and PTP-BAS, capable of interacting with the cytosolic carboxyl terminal 15 amino acid-domain of Fas/CD95, which is a negative regulatory domain (C-terminal 15 amino acids) of Fas/CD95 [30], shows its highest expression in tissues and cell lines that are relatively resistant to Fas/CD95-mediated cytotoxicity [110, 111]. FAP-1 is one of the largest known non-receptor protein-tyrosine phosphatases PTPases (about 250 kDa), comprising 2485 residues [112], and is mutated in a significant number of colorectal tumors [113, 114]. There are three major structural characteristics of FAP-1 action: a leucine zipper, a membrane-binding domain, and 6 PDZ domains [110]. The binding of the third PDZ domain (PDZ3) of FAP-1 to the inhibitory domain of Fas/CD95 [115] could be the underlying basis for the action of FAP-1 as a negative regulator of Fas/CD95-mediated apoptosis. Because FAP-1 negatively regulates Fas/CD95-mediated apoptosis in several tumors, including pancreatic adenocarcinoma [116, 117] and melanoma [118]; it has been suggested to positively regulate tumorigenesis, thus becoming a potential therapeutic target [119]. Gene transfer-mediated elevations in FAP-1 partially abolish Fas/CD95-induced apoptosis in T-cell leukemia Jurkat cells [110, 111] as well as in other cancer cells, including ovarian, pancreatic, and colon cancer cells [111, 116, 120, 121]. FAP-1 is also suggested to inhibit Fas/CD95-mediated apoptosis in colon cancer [121], head and neck cancer [122], hepatocellular carcinoma [123], and ovarian cancer [120]. In addition, FAP-1 is highly expressed in Ewing's sarcoma [124] and has been identified as a target of EWS-FL1, modulating Ewing's sarcoma tumorigenesis [125]. Silencing FAP-1 expression increases the efficacy of chemotherapy for colon carcinoma with oxaliplatin [126]. miR-200c microRNA regulates Fas/CD95-mediated apoptosis by targeting FAP-1 [127], which could explain the reduction in sensitivity of cells to Fas/CD95-mediated apoptosis observed in the context of reduced miR-200 expression during tumor progression. Interaction of FAP-1 with Fas/CD95 inhibits Fas/CD95 export to the cell surface, thus reducing cell surface Fas/CD95 levels, and increases the intracellular pool of Fas/CD95 within the cytoskeleton network [118], as well as the co-localization of Fas/CD95-FAP-1 in the Golgi complex [116], hence preventing translocation of Fas/CD95 from intracellular stores to the cell surface. In contrast, dynamin-2 facilitates Fas/CD95 protein translocation from the Golgi apparatus via the trans-Golgi network to the cell surface [128]. Interestingly, FasL/CD95L has been shown to induce tyrosine phosphorylation of Fas/CD95 in astrocytoma cells, and FAP-1 dephosphorylates Tyr-275 in the C-terminus of the mature Fas/CD95 form [129]. Mutation in amino acid 275 of mature Fas/CD95 results in decreased association of Fas/CD95 with FAP-1, and greater export of Fas/CD95 to the cell surface in melanomas and normal fibroblasts [118]. On the other hand, recent evidence has shown that autophagy modulates Fas/CD95-induced cell death through the selective autophagy-mediated degradation of FAP-1 via its interaction with the adapter protein p62/Sequestosome-1 (SQSTM1) in Fas/CD95-mediated cell death [130]. These data, together with those described in the previous section, further support that reversible phosphorylation can regulate Fas/CD95 function [91, 96, 97, 100, 131–133].

9.4.2 FAIM

Fas **a**poptosis **i**nhibitory **m**olecule (FAIM) was first cloned as an evolutionary conserved protein that antagonizes Fas/CD95-mediated apoptosis of mature B cells, through a differential display strategy to detect cDNAs present in B cells rendered Fas/CD95 resistant, but absent in those rendered Fas/CD95 sensitive [134]. FAIM exists in two alternatively spliced forms: the broadly expressed FAIM-S and the tissue-specific FAIM-L [135–137]. FAIM seems to act upstream of Akt during T-cell receptor (TCR) signalling and overexpression of FAIM leads to increased amount of Akt in lipid rafts and thereby its activation [138]. Thus, FAIM seems to modulate the localization of Akt to lipid rafts, but no interaction between FAIM and Akt has been detected following co-immunoprecipitation experiments [138]. In addition, $faim^{-/-}$ B cells and thymocytes exhibit increased sensitivity to Fas/CD95-triggered apoptosis in vitro, and $faim^{-/-}$ mice show exacerbated liver damage in response to Fas/CD95 engagement in vivo [139]. The lack of FAIM results in decreased expression of c-FLIP$_L$ (about 55 kDa), the long isoform of c-FLIP [140], and c-FLIP$_R$ (about 24 kDa), the only short c-FLIP isoform expressed in mice [141], as well as in increased association, and subsequent activation, of caspase-8 with Fas/CD95 [139]. Genetic deletion of *faim* also results in elevated levels of apoptotic molecules such as Nur77, Bak and Bax, which have been involved in thymocyte apoptosis [138]. FAIM has been shown to play a major role in modulating TCR-induced and Fas/CD95-mediated apoptosis of thymocytes [138], as well as in neuron protection [142] and cell death in non-small lung cancer [143] and multiple myeloma [144]. The anti-apoptotic protein FAIM is a target for miR-133b, which in turn is suggested to have a role in prostate cancer [145].

9.4.3 Nucleolin

Following screenings of primary lymphoma cell extracts for Fas/CD95-associated proteins that have the potential to regulate Fas/CD95 signalling, an activation-resistant Fas/CD95 complex selectively included nucleolin [146]. Nucleolin-Fas/CD95 complexes were detected in B-cell lymphoma cells and primary tissues, but not in B-lymphocytes from healthy donors. Cell surface nucleolin binds Fas/CD95 and prevents induction of Fas/CD95-mediated apoptosis by inhibiting ligand binding in B-cell lymphomas [146]. Nucleolin knockdown sensitized BJAB human Burkitt B-lymphoma cells to FasL/CD95L- and Fas/CD95 agonistic antibody-induced apoptosis through enhanced ligand binding, suggesting that nucleolin blocks the FasL/CD95L–Fas/CD95 interaction. Nucleolin is a multifunctional nucleolar phosphoprotein that was first identified in ribosomal RNA processing, but its localization is altered in highly proliferating cells, being translocated into the cytoplasm and onto the plasma membrane, where it exerts pro-survival functions, including stabilization of Bcl-2, Bcl-x$_L$, and IL-2 mRNAs [147–151]. Nucleolin is highly expressed on the surface of several types of cancer cells, where it has been shown to serve as a receptor for hepatocyte growth factor and P-selectin, as well as a transport protein [152–154]. Extranuclear nucleolin is also involved in regulating multiple apoptosis-related molecules contributing to the survival and anti-apoptotic pathways of cancer cells [155, 156]. Nucleolin expression is suggested to be regulated by miR-194 and miR-206 [157]. In addition, nucleolin expression is positively regulated by human antigen R (HuR) and negatively regulated via competition with miR-494 [158].

9.4.4 CD74

Berkova et al. [159] have recently found that the B-lymphoma cell line BJAB with suppressed CD74, a MHC class II chaperone [160] that has been implicated in malignant B-cell proliferation and survival [161, 162], is more sensitive to FasL/CD95L-induced apoptosis and Fas/CD95 signalling-dependent chemotherapies, such as edelfosine (aka ET-18-OCH_3) and doxorubicin, than control CD74-expressing cells. Expression of full-length CD74 in liver protected mice from a lethal challenge with agonistic anti-Fas/CD95 antibody Jo2, whereas the absence of CD74 promoted Fas/CD95 upregulation at the cell surface and increased cleavage/activation of procaspase-8 [159]. Pretreatment with the fully humanized anti-CD74 monoclonal antibody milatuzumab sensitized BJAB cells to Fas/CD95-mediated apoptosis [161]. These data suggest that CD74 modulates Fas/CD95 signalling in lymphomas by decreasing the levels of Fas/CD95 receptor on the cell surface through mechanisms that still remain unclear [159]. Specific targeting of the CD74 on the cell surface seems to sensitize CD74-expressing cancer cells to Fas/CD95-mediated apoptosis, and thus this could be an approach to increase effectiveness of Fas/CD95-mediated chemotherapy regimens for hematologic malignancies. A number of trials testing different treatment schedules of milatuzumab in different hematologic malignancies, including chronic lymphocytic leukemia (CLL), non-Hodgkin lymphoma (NHL), mantle cell lymphoma (MCL), and multiple myeloma (MM), are underway and show no severe adverse effects [163–165]. CD74 expression is rather limited in normal human tissues, but it was found to be overexpressed in over 85% of NHL, CLL and a majority of MM cells [161, 166, 167]. Cell surface levels of CD74 are higher in CLL patient-derived B cells than in normal B cells, and CD74 activation by macrophage migration inhibitory factor (MIF) activates NF-κB and induces secretion of IL-8, which promotes cell survival and tumor progression [167, 168]. MIF fosters cell survival and proliferation [169] and has been shown to be a ligand of CD74 [170], which generates a complex with CD44 acting as a receptor for MIF, and where CD44 is an integral member of the CD74 receptor complex required for signal transduction [171]. Thus, CD74-mediated proliferative and pro-survival signalling can initiate or contribute to pro-carcinogenic events and enhance the survival of cancer cells. CD74 expression has been associated with poor prognostic markers in breast cancer [172], but intriguingly, recent reports have also associated CD74 expression with a favorable survival for melanoma [173] and mesothelioma [174]. Engagement of CD74 leads to the activation of extracellular signal-regulated kinase-1/2 (ERK1/2) MAP kinase (MAPK) cascade and cell proliferation [170]. CD74 is internalized from the plasma membrane into the endocytic compartment, where intramembrane cleavage releases the intracellular cytosolic domain (CD74-ICD) that enters the nucleus and activates NF-κB p65/RelA, controlling B cell differentiation [160, 175]. In addition, CD74-ICD promotes the expression of TAp63 transcription factor, which subsequently upregulates Bcl-2 and promotes survival of B cells [176].

Accumulating evidence suggests that CD74 is a novel target for immunotherapy of neoplasms expressing this antigen. Anti-CD74 naked antibody or conjugated to isotypes, drugs or toxins synergizes with other chemotherapeutic agents and elicits significant antitumor effects in vitro and in vivo. In this regard, in vitro and preclinical data show that the humanized antibody milatuzumab, alone or in combination therapy with additional anticancer agents, is a promising approach to treat B-cell malignancies, including NHL, CLL, MCL, and MM [164, 177–184]. Because CD74 regulates Fas/CD95 death receptor signalling by decreasing the levels of Fas/CD95 on the cell surface [159], with a major role in B-cell malignancies, and co-clustering of Fas/CD95 and lipid rafts have been involved in a novel approach for the treatment of some B-cell malignancies [185–187], it is tempting to envisage a putative combination therapy involving agents that affect both phenomena. In this regard, the ether lipid edelfosine has been found to induce Fas/CD95-mediated apoptosis in a wide number of hematological cancer cells through the recruitment of Fas/CD95 in raft platforms [21, 185–188], and recent evidence shows that the B-lymphoma BJAB cells lacking CD74 are sensitized to edelfosine [159].

9.5 Compartmentalization of Fas/CD95 Apoptotic Signalling in Lipid Rafts

With the advent of the second millennium, it was found that apoptosis mediated by the death receptor Fas/CD95 involved its recruitment in specific domains at the plasma membrane, particularly in clusters of cholesterol- and sphingolipid-rich membrane domains, termed lipid rafts [21, 188–192]. The apoptosis response induced by a synthetic ether lipid called edelfosine was mediated by the recruitment of Fas/CD95 death receptor in lipid rafts, and the disruption of raft domains by cholesterol depletion led to the inhibition of apoptosis [21], thus leading to the first compelling evidence for the involvement of lipid rafts in Fas/CD95-mediated apoptosis. Edelfosine is considered the prototype of a family of synthetic antitumor drugs collectively known as alkylphospholipid analogs [193–195], and it is a stark example of how a chemical tool can reveal novel molecular processes in cell death regulation. Soon after the finding of the edelfosine-induced Fas/CD95 recruitment in rafts [21], the natural ligand FasL/CD95L was also found to promote Fas/CD95 clustering in lipid rafts [196]. Thus, it seems clear that the antitumor drug edelfosine makes use of physiological processes, exacerbating them and offering new ways to promote cell death in cancer cells. Later on, we also found that the adaptor protein FADD and procaspase-8 were also recruited into lipid rafts, forming the DISC, as well as additional downstream signalling molecules during the apoptotic response induced by edelfosine [185, 188, 197, 198]. Taken together, these data led to the conclusion that lipid rafts act as scaffolds where molecules of the Fas/CD95 signalling pathway are concentrated, providing a limited physical space where protein–protein interactions are highly facilitated, thus forming a kind of a linchpin from which a potent death signal is launched. On these grounds, the co-clustering of lipid rafts and Fas/CD95 signalling provides a new framework in the triggering of death receptor-mediated apoptosis.

Redistribution of Fas/CD95 in lipid rafts together with downstream signalling molecules lead to a new concept of apoptosis regulation by membrane compartmentalization. Thus, redistribution of death receptors and signalling molecules in lipid rafts and non-raft regions may regulate different signalling responses, segregating molecules with opposite functional activities and putting together molecules that share and yield the same final outcome. Thus, recruitment of death receptors and downstream signalling molecules in lipid rafts could potentiate protein–protein interactions and signalling cross talk, which ultimately would lead to the triggering of cell death signalling. In this regard, the recruitment of death receptors and downstream apoptotic signalling molecules in clustered raft platforms has led us to coin the word CASMER as an acronym for "**c**luster of **a**poptotic **s**ignalling **m**olecule-**e**nriched **r**afts" [22, 27, 28, 188, 198, 199]. CASMER refers to the recruitment of death receptors together with downstream apoptotic signalling molecules in clustered rafts or raft platforms [22, 27]. CASMER represents a novel raft-based supramolecular entity, acting as death-promoting platforms where death receptors and downstream signalling molecules are brought together, thus facilitating protein–protein interactions (Fig. 9.3). CASMER formation represents a way to regulate apoptosis by creating a kind of large islands enriched in pro-apoptotic molecules, from which apoptotic signalling is launched. Fas/CD95-DISC assembly in lipid rafts has been visualized by electron microscopy [198] (Fig. 9.4). Moreover, the edelfosine-induced recruitment of Bid in lipid rafts further highlights the importance of CASMERs in cell death modulation by acting as linkers between the extrinsic death receptor- and intrinsic mitochondria-related signalling pathways in apoptosis [28, 185, 188, 199, 200].

Because death receptors can lead to either cell death or survival signalling, it is tempting to envisage that the above compartmentalization of signalling pathways in lipid rafts could be critical to promote either an apoptotic or a non-apoptotic response, and therefore lipid rafts might play a key role in determining the final outcome, cell death or survival.

Moderate traumatic brain injury has been shown to result in rapid recruitment of tumor necrosis factor receptor 1 (TNFR1) to lipid rafts, altered associations with signalling intermediates and subsequent recruitment of caspase-8, leading to apoptosis [201]. Tumor necrosis factor (TNF)-related apoptosis ligand (TRAIL) has

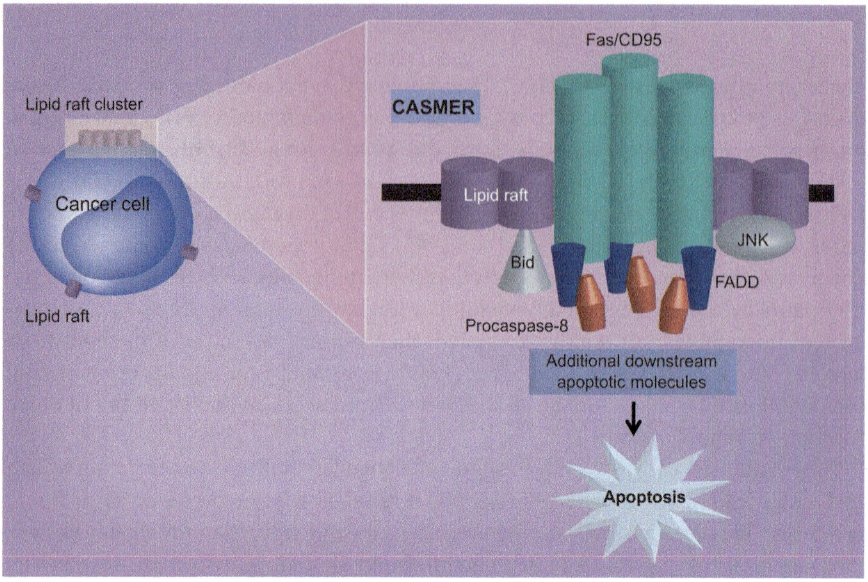

Fig. 9.3 CASMER formation. A number of apoptotic signalling molecules, including CD95, FADD and procaspase-8, forming the DISC, and downstream apoptotic signalling molecules are recruited and brought together in close proximity in large lipid raft platforms or raft clusters to generate the CASMER supramolecular entity. See text for further details. (From [27], © Future Science Group)

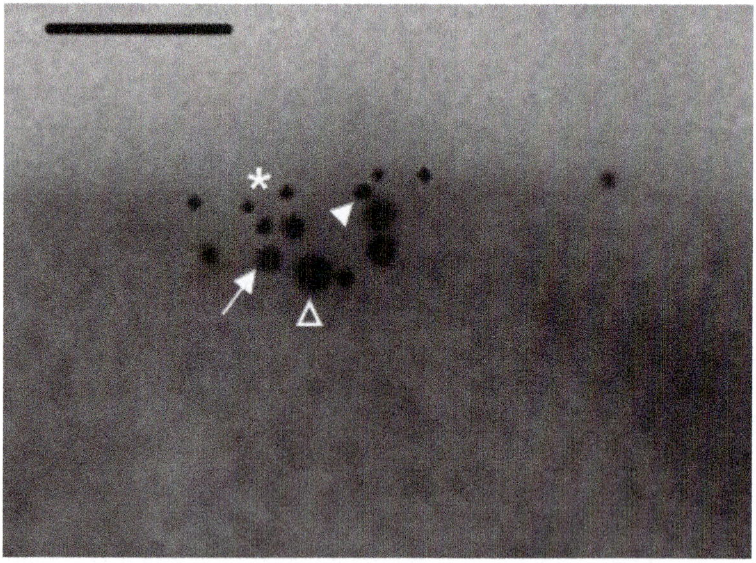

Fig. 9.4 Visualization of DISC in a lipid raft platform. Electron microscopy image of edelfosine-treated Jurkat cells showing DISC formation in lipid rafts. Sections of edelfosine-treated cells were labeled with the raft marker GM1 using cholera toxin B subunit (6-nm gold) (*asterisk*), anti-Fas/CD95 antibody (10-nm) (*closed arrowhead*), anti-FADD antibody (15-nm) (*arrow*), and anti-procaspase-8 antibody (20-nm) (*open arrowhead*). Lipid rafts were labeled on the external face of the membrane, whereas DISC components were located in the internal face of raft-enriched membrane domains. Bar, 400 nm. (From [198], © Public Library of Science)

been shown to induce apoptosis in TRAIL-sensitive non-small cell lung carcinoma (NSCLC) cells through the induction of DISC assembly in lipid rafts of plasma membrane, leading to caspase-8 activation and subsequent apoptosis [202]. In contrast, the formation of DISC in the non-raft phase of the plasma membrane leads to the inhibition of caspase-8 cleavage and the activation of the survival NF-κB and ERK1/2 signalling pathways in TRAIL-resistant NSCLC cells [202]. This DISC assembly in non-rafts is suggested to be mediated by receptor-interacting protein (RIP) and c-FLIP. Selective knockdown of either RIP or c-FLIP with interfering RNA leads to redistribution of DISC from non-raft to raft membrane domains following TRAIL incubation, thereby switching the DISC downstream signals from NF-κB and ERK1/2-mediated survival to caspase-8-initiated apoptosis [202]. In this regard, the treatment of NSCLC A549 cells with cis-diaminedichloroplatinum II (CDDP or cisplatin) decreased c-FLIP expression, enhanced TRAIL-induced apoptosis, and redistributed DISC in rafts [202]. TRAIL-induced redistribution of death receptors DR4 and DR5 in lipid rafts contributed to the sensitivity to TRAIL in the TRAIL-sensitive NSCLC H460 cell line [203]. These data support that chemotherapeutic agents that enhance TRAIL-DISC redistribution in lipid rafts potentiate the apoptotic effect of TRAIL in cancer cells [202]. However, the lack of death receptor redistribution in lipid rafts negatively impacts DISC assembly, which at least partially leads to the development of acquired resistance to death receptors in distinct tumor cells [204]. On these grounds, it could be envisaged that location of a death receptor in lipid rafts could lead to a DISC-mediated apoptosis, likely through CASMER formation, whereas RIP and c-FLIP-mediated assembly of the DISC in non-rafts could represent a critical upstream event in death receptor resistance and the triggering of non-apoptotic responses. Thus, death receptor distribution within the plasma membrane may have a pivotal impact on modulation of cell sensitivity/resistance to apoptotic signals.

9.6 Ceramide and Lipid Rafts

The early noughties were really a time of burst of activity and advances in raft and Fas/CD95 studies. Thus, in the early 2000s, the physiological lipid molecule ceramide was involved in the clustering of Fas/CD95 into ceramide-rich rafts [191, 192, 205, 206]. Addition of natural C16-ceramide completely restored the apoptotic response to agonistic anti-Fas/CD95 antibody in acid sphingomyelinase$^{-/-}$ hepatocytes, but per se did not trigger Fas/CD95 clustering or induce apoptosis in the absence of an agonist anti-Fas/CD95 antibody or FasL/CD95L [191, 206]. Thus, ceramide seems to act as a mediator of the death receptor clustering process, amplifying the primary Fas/CD95 signalling events, but not as an initiator of the process. The current view agrees with the following sequence of events: upon FasL/CD95L stimulation, the FasL/CD95L-Fas/CD95 complexes are suggested to be translocated into small membrane rafts, leading to a primary formation of the DISC and a subsequent and slight caspase-8 activation, which in turn activates caspase-7, leading to the proteolytic activation of acid sphingomyelinase and its translocation to small lipid rafts on the plasma membrane, where sphingomyelinase generates ceramide from raft-located sphingomyelin, thus promoting lipid raft coalescence [12, 191, 192, 205, 207, 208]. Direct incorporation of ceramide and enzymatic hydrolysis of sphingomyelin by sphingomyelinase have been shown to promote the enlargement of the initial ordered domains in model raft membranes [209, 210], suggesting the clustering and coalescence of small raft domains to form large raft platforms. Because sphingomyelin is highly abundant in rafts, in as much as 70% of all cellular sphingomyelin [211], the generated ceramide might promote coalescence of elementary rafts [212]. On these grounds, sphingomyelinase and ceramide serve to amplify the signalling of Fas/CD95 at the membrane level after the initial FasL/CD95L–Fas/CD95 interaction, leading to the formation of large patches containing FasL/CD95L-Fas/CD95 complexes that would further potentiate DISC formation and Fas/CD95 signalling. This notion is supported by biophysical studies showing that, by increasing membrane order, ceramide reduces the lateral diffusion of membrane proteins and lipids, leading to their trapping and clustering [213]. However, ceramide does not alter the preferred localization of the Fas/CD95 transmembrane domain in liquid disordered non-raft membrane region, and thereby neither the Fas/CD95 transmembrane domain membrane organization nor its conformation is affected by ceramide [214]. Nevertheless, diffusion of Fas/CD95 oligomer would be reduced in membrane domains containing ceramide, thus minimizing receptor translocation out of ceramide-rich domains [214], and favoring the formation of large and stable apoptotic Fas/CD95 clusters that could enhance apoptosis signalling.

On the other hand, ceramide has been reported to recruit a reduced number of sphingomyelin molecules forming very small highly ordered gel domains, surrounded by liquid-ordered phase rafts, without the formation of large platforms or the coalescence of small rafts [215]. Thus, ceramide has been shown to induce neither the formation of large platforms in raft model membranes nor raft coalescence, but instead it may induce the formation of small gel nanodomains, which could lead to strong changes in the membrane biophysical properties [215]. Because lipid rafts are rich in cholesterol, and cholesterol and ceramide compete for association with sphingomyelin, driving the formation of liquid-ordered and gel phases respectively, it might be suggested that ceramide/sphingomyelin-rich domains should be in a gel-like phase and exclude cholesterol, thus leading to raft collapse rather than to raft coalescence [215]. The above changes would likely lead to a severe reorganization of the membrane domain with consequences in cell signalling. The competition between ceramide and cholesterol in their association with rafts, together with the fact that ceramide displaces sterols from rafts [216–218], is likely to have a marked effect on raft structure and function, altering liquid ordered properties as well as molecular composition, including the lipid raft proteome. Taken together, these results suggest the presence of distinct membrane domains, either more enriched in ceramide or in cholesterol that could lead to distinct protein composition and function.

Interestingly, incubation of tumor cells with the synthetic ether lipid edelfosine has been shown to promote Fas/CD95 clustering and recruitment in lipid rafts, as well as subsequent apoptosis, independently of FasL/CD95L or agonist Fas/CD95 antibody, in the absence of sphingomyelinase activation and ceramide generation [21, 188, 189]. Further studies showed that raft disruption by cholesterol depletion inhibited drug-mediated killing in cancer cells, while cholesterol replenishment restored cancer cell ability to undergo drug-induced apoptosis [186]. Ceramide addition displaced cholesterol from rafts, and inhibited edelfosine-induced apoptosis [186]. These results suggest that cholesterol-rich lipid rafts play a major role in Fas/CD95-mediated apoptosis, and particularly in cancer chemotherapy.

9.7 S-Palmitoylation and Additional Posttranslational Modifications or Signatures Regulating Fas/CD95 Localization in Lipid Rafts

A number of posttranslational modifications and signatures have been found to affect Fas/CD95 recruitment in lipid rafts (Fig. 9.1). S-palmitoylation of Fas/CD95 in the membrane proximal intracellular region at the cysteine residue 199 for human (Fig. 9.1) and 194 for mouse Fas/CD95 is required for the localization of the death receptor in lipid rafts [219, 220]. S-palmitoylation leads to the formation of sodium dodecyl sulfate (SDS)-stable Fas/CD95 aggregates that accumulate in lipid rafts, due in part to an increase in the amount of FADD and processed caspase-8 [220]. These SDS-stable Fas/CD95 aggregates, which are SDS- and β-mercaptoethanol-resistant on SDS–polyacrylamide gel electrophoresis migrate in the range of 90–200 kDa depending on the cell type [42, 221]. Inhibition of protein palmitoylation with the palmitate analog 13-oxypalmitate [222] inhibits the incorporation of [^{3}H]palmitate into Fas/CD95 and cell death after FasL/CD95L engagement [219]. The palmitoylation inhibitor 2-bromo-palmitic acid inhibits Fas/CD95 internalization and formation of SDS-stable Fas/CD95 aggregates [220]. This thioester linkage of the 16-carbon saturated fatty acid palmitate to cysteine residues (S-palmitoylation) is a reversible posttranslational modification catalyzed by membrane-bound palmitoyl acyltransferases [223], and regulates raft affinity for the majority of integral raft proteins [224]. Reversible S-palmitoylation is dynamically regulated by two opposing types of enzymes that add (palmitoyl acyltransferases) or remove (acyl protein thioesterases) palmitate from proteins, thus allowing proteins to shuttle between intracellular membrane compartments [225]. The palmitoyl acyltransferase DHHC(aspartate-histidine-histidine-cysteine)7 has recently been found to regulate Fas/CD95 palmitoylation and stability [226].

On the other hand, additional signatures for Fas/CD95 localization in lipid rafts include nitric oxide (NO)-induced S-nitrosylation at cysteine 304 [227], and a lysine-rich region (LRR) in the cytoplasmic membrane-proximal region of Fas/CD95 [228] (Fig. 9.1).

Another modification affecting Fas/CD45 death receptor-induced apoptosis is sialylation [229–231]. The ST6Gal-I sialyltransferase, which is dynamically regulated in immune and cancer cells, adds an α2-6 linked sialic acid to Fas/CD95, thus inhibiting receptor internalization and DISC formation and shutting off apoptosis [232]. On the other hand, the addition of this sugar does not simply inhibit apoptosis, but also promotes survival signalling [232]. In this regard, it has been found and suggested that plasma membrane-localized Fas/CD95 may send pro-survival signals, whereas receptor internalization is required for apoptosis induction [233–236]. Thus, the α2-6 sialylation-dependent retention of Fas/CD95 at the cell surface could serve as a mechanism to control the switch between cell survival and cell death, and could regulate: (a) Fas/CD95 clustering, (b) receptor tertiary conformation, and/or (c) localization of the receptor to lipid rafts [232].

9.8 Signalling Pathways and Proteins Affecting Fas/CD95 Recruitment in Lipid Rafts

Despite little is still known about the molecular mechanisms regulating the recruitment of Fas/CD95 in lipid rafts, some insights involving signalling pathways and proteins have been achieved and discussed below.

9.8.1 PI3K/Akt Signalling

The PI3K/Akt pathway is pivotal for cell survival [237], and has a multiple-step activation process [238–240]. Akt is recruited to the plasma membrane through interaction of its pleckstrin homology (PH) domain with phosphatidylinositol-3,4,5-trisphosphate (PIP3), generated by phosphatidylinositol 3-kinase (PI3K)-mediated phosphatidylinositol-4,5-bisphosphate (PIP2) phosphorylation. Then, Akt is activated at the plasma membrane through phosphorylation at two key residues, Thr308 by phosphoinositide-dependent kinase 1 (PDK1), and Ser473 by mammalian target of rapamycin (mTOR) [240–242]. Membrane domains, likely lipid rafts, have been shown to play a crucial role in the triggering of the PI3K/Akt signalling pathway by facilitating Akt recruitment and activation in the plasma membrane [243–248]. A number of mechanisms, including JNK signalling, reactive oxygen species, and actin cytoskeleton, have been proposed to be involved in Fas/CD95 clustering in rafts [28, 33, 219, 228], but strong evidence suggests that PI3K/Akt signalling can play a major role in modulating Fas/CD95 localization in lipid rafts [249]. Inhibition of PI3K signalling induces the rapid formation of Fas/CD95 clusters and the redistribution of Fas/CD95 into lipid rafts [249]. Interestingly, the ether lipid edelfosine displaces PI3K/Akt signalling from lipid rafts in human mantle cell lymphoma cells, thus preventing its proper activation [250]. The alkylphospholipid analogs edelfosine and perifosine inhibit Akt signalling and promote Fas/CD95 recruitment into rafts [185, 187, 250], further supporting the involvement of PI3K/Akt signalling inhibition in Fas/CD95-raft co-clustering and subsequent cell killing. The PI3K/Akt signalling pathway is constitutively activated in many tumor cells, and one of its actions in promoting cell survival might include the inhibition of Fas/CD95 clustering in rafts required for apoptosis triggering, in addition to the well-known effects in suppressing apoptosis by phosphorylation of pro-apoptotic proteins, such as Bad (Bcl-2-associated death promoter) and procaspase-9 [251]. In this regard, CD3-mediated PI3K activation in Th2 cells blocks Fas/CD95 aggregation and procaspase-8 cleavage through the effects of PI3K upon actin cytoskeleton, thus affecting Fas/CD95 lateral diffusion and aggregation [252, 253]. The alkylphospholipid perifosine induces apoptosis in CEM-R (R, resistant), a variant of the T-lymphoblastic CEM cell line characterized by both overexpression of P-glycoprotein and constitutive PI3K/Akt signalling upregulation, involving JNK, lipid rafts and a rapid and complete dephosphorylation of Akt at Ser473, whereas slight phosphorylation of Thr308 was still observable [254]. Similarly, edelfosine induces a total dephosphorylation of Akt at Ser473, while Thr308 phosphorylation was still detected in mantle cell lymphoma cells [250].

9.8.2 Semaphorin 3A

Semaphorin 3A (Sema3A), a prototype member of secreted semaphorins of class 3, has been shown to trigger a pro-apoptotic program that sensitizes leukemic T cells to Fas/CD95-mediated apoptosis, through translocation of Fas/CD95 into lipid raft microdomains before binding with agonistic antibody or FasL/CD95L [255]. Sema3A coreceptor neuropilin-1 (NP-1) is mostly located in lipid rafts, whereas Fas/CD95 is not found in rafts in unstimulated T-cell leukemia Jurkat cells, but following a 60-min treatment with Sema3A, a marked proportion of Fas/CD95 as well as plexin-A1 are recruited into lipid rafts, thus co-localizing plexin-A1 and NP1 with Fas/CD95 in Sema3A-treated Jurkat cells as assessed by immunofluorescence microscopy [255]. Furthermore, Sema3A-induced translocation of Fas/CD95 to lipid rafts requires actin cytoskeleton, and the actin-linking protein ezrin as well as the actin dynamics regulatory proteins, such as RhoA and RhoGDI, are redistributed to lipid rafts upon Sema3A stimulation [255]. These data show that Sema3A/NP1/plexin signalling rearranges membrane rafts, promoting Fas/CD95 clustering and redistribution in raft domains. The transient axonal glycoprotein-1 (TAG-1), also known as contactin-2 (CNTN2), a 135 kDa GPI-anchored protein that is expressed on neurons and glial cells, plays a central role in the localization of NP-1 in lipid rafts and in the trafficking of NP-1 into distinct endocytic pathways, which appears necessary for Sema3A signal generation [256].

9.9 Chemotherapy and Lipid Raft-Mediated Fas/CD95 Apoptotic Signalling in Cancer

At the end of 2001, we found that the ether lipid edelfosine induced apoptosis through the recruitment and clustering of Fas/CD95 death receptor in lipid rafts [21]. This was the first time that an antitumor drug was found to promote cell death through this raft-Fas/CD95 clustering and opened up a novel raft-mediated mechanism by which an anticancer drug could lead to tumor cell demise, thus constituting the first evidence for the involvement of membrane rafts in cancer chemotherapy and the beginning of a new avenue for cancer treatment. Since this seminal publication, there have been an increasing number of reports in the literature showing that different antitumor drugs promote recruitment of death receptors in lipid rafts. Table 9.1 shows an update of the distinct antitumor drugs that have been reported so far to promote death receptor recruitment in rafts.

Because edelfosine-induced apoptosis is independent of FasL/CD95L [188, 189], the synthetic ether lipid edelfosine seems to put in motion and exacerbate a series of physiological processes that otherwise would remain dormant in the cancer cell, thus offering a novel way to promote cell death in tumor cells. Moreover, edelfosine was found to promote recruitment of Fas/CD95 in rafts and subsequent apoptosis in a number of cells that were resistant to the action of FasL/CD95L. On these grounds, it might be envisaged that pharmacological activation of Fas/CD95 system might bypass certain processes that could block the physiological death receptor stimulation, thus leading to a better response in cells showing resistance to Fas/CD95 death receptor triggering. As shown in Table 9.1, additional studies have shown that an increasing number of antitumor agents promote apoptosis, at least in part, through the recruitment of death receptors in lipid rafts. However, so far, edelfosine can be considered as the lead compound and gold standard in the search for chemical agents promoting Fas/CD95 system recruitment in rafts.

Recruitment in lipid rafts of additional death receptors other than Fas/CD95, such as TNFR1 (CD120a) [28, 201, 257] and the TRAIL receptors TRAIL-R1 (DR4) and TRAIL-R2 (DR5) [28, 185, 258], has been shown to be required to initiate apoptosis. Interestingly, fluorescence resonance energy transfer (FRET) experiments have shown a molecular interaction between ganglioside GM3, abundant in lymphoid cells and lipid rafts [259–262], and DR4 that was related to TRAIL susceptibility of B-cell cancer cells, whereas this association was negligible in non-transformed cells [258].

Cisplatin has been previously shown to induce Fas/CD95 redistribution in lipid rafts and to potentiate Fas/CD95-induced apoptosis in HT29 human colon cancer cells [263]. Interestingly, cisplatin was shown to inhibit Na^+/H^+ membrane exchanger-1 (NHE1), leading to intracellular acidification and acidic sphingomyelinase (aSMase) activation, which was concomitant with an increase in membrane fluidity and aggregation of membrane lipid rafts in HT-29 human colon cancer cells [264]. In addition, cisplatin augments Fas/CD95-mediated apoptosis through lipid rafts in WR19L mouse T-cell lymphoma cells [265]. Altogether, these findings sug-

Table 9.1 Recruitment of death receptors and downstream signalling molecules into lipid rafts by anticancer drugs or chemical entities in cancer cells

Anticancer drug	Cancer cells	Death receptors (and downstream signalling molecules) recruited in rafts	References
Akt signalling inhibition (Akt inh-VIII)	Jurkat	Fas/CD95	[286]
Anandamide	Mz-ChA-1	Fas/CD95	[287]
Aplidin	Jurkat	Fas/CD95, DR5, TNF-R1 (FADD, procaspase-8, procaspase-10, JNK, Bid)	[28]
Avicin D	Jurkat	Fas/CD95 (FADD, procaspase-8, procaspase-7, Bid)	[288]
Bufalin	MCF-7, MDA-MB-231	DR4, DR5	[289]
Cationic amphipathic lytic peptide, KLA (HHHHHKLAKL AKKLAKLAKC)	LNCaP	DR5	[290]
Ceramide[a]	Jurkat	Fas/CD95	[191, 192, 207]
Cisplatin	HT-29	Fas/CD95 (FADD, procaspase-8)	[263]
Cisplatin, platinum(IV) complex LA-12	PC-3	DR4, DR5	[291]
	HCT116	DR4, DR5	
Cryptocaryone	PC-3	Fas/CD95, DR4, DR5 (FADD, procaspase-8)	[292]
Depsipeptide FR901228	DU-145	DR4, DR5	[293]
Doxorubicin coupled to cell penetrating peptides (Dox-CPPs)	MDA-MB-231	DR4, DR5	[294]
Edelfosine	Jurkat	Fas/CD95 (FADD, procaspase-8, procaspase-10, JNK, Bid)	[21, 188, 198]
	MM144	Fas/CD95, DR4, DR5, TNF-R1 (FADD, procaspase-8, procaspase-9, procaspase-10, JNK, Bid, cytochrome *c*, APAF-1)	[185, 186, 199]
Epirubicin	MGC-803	DR4, DR5	[295]
Oxaliplatin	MGC-803	DR4, DR5	[296]
Perifosine	MM144	Fas/CD95, DR4, DR5 (FADD, procaspase-8, Bid)	[185]

(continued)

Table 9.1 (continued)

Anticancer drug	Cancer cells	Death receptors (and downstream signalling molecules) recruited in rafts	References
PI3K signalling inhibition (LY294002, wortmannin)	Jurkat, CEM	Fas/CD95	[249, 286]
Quercetin	HT-29	DR4, DR5	[297]
Resveratrol	HT-29	Fas/CD95, DR4, DR5 (FADD, procaspase-8)	[298]
	Jurkat	Fas/CD95, DR5 (FADD, procaspase-8, procaspase-10, JNK, Bid)	[200]
	MM144	Fas/CD95, DR4, DR5 (FADD, procaspase-8, procaspase-10, JNK, Bid)	[200]
	SW480	CD95 (FADD, procaspase-8)	[299]
Rituximab	Ramos	Fas/CD95 (FADD, procaspase-8)	[300]
Stichoposide D	K562, HL-60, primary human leukemia cells	Fas/CD95 (ceramide synthase 6, p38 kinase, caspase-8)	[301]
TSWU-BR23 (a synthetic bichalcone analog)	HT-29	Fas/CD95	[302]
Ultraviolet light	M624	Fas/CD95 (FADD, procaspase-8)	[303]
Ursodeoxycholic acid (UDCA)	SNU601, SNU638	DR5, Fas/CD95	[304, 305]

CEM, human acute T-cell leukemia cell line; DR4, death receptor 4 (also known as TRAIL receptor 1);DR5, death receptor 5 (also known as TRAIL receptor 2); DU-145, human prostate cancer cell line; HCT116, human colon carcinoma cell line; HL-60, human myeloid leukemia cell line; HT-29, human colon carcinoma cell line; Jurkat, human acute T-cell leukemia cell line; K562, human chronic myelogenous leukemia cell line; LNCaP, human prostate cancer cell line; M624, human melanoma cell line; MCF-7, human breast cancer cell line; MDA-MB-231, human breast cancer cell line; MGC-803, human gastric carcinoma cell line; MM144, human multiple myeloma cell line; Mz-ChA-1 cells, human cholangiocarcinoma cell line; PC-3, human prostate cancer cell line; Ramos, human Burkitt's lymphoma cell line; SNU601, human gastric cancer cell line; SNU638, human gastric cancer cell line; SW480, human colon carcinoma cell line; TSWU-BR23, (E)-1-(3-((4-(4-acetylphenyl)piperazin-1-yl)methyl)-4-hydroxy-5-methoxyphenyl)-3-(pyridin-3-yl)prop-2-en-1-one.

[a]Acting not as an inducer, but as an amplifier of a previous triggering of Fas/CD95 response by its cognate ligand or agonistic antibodies

gest that the apoptotic pathway triggered by cisplatin involves a very early NHE1-dependent intracellular acidification leading to aSMase activation and changes in membrane fluidity that might affect lateral diffusion of membrane proteins. In addition, early after the onset of cisplatin treatment, ezrin co-localized with Fas/CD95 at the cell membrane and was redistributed with Fas/CD95, FADD and procaspase-8 into membrane lipid rafts, together with an early small GTPase RhoA activation, Rho kinase (ROCK)-dependent ezrin phosphorylation and actin microfilaments remodeling [266]. Interestingly, Fas/CD95 silencing by RNA interference abrogates cisplatin-induced ROCK-dependent ezrin phosphorylation, actin reorganization and apoptosis, thus suggesting that Fas/CD95 is a key regulator of cisplatin-induced actin remodeling and apoptosis [266].

It is worth to note that the initial redistribution of Fas/CD95 in lipid rafts not only facilitates caspase-8 activation and apoptosis, but in turn could be favored by a caspase-8-mediated positive feed-forward loop, involving ceramide formation through caspase-8-activated aSMase that promotes the capping of Fas/CD95 in large patches in the plasma membrane [2, 189, 191, 192, 207]. The latter process is supported by a reduction in Fas/CD95–lipid raft association and Fas/CD95 capping in sphingomyelin synthase-defective cells [267].

As mentioned above, despite FasL/CD95L induces translocation to rafts and activation of Fas/CD95-mediated apoptosis, it is clear that Fas/CD95 translocation to lipid rafts and Fas/CD95-mediated apoptosis can proceed in the absence of its physiological ligand [28, 32–34, 188, 189, 269, 268]. This is of particular importance in cancer chemotherapy, raising the possibility to modulate cell death pharmacologically. Importantly, the antitumor drug edelfosine is taken up in a rather selective way by cancer cells [185, 188, 270], and once inside the cancer cell the ether lipid drug initiates a series of not yet well characterized processes leading to the recruitment of Fas/CD95 and downstream signalling molecules in lipid rafts, followed by the formation of DISC and the triggering of apoptosis independently of FasL/CD95L [28, 185, 188, 199]. Thus, edelfosine kills tumor cells from within the cell, and this aspect is of major importance because it avoids the necessity to activate death receptor-mediated apoptosis through the use of the cognate ligand, which could lead to the death of normal cells and therefore to severe side effects to normal tissues. As a matter of fact, systemic administration of TNF causes a severe inflammatory response syndrome that resembles septic shock [271], and administration of agonistic antibody to Fas in mice is lethal because of liver failure through massive hepatocyte apoptosis [272, 273], thus hampering the clinical usefulness of exogenous activation of some death receptors, particularly TNF and Fas/CD95, and making clinicians and researchers to be aware and conscious about putative problems that might arise following death receptor-targeted therapy [33, 274–276]. However, TRAIL is the ligand that has sparked growing interest in cancer therapy due to its ability to selectively trigger cell death in cancer cells, but not in normal cells, and to its lack of significant toxicity in animal models [276–281], in spite of the fact that TRAIL has been reported to induce apoptosis in human hepatocytes [282].

As mentioned above, the rather selective uptake of edelfosine in cancer cells leading to their cell death, while sparing normal cells, together with the intracellular activation of Fas/CD95, as opposed to exogenous activation through its cognate ligand, is crucial to avoid the side effects that could be raised by a systemic exogenous activation of Fas/CD95. Thus, edelfosine oral administration in murine animal models lacked any significant toxicity [193, 283], pointing out the notion that a selective activation of Fas/CD95 from within the cell is a promising approach to implement Fas/CD95-targeted therapies in the treatment of cancer. In addition, the recruitment of death receptors and downstream signalling molecules into lipid rafts induced by edelfosine, including Fas/CD95 and TRAIL receptors [185, 186], not only leads to apoptosis, but also facilitates and potentiates further induction of apoptosis by the subsequent addition of their respective ligands. Thus, pretreatment of multiple myeloma MM144 cells with edelfosine potentiated significantly the antitumor responses to the extracellular engagement of death receptors by the action of their ligands (FasL/CD95L and TRAIL) or the agonistic cytotoxic anti-Fas/CD95 CH-11 antibody [185]. In this regard, edelfosine has also been reported to enhance TRAIL-mediated apoptosis in gastric cells by DR5 upregulation in lipid rafts [284]. On the other hand, incubation of LM7 and CCH-OS-D osteosarcoma cells with histone deacetylase inhibitor MS-275 increased the localization of Fas/CD95 in lipid rafts, likely through downregulation of c-FLIP, and sensitizes these cells to FasL/CD95L-induced apoptosis [285].

9.10 Concluding Remarks

Following the first identification of the recruitment of Fas/CD95 in lipid rafts as a major regulatory step in the induction of death receptor-mediated apoptosis, which in turn could be pharmacologically modulated [21], further insights in characterizing this pro-apoptotic process have been provided in the last 15 years. Additional downstream signalling molecules can also be recruited into lipid rafts together with the death receptor, thus forming the DISC at the raft domain and facilitating interaction with other signalling routes leading to an affective apoptosis [185, 188, 198, 199]. This concentration of death receptors and downstream signalling molecules in raft platforms facilitates and potentiates protein–protein interactions. This accumulation of death receptors and downstream signalling molecules in raft clusters led to the concept of CASMER as a cluster of rafts enriched in apoptotic signalling molecules [12, 22, 23, 25, 27, 28], which serves as a linchpin from which apoptotic signals are launched. Thus, CASMERs act as hubs in death receptor-mediated apoptosis, and their formation represents a new and promising target in cancer chemotherapy. Our data suggest that the sorting and concentration of apoptotic molecules in lipid rafts, being segregated from survival signalling molecules, promote a dramatic local change in the apoptosis/survival signalling ratio in a specific and restricted area that eventually triggers a cell death response [24]. Direct activation of the cancer cell apoptotic machinery constitutes an appealing approach to kill cancer cells, and the formation of CASMERs is an elegant and efficient way to turn a dispersed array of apoptotic molecules into a more compact and tight pro-apoptotic area where molecules are highly facilitated to interact each other, thus resulting in a much easier and efficient way to trigger and transmit pro-apoptotic signal transduction. The notion of the formation of CASMERs, highlighting the importance of lipid rafts in generating specific areas of cell membrane enriched in pro-apoptotic signalling molecules, represents an innovative paradigm shift in cancer therapy, so far more focused in inhibiting survival pathways than in potentiating the activity of pro-apoptotic routes leading to cancer cell self-destruction.

The fact that Fas/CD95 can also trigger non-apoptotic signalling, including survival or proliferation signalling, makes the unveiling of the mechanisms responsible for the switch to either cell death or cell survival/proliferation an urgent issue to deal with. Although these mechanisms are not yet well understood, a putative rationale might lie in the localization of Fas/CD95 in specific membrane domains where it might interact with either pro-apoptotic or pro-survival downstream signalling molecules, thus leading to opposite outcomes. On these grounds, modulation of survival and apoptotic signalling through rafts could be a promising and appealing approach in cancer therapy, and increasing evidence shows the potential of rafts as a novel therapeutic target in cancer therapy [12, 23, 24, 33].

What are the mechanisms involved in the recruitment of Fas/CD95 and downstream signalling molecules in lipid rafts? What are the mechanisms that switch Fas/CD95 from a pro-apoptotic (tumor suppressor) to a pro-survival (tumor promoter) signalling? Do these switches on the involvement of Fas/CD95 in apoptosis or survival signalling require different raft platforms? These are some questions that should be answered in the upcoming years to fully understand the role of Fas/CD95 and lipid rafts in determining cell fate decision, which should be of paramount importance for the development of novel anticancer therapies.

Acknowledgments This work was supported by grants from the Spanish Ministerio de Economia y Competitividad (SAF2014-59716-R), European Community's Seventh Framework Programme FP7-2007-2013 (grant HEALTH-F2-2011-256986, PANACREAS), and Red Temática de Investigación Cooperativa en Cáncer, Instituto de Salud Carlos III, cofunded by the Fondo Europeo de Desarrollo Regional of the European Union (RD12/0036/0065).

References

1. Nagata S, Golstein P (1995) The Fas death factor. Science 267(5203):1449–1456
2. Wajant H (2014) Principles and mechanisms of CD95 activation. Biol Chem 395(12):1401–1416. doi:10.1515/hsz-2014-0212. /j/bchm.just-accepted/hsz-2014-0212/hsz-2014-0212.xml [pii]
3. Roths JB, Murphy ED, Eicher EM (1984) A new mutation, gld, that produces lymphoproliferation and autoimmunity in C3H/HeJ mice. J Exp Med 159(1):1–20
4. Matsuzawa A, Moriyama T, Kaneko T, Tanaka M, Kimura M, Ikeda H, Katagiri T (1990) A new allele of the lpr locus, lprcg, that complements the gld gene in induction of lymphadenopathy in the mouse. J Exp Med 171(2):519–531
5. Watanabe-Fukunaga R, Brannan CI, Copeland NG, Jenkins NA, Nagata S (1992) Lymphoproliferation disorder in mice explained by defects in Fas antigen that mediates apoptosis. Nature 356(6367):314–317. doi:10.1038/356314a0

6. Sneller MC, Straus SE, Jaffe ES, Jaffe JS, Fleisher TA, Stetler-Stevenson M, Strober W (1992) A novel lymphoproliferative/autoimmune syndrome resembling murine lpr/gld disease. J Clin Invest 90(2):334–341. doi:10.1172/JCI115867
7. Rieux-Laucat F, Le Deist F, Hivroz C, Roberts IA, Debatin KM, Fischer A, de Villartay JP (1995) Mutations in Fas associated with human lymphoproliferative syndrome and autoimmunity. Science 268(5215):1347–1349
8. Fisher GH, Rosenberg FJ, Straus SE, Dale JK, Middleton LA, Lin AY, Strober W, Lenardo MJ, Puck JM (1995) Dominant interfering Fas gene mutations impair apoptosis in a human autoimmune lymphoproliferative syndrome. Cell 81(6):935–946
9. Drappa J, Vaishnaw AK, Sullivan KE, Chu JL, Elkon KB (1996) Fas gene mutations in the Canale-Smith syndrome, an inherited lymphoproliferative disorder associated with autoimmunity. N Engl J Med 335(22):1643–1649
10. Sneller MC, Wang J, Dale JK, Strober W, Middelton LA, Choi Y, Fleisher TA, Lim MS, Jaffe ES, Puck JM, Lenardo MJ, Straus SE (1997) Clinical, immunologic, and genetic features of an autoimmune lymphoproliferative syndrome associated with abnormal lymphocyte apoptosis. Blood 89(4):1341–1348
11. Shah S, Wu E, Rao VK, Tarrant TK (2014) Autoimmune lymphoproliferative syndrome: an update and review of the literature. Curr Allergy Asthma Rep 14(9):462. doi:10.1007/s11882-014-0462-4
12. Gajate C, Mollinedo F (2015) Lipid raft-mediated Fas/CD95 apoptotic signaling in leukemic cells and normal leukocytes and therapeutic implications. J Leukoc Biol 98(5):739–759. doi:10.1189/jlb.2MR0215-055R. jlb.2MR0215-055R [pii]
13. Li-Weber M, Krammer PH (2003) Function and regulation of the CD95 (APO-1/Fas) ligand in the immune system. Semin Immunol 15(3):145–157
14. Lambert C, Landau AM, Desbarats J (2003) Fas-beyond death: a regenerative role for Fas in the nervous system. Apoptosis 8(6):551–562. doi:10.1023/A:1026113222478. 5150569 [pii]
15. Strasser A, Jost PJ, Nagata S (2009) The many roles of FAS receptor signaling in the immune system. Immunity 30(2):180–192. doi:10.1016/j.immuni.2009.01.001. S1074-7613(09)00069-7 [pii]
16. Kleber S, Sancho-Martinez I, Wiestler B, Beisel A, Gieffers C, Hill O, Thiemann M, Mueller W, Sykora J, Kuhn A, Schreglmann N, Letellier E, Zuliani C, Klussmann S, Teodorczyk M, Grone HJ, Ganten TM, Sultmann H, Tuttenberg J, von Deimling A, Regnier-Vigouroux A, Herold-Mende C, Martin-Villalba A (2008) Yes and PI3K bind CD95 to signal invasion of glioblastoma. Cancer Cell 13(3):235–248. doi:10.1016/j.ccr.2008.02.003. S1535-6108(08)00043-3 [pii]
17. Chen L, Park SM, Tumanov AV, Hau A, Sawada K, Feig C, Turner JR, YX F, Romero IL, Lengyel E, Peter ME (2010) CD95 promotes tumour growth. Nature 465(7297):492–496. doi:10.1038/nature09075
18. Steller EJ, Borel Rinkes IH, Kranenburg O (2011) How CD95 stimulates invasion. Cell Cycle 10(22):3857–3862. doi:10.4161/cc.10.22.18290
19. Peter ME, Hadji A, Murmann AE, Brockway S, Putzbach W, Pattanayak A, Ceppi P (2015) The role of CD95 and CD95 ligand in cancer. Cell Death Differ 22(4):549–559. doi:10.1038/cdd.2015.3. cdd20153 [pii]
20. Brint E, O'Callaghan G, Houston A (2013) Life in the Fas lane: differential outcomes of Fas signaling. Cell Mol Life Sci 70(21):4085–4099. doi:10.1007/s00018-013-1327-z
21. Gajate C, Mollinedo F (2001) The antitumor ether lipid ET-18-OCH_3 induces apoptosis through translocation and capping of Fas/CD95 into membrane rafts in human leukemic cells. Blood 98(13):3860–3863
22. Mollinedo F, Gajate C (2010) Lipid rafts and clusters of apoptotic signaling molecule-enriched rafts in cancer therapy. Future Oncol 6(5):811–821
23. Mollinedo F, Gajate C (2015) Lipid rafts as major platforms for signaling regulation in cancer. Adv Biol Regul 57:130–146. doi:10.1016/j.jbior.2014.10.003. S2212-4926(14)00058-X [pii]

24. Gajate C, Mollinedo F (2014) Lipid rafts, endoplasmic reticulum and mitochondria in the antitumor action of the alkylphospholipid analog edelfosine. Anticancer Agents Med Chem 14(4):509–527. ACAMC-EPUB-59567 [pii]
25. Gajate C, Mollinedo F (2015) Lipid rafts and raft-mediated supramolecular entities in the regulation of CD95 death receptor apoptotic signaling. Apoptosis 20(5):584–606. doi:10.1007/s10495-015-1104-6
26. Pike LJ (2006) Rafts defined: a report on the keystone symposium on lipid rafts and cell function. J Lipid Res 47(7):1597–1598
27. Mollinedo F, Gajate C (2010) Lipid rafts, death receptors and CASMERs: new insights for cancer therapy. Future Oncol 6(4):491–494
28. Gajate C, Mollinedo F (2005) Cytoskeleton-mediated death receptor and ligand concentration in lipid rafts forms apoptosis-promoting clusters in cancer chemotherapy. J Biol Chem 280(12):11641–11647. doi:10.1074/jbc.M411781200. M411781200 [pii]
29. Itoh N, Yonehara S, Ishii A, Yonehara M, Mizushima S, Sameshima M, Hase A, Seto Y, Nagata S (1991) The polypeptide encoded by the cDNA for human cell surface antigen Fas can mediate apoptosis. Cell 66(2):233–243. doi:10.1016/0092-8674(91)90614-5. [pii]
30. Itoh N, Nagata S (1993) A novel protein domain required for apoptosis. Mutational analysis of human Fas antigen. J Biol Chem 268(15):10932–10937
31. Nagata S (1997) Apoptosis by death factor. Cell 88(3):355–365
32. Mollinedo F, Gajate C (2006) FasL-independent activation of Fas. In: Wajant H (ed) Fas signaling (Chapter 2). Landes Bioscience and Springer Science, Georgetown, pp 13–27
33. Mollinedo F, Gajate C (2006) Fas/CD95 death receptor and lipid rafts: new targets for apoptosis-directed cancer therapy. Drug Resist Updat 9(1–2):51–73. doi:10.1016/j.drup.2006.04.002
34. Mollinedo F (2008) Death receptors in multiple myeloma and therapeutic opportunities. In: Lonial S (ed) Myeloma therapy. Pursuing the plasma cell (Chapter 25). Humana Press, Totowa, pp 393–419
35. Chinnaiyan AM, O'Rourke K, Tewari M, Dixit VM (1995) FADD, a novel death domain-containing protein, interacts with the death domain of Fas and initiates apoptosis. Cell 81(4):505–512. 0092-8674(95)90071-3 [pii]
36. Dickens LS, Powley IR, Hughes MA, MacFarlane M (2012) The 'complexities' of life and death: death receptor signalling platforms. Exp Cell Res 318(11):1269–1277. doi:10.1016/j.yexcr.2012.04.005. S0014-4827(12)00188-7 [pii]
37. Siegel RM, Chan FK, Chun HJ, Lenardo MJ (2000) The multifaceted role of Fas signaling in immune cell homeostasis and autoimmunity. Nat Immunol 1(6):469–474
38. Chan FK, Chun HJ, Zheng L, Siegel RM, Bui KL, Lenardo MJ (2000) A domain in TNF receptors that mediates ligand-independent receptor assembly and signaling. Science 288(5475):2351–2354
39. Scott FL, Stec B, Pop C, Dobaczewska MK, Lee JJ, Monosov E, Robinson H, Salvesen GS, Schwarzenbacher R, Riedl SJ (2009) The Fas-FADD death domain complex structure unravels signalling by receptor clustering. Nature 457(7232):1019–1022. doi:10.1038/nature07606. nature07606 [pii]
40. Boldin MP, Goncharov TM, Goltsev YV, Wallach D (1996) Involvement of MACH, a novel MORT1/FADD-interacting protease, in Fas/APO-1- and TNF receptor-induced cell death. Cell 85(6):803–815
41. Ashkenazi A, Dixit VM (1998) Death receptors: signaling and modulation. Science 281(5381):1305–1308
42. Kischkel FC, Hellbardt S, Behrmann I, Germer M, Pawlita M, Krammer PH, Peter ME (1995) Cytotoxicity-dependent APO-1 (Fas/CD95)-associated proteins form a death-inducing signaling complex (DISC) with the receptor. EMBO J 14(22):5579–5588
43. Holler N, Zaru R, Micheau O, Thome M, Attinger A, Valitutti S, Bodmer JL, Schneider P, Seed B, Tschopp J (2000) Fas triggers an alternative, caspase-8-independent cell death pathway using the kinase RIP as effector molecule. Nat Immunol 1(6):489–495

44. Pietkiewicz S, Eils R, Krammer PH, Giese N, Lavrik IN (2015) Combinatorial treatment of CD95L and gemcitabine in pancreatic cancer cells induces apoptotic and RIP1-mediated necroptotic cell death network. Exp Cell Res 339(1):1–9. doi:10.1016/j.yexcr.2015.10.005. S0014-4827(15)30110-5 [pii]
45. Towns R, Pietropaolo M, Wiley JW (2008) Stimulation of autophagy by autoantibody-mediated activation of death receptor cascades. Autophagy 4(5):715–716. 6336 [pii]
46. Zhang Y, Wu Y, Cheng Y, Zhao Z, Tashiro S, Onodera S, Ikejima T (2008) Fas-mediated autophagy requires JNK activation in HeLa cells. Biochem Biophys Res Commun 377(4):1205–1210. doi:10.1016/j.bbrc.2008.10.151. S0006-291X(08)02123-2 [pii]
47. Park MA, Reinehr R, Haussinger D, Voelkel-Johnson C, Ogretmen B, Yacoub A, Grant S, Dent P (2010) Sorafenib activates CD95 and promotes autophagy and cell death via Src family kinases in gastrointestinal tumor cells. Mol Cancer Ther 9(8):2220–2231. doi:10.1158/1535-7163.MCT-10-0274. 1535-7163.MCT-10-0274 [pii]
48. Landowski TH, Qu N, Buyuksal I, Painter JS, Dalton WS (1997) Mutations in the Fas antigen in patients with multiple myeloma. Blood 90(11):4266–4270
49. Boldrini L, Loggini B, Gisfredi S, Zucconi Y, Baldinotti F, Fogli A, Simi P, Cervadoro G, Barachini P, Basolo F, Pingitore R, Fontanini G (2003) Mutations of Fas (APO-1/CD95) and p53 genes in nonmelanoma skin cancer. J Cutan Med Surg 7(2):112–118. doi:10.1007/s10227-002-0105-6
50. Peter ME, Legembre P, Barnhart BC (2005) Does CD95 have tumor promoting activities? Biochim Biophys Acta 1755(1):25–36. doi:10.1016/j.bbcan.2005.01.001
51. Tauzin S, Debure L, Moreau JF, Legembre P (2012) CD95-mediated cell signaling in cancer: mutations and post-translational modulations. Cell Mol Life Sci 69(8):1261–1277. doi:10.1007/s00018-011-0866-4
52. Moller P, Koretz K, Leithauser F, Bruderlein S, Henne C, Quentmeier A, Krammer PH (1994) Expression of APO-1 (CD95), a member of the NGF/TNF receptor superfamily, in normal and neoplastic colon epithelium. Int J Cancer 57(3):371–377
53. Lebel M, Bertrand R, Mes-Masson AM (1996) Decreased Fas antigen receptor expression in testicular tumor cell lines derived from polyomavirus large T-antigen transgenic mice. Oncogene 12(5):1127–1135
54. Shin EC, Shin JS, Park JH, Kim JJ, Kim H, Kim SJ (1998) Expression of Fas-related genes in human hepatocellular carcinomas. Cancer Lett 134(2):155–162. S0304-3835(98)00251-1 [pii]
55. Ramenghi U, Bonissoni S, Migliaretti G, DeFranco S, Bottarel F, Gambaruto C, DiFranco D, Priori R, Conti F, Dianzani I, Valesini G, Merletti F, Dianzani U (2000) Deficiency of the Fas apoptosis pathway without Fas gene mutations is a familial trait predisposing to development of autoimmune diseases and cancer. Blood 95(10):3176–3182
56. Maas S, Warskulat U, Steinhoff C, Mueller W, Grimm MO, Schulz WA, Seifert HH (2004) Decreased Fas expression in advanced-stage bladder cancer is not related to p53 status. Urology 63(2):392–397. doi:10.1016/j.urology.2003.08.023. S0090429503009129 [pii]
57. Rodriguez-Pinilla M, Rodriguez-Peralto JL, Hitt R, Sanchez JJ, Sanchez-Verde L, Alameda F, Ballestin C, Sanchez-Cespedes M (2005) beta-Catenin, Nf-kappaB and FAS protein expression are independent events in head and neck cancer: study of their association with clinical parameters. Cancer Lett 230(1):141–148. doi:10.1016/j.canlet.2004.12.045. S0304-3835(05)00008-X [pii]
58. Zhou Z, Lafleur EA, Koshkina NV, Worth LL, Lester MS, Kleinerman ES (2005) Interleukin-12 up-regulates Fas expression in human osteosarcoma and Ewing's sarcoma cells by enhancing its promoter activity. Mol Cancer Res 3(12):685–691. doi:10.1158/1541-7786.MCR-05-0092. 3/12/685 [pii]
59. van Blitterswijk WJ, Klarenbeek JB, van der Luit AH, Alderliesten MC, van Lummel M, Verheij M (2009) Fas/CD95 down-regulation in lymphoma cells through acquired alkyl-lysophospholipid resistance: partial role of associated sphingomyelin deficiency. Biochem J 425(1):225–234

60. Hoogwater FJ, Steller EJ, Westendorp BF, Borel Rinkes IH, Kranenburg O (2012) CD95 signaling in colorectal cancer. Biochim Biophys Acta 1826(1):189–198. doi:10.1016/j.bbcan.2012.03.007
61. Fouque A, Debure L, Legembre P (2014) The CD95/CD95L signaling pathway: a role in carcinogenesis. Biochim Biophys Acta 1846(1):130–141. doi:10.1016/j.bbcan.2014.04.007
62. Legembre P, Schickel R, Barnhart BC, Peter ME (2004) Identification of SNF1/AMP kinase-related kinase as an NF-kappaB-regulated anti-apoptotic kinase involved in CD95-induced motility and invasiveness. J Biol Chem 279(45):46742–46747. doi:10.1074/jbc.M404334200. M404334200 [pii]
63. Legembre P, Barnhart BC, Peter ME (2004) The relevance of NF-kappaB for CD95 signaling in tumor cells. Cell Cycle 3(10):1235–1239
64. Peter ME, Budd RC, Desbarats J, Hedrick SM, Hueber AO, Newell MK, Owen LB, Pope RM, Tschopp J, Wajant H, Wallach D, Wiltrout RH, Zornig M, Lynch DH (2007) The CD95 receptor: apoptosis revisited. Cell 129(3):447–450
65. Guicciardi ME, Gores GJ (2009) Life and death by death receptors. FASEB J 23(6):1625–1637. doi:10.1096/fj.08-111005. fj.08-111005 [pii]
66. Zhang Y, Liu Q, Zhang M, Yu Y, Liu X, Cao X (2009) Fas signal promotes lung cancer growth by recruiting myeloid-derived suppressor cells via cancer cell-derived PGE2. J Immunol 182(6):3801–3808. doi:10.4049/jimmunol.0801548. 182/6/3801 [pii]
67. Ametller E, Garcia-Recio S, Costamagna D, Mayordomo C, Fernandez-Nogueira P, Carbo N, Pastor-Arroyo EM, Gascon P, Almendro V (2010) Tumor promoting effects of CD95 signaling in chemoresistant cells. Mol Cancer 9:161. doi:10.1186/1476-4598-9-161. 1476-4598-9-161 [pii]
68. Lai YJ, Lin VT, Zheng Y, Benveniste EN, Lin FT (2010) The adaptor protein TRIP6 antagonizes Fas-induced apoptosis but promotes its effect on cell migration. Mol Cell Biol 30(23):5582–5596. doi:10.1128/MCB.00134-10
69. Nijkamp MW, Hoogwater FJ, Steller EJ, Westendorp BF, van der Meulen TA, Leenders MW, Borel Rinkes IH, Kranenburg O (2010) CD95 is a key mediator of invasion and accelerated outgrowth of mouse colorectal liver metastases following radiofrequency ablation. J Hepatol 53(6):1069–1077. doi:10.1016/j.jhep.2010.04.040. S0168-8278(10)00689-6 [pii]
70. Yuan K, Jing G, Chen J, Liu H, Zhang K, Li Y, Wu H, McDonald JM, Chen Y (2011) Calmodulin mediates Fas-induced FADD-independent survival signaling in pancreatic cancer cells via activation of Src-extracellular signal-regulated kinase (ERK). J Biol Chem 286(28):24776–24784. doi:10.1074/jbc.M110.202804. M110.202804 [pii]
71. Barnhart BC, Legembre P, Pietras E, Bubici C, Franzoso G, Peter ME (2004) CD95 ligand induces motility and invasiveness of apoptosis-resistant tumor cells. EMBO J 23(15):3175–3185. doi:10.1038/sj.emboj.7600325
72. Li H, Fan X, Stoicov C, Liu JH, Zubair S, Tsai E, Ste Marie R, Wang TC, Lyle S, Kurt-Jones E, Houghton J (2009) Human and mouse colon cancer utilizes CD95 signaling for local growth and metastatic spread to liver. Gastroenterology 137(3):934–944, 944 e931–934. doi:10.1053/j.gastro.2009.06.004. S0016-5085(09)00912-3 [pii]
73. Steller EJ, Ritsma L, Raats DA, Hoogwater FJ, Emmink BL, Govaert KM, Laoukili J, Rinkes IH, van Rheenen J, Kranenburg O (2011) The death receptor CD95 activates the cofilin pathway to stimulate tumour cell invasion. EMBO Rep 12(9):931–937. doi:10.1038/embor.2011.129. embor2011129 [pii]
74. O'Brien D, O'Connor T, Shanahan F, O'Connell J (2002) Activation of the p38 MAPK and ERK1/2 pathways is required for Fas-induced IL-8 production in colonic epithelial cells. Ann N Y Acad Sci 973:161–165
75. Seko Y, Kayagaki N, Seino K, Yagita H, Okumura K, Nagai R (2002) Role of Fas/FasL pathway in the activation of infiltrating cells in murine acute myocarditis caused by Coxsackievirus B3. J Am Coll Cardiol 39(8):1399–1403. S073510970201776X [pii]
76. Park DR, Thomsen AR, Frevert CW, Pham U, Skerrett SJ, Kiener PA, Liles WC (2003) Fas (CD95) induces proinflammatory cytokine responses by human monocytes and monocyte-derived macrophages. J Immunol 170(12):6209–6216

77. Ma Y, Liu H, Tu-Rapp H, Thiesen HJ, Ibrahim SM, Cole SM, Pope RM (2004) Fas ligation on macrophages enhances IL-1R1-Toll-like receptor 4 signaling and promotes chronic inflammation. Nat Immunol 5(4):380–387. doi:10.1038/ni1054. ni1054 [pii]
78. Palao G, Santiago B, Galindo MA, Rullas JN, Alcami J, Ramirez JC, Pablos JL (2006) Fas activation of a proinflammatory program in rheumatoid synoviocytes and its regulation by FLIP and caspase 8 signaling. Arthritis Rheum 54(5):1473–1481. doi:10.1002/art.21768
79. Perl M, Chung CS, Perl U, Lomas-Neira J, de Paepe M, Cioffi WG, Ayala A (2007) Fas-induced pulmonary apoptosis and inflammation during indirect acute lung injury. Am J Respir Crit Care Med 176(6):591–601. doi:10.1164/rccm.200611-1743OC
80. Lee SM, Kim EJ, Suk K, Lee WH (2011) Stimulation of Fas (CD95) induces production of pro-inflammatory mediators through ERK/JNK-dependent activation of NF-kappaB in THP-1 cells. Cell Immunol 271(1):157–162. doi:10.1016/j.cellimm.2011.06.019. S0008-8749(11)00157-2 [pii]
81. Becker KA, Henry B, Ziobro R, Tummler B, Gulbins E, Grassme H (2012) Role of CD95 in pulmonary inflammation and infection in cystic fibrosis. J Mol Med (Berl) 90(9):1011–1023. doi:10.1007/s00109-012-0867-2
82. Poissonnier A, Sanseau D, Le Gallo M, Malleter M, Levoin N, Viel R, Morere L, Penna A, Blanco P, Dupuy A, Poizeau F, Fautrel A, Seneschal J, Jouan F, Ritz J, Forcade E, Rioux N, Contin-Bordes C, Ducret T, Vacher AM, Barrow PA, Flynn RJ, Vacher P, Legembre P (2016) CD95-mediated calcium signaling promotes T helper 17 trafficking to inflamed organs in lupus-prone mice. Immunity 45(1):209–223. doi:10.1016/j.immuni.2016.06.028
83. Desbarats J, Birge RB, Mimouni-Rongy M, Weinstein DE, Palerme JS, Newell MK (2003) Fas engagement induces neurite growth through ERK activation and p35 upregulation. Nat Cell Biol 5(2):118–125
84. Zuliani C, Kleber S, Klussmann S, Wenger T, Kenzelmann M, Schreglmann N, Martinez A, del Rio JA, Soriano E, Vodrazka P, Kuner R, Groene HJ, Herr I, Krammer PH, Martin-Villalba A (2006) Control of neuronal branching by the death receptor CD95 (Fas/Apo-1). Cell Death Differ 13(1):31–40. doi:10.1038/sj.cdd.4401720. 4401720 [pii]
85. Beier CP, Kolbl M, Beier D, Woertgen C, Bogdahn U, Brawanski A (2007) CD95/Fas mediates cognitive improvement after traumatic brain injury. Cell Res 17(8):732–734. doi:10.1038/cr.2007.60. cr200760 [pii]
86. Alderson MR, Armitage RJ, Maraskovsky E, Tough TW, Roux E, Schooley K, Ramsdell F, Lynch DH (1993) Fas transduces activation signals in normal human T lymphocytes. J Exp Med 178(6):2231–2235
87. Desbarats J, Newell MK (2000) Fas engagement accelerates liver regeneration after partial hepatectomy. Nat Med 6(8):920–923. doi:10.1038/78688
88. Shinohara H, Yagita H, Ikawa Y, Oyaizu N (2000) Fas drives cell cycle progression in glioma cells via extracellular signal-regulated kinase activation. Cancer Res 60(6):1766–1772
89. Toyoshima F, Moriguchi T, Nishida E (1997) Fas induces cytoplasmic apoptotic responses and activation of the MKK7-JNK/SAPK and MKK6-p38 pathways independent of CPP32-like proteases. J Cell Biol 139(4):1005–1015
90. Kober AM, Legewie S, Pforr C, Fricker N, Eils R, Krammer PH, Lavrik IN (2011) Caspase-8 activity has an essential role in CD95/Fas-mediated MAPK activation. Cell Death Dis 2:e212. doi:10.1038/cddis.2011.93
91. Sancho-Martinez I, Martin-Villalba A (2009) Tyrosine phosphorylation and CD95: a FAScinating switch. Cell Cycle 8(6):838–842
92. Letellier E, Kumar S, Sancho-Martinez I, Krauth S, Funke-Kaiser A, Laudenklos S, Konecki K, Klussmann S, Corsini NS, Kleber S, Drost N, Neumann A, Levi-Strauss M, Brors B, Gretz N, Edler L, Fischer C, Hill O, Thiemann M, Biglari B, Karray S, Martin-Villalba A (2010) CD95-ligand on peripheral myeloid cells activates Syk kinase to trigger their recruitment to the inflammatory site. Immunity 32(2):240–252. doi:10.1016/j.immuni.2010.01.011. S1074-7613(10)00041-5 [pii]

93. Kreuz S, Siegmund D, Rumpf JJ, Samel D, Leverkus M, Janssen O, Hacker G, Dittrich-Breiholz O, Kracht M, Scheurich P, Wajant H (2004) NFkappaB activation by Fas is mediated through FADD, caspase-8, and RIP and is inhibited by FLIP. J Cell Biol 166(3):369–380
94. Wajant H, Pfizenmaier K, Scheurich P (2003) Non-apoptotic Fas signaling. Cytokine Growth Factor Rev 14(1):53–66. S1359610102000722 [pii]
95. Eischen CM, Dick CJ, Leibson PJ (1994) Tyrosine kinase activation provides an early and requisite signal for Fas-induced apoptosis. J Immunol 153(5):1947–1954
96. Schlottmann KE, Gulbins E, Lau SM, Coggeshall KM (1996) Activation of Src-family tyrosine kinases during Fas-induced apoptosis. J Leukoc Biol 60(4):546–554
97. Atkinson EA, Ostergaard H, Kane K, Pinkoski MJ, Caputo A, Olszowy MW, Bleackley RC (1996) A physical interaction between the cell death protein Fas and the tyrosine kinase p59fynT. J Biol Chem 271(11):5968–5971
98. Daigle I, Yousefi S, Colonna M, Green DR, Simon HU (2002) Death receptors bind SHP-1 and block cytokine-induced anti-apoptotic signaling in neutrophils. Nat Med 8(1):61–67. doi:10.1038/nm0102-61. nm0102-61 [pii]
99. Reinehr R, Schliess F, Haussinger D (2003) Hyperosmolarity and CD95L trigger CD95/EGF receptor association and tyrosine phosphorylation of CD95 as prerequisites for CD95 membrane trafficking and DISC formation. FASEB J 17(6):731–733. doi:10.1096/fj.02-0915fje
100. Chakrabandhu K, Huault S, Durivault J, Lang K, Ta Ngoc L, Bole A, Doma E, Derijard B, Gerard JP, Pierres M, Hueber AO (2014) An evolution-guided analysis reveals a multi-signaling regulation of Fas by tyrosine phosphorylation and its implication in human cancers. PLoS Biol 14(3):e1002401. doi:10.1371/journal.pbio.1002401. PBIOLOGY-D-15-02701 [pii]
101. Lavrik IN (2010) Systems biology of apoptosis signaling networks. Curr Opin Biotechnol 21(4):551–555. doi:10.1016/j.copbio.2010.07.001. S0958-1669(10)00120-5 [pii]
102. Toivonen HT, Meinander A, Asaoka T, Westerlund M, Pettersson F, Mikhailov A, Eriksson JE, Saxen H (2011) Modeling reveals that dynamic regulation of c-FLIP levels determines cell-to-cell distribution of CD95-mediated apoptosis. J Biol Chem 286(21):18375–18382. doi:10.1074/jbc.M110.177097. M110.177097 [pii]
103. Safa AR (2012) c-FLIP, a master anti-apoptotic regulator. Exp Oncol 34(3):176–184
104. Lavrik IN (2014) Systems biology of death receptor networks: live and let die. Cell Death Dis 5:e1259. cddis2014160 [pii]
105. Dutton A, Young LS, Murray PG (2006) The role of cellular FLICE inhibitory protein (c-FLIP) in the pathogenesis and treatment of cancer. Expert Opin Ther Targets 10(1):27–35. doi:10.1517/14728222.10.1.27
106. Bai M, Papoudou-Bai A, Kitsoulis P, Horianopoulos N, Kamina S, Agnantis NJ, Kanavaros P (2005) Cell cycle and apoptosis deregulation in classical Hodgkin lymphomas. In Vivo 19(2):439–453
107. Nikoletopoulou V, Markaki M, Palikaras K, Tavernarakis N (2013) Crosstalk between apoptosis, necrosis and autophagy. Biochim Biophys Acta 1833(12):3448–3459. doi:10.1016/j.bbamcr.2013.06.001
108. Shirley S, Micheau O (2013) Targeting c-FLIP in cancer. Cancer Lett 332(2):141–150. doi:10.1016/j.canlet.2010.10.009
109. Kummer JA, Micheau O, Schneider P, Bovenschen N, Broekhuizen R, Quadir R, Strik MC, Hack CE, Tschopp J (2007) Ectopic expression of the serine protease inhibitor PI9 modulates death receptor-mediated apoptosis. Cell Death Differ 14(8):1486–1496. doi:10.1038/sj.cdd.4402152. 4402152 [pii]
110. Sato T, Irie S, Kitada S, Reed JC (1995) FAP-1: a protein tyrosine phosphatase that associates with Fas. Science 268(5209):411–415
111. Li Y, Kanki H, Hachiya T, Ohyama T, Irie S, Tang G, Mukai J, Sato T (2000) Negative regulation of Fas-mediated apoptosis by FAP-1 in human cancer cells. Int J Cancer 87(4):473–479
112. Alonso A, Sasin J, Bottini N, Friedberg I, Osterman A, Godzik A, Hunter T, Dixon J, Mustelin T (2004) Protein tyrosine phosphatases in the human genome. Cell 117(6):699–711. doi:10.1016/j.cell.2004.05.018. S0092867404005343 [pii]

113. Wang Z, Shen D, Parsons DW, Bardelli A, Sager J, Szabo S, Ptak J, Silliman N, Peters BA, van der Heijden MS, Parmigiani G, Yan H, Wang TL, Riggins G, Powell SM, Willson JK, Markowitz S, Kinzler KW, Vogelstein B, Velculescu VE (2004) Mutational analysis of the tyrosine phosphatome in colorectal cancers. Science 304(5674):1164–1166. doi:10.1126/science.1096096. 304/5674/1164 [pii]
114. Villa F, Deak M, Bloomberg GB, Alessi DR, van Aalten DM (2005) Crystal structure of the PTPL1/FAP-1 human tyrosine phosphatase mutated in colorectal cancer: evidence for a second phosphotyrosine substrate recognition pocket. J Biol Chem 280(9):8180–8187. doi:10.1074/jbc.M412211200. M412211200 [pii]
115. Yanagisawa J, Takahashi M, Kanki H, Yano-Yanagisawa H, Tazunoki T, Sawa E, Nishitoba T, Kamishohara M, Kobayashi E, Kataoka S, Sato T (1997) The molecular interaction of Fas and FAP-1. A tripeptide blocker of human Fas interaction with FAP-1 promotes Fas-induced apoptosis. J Biol Chem 272(13):8539–8545
116. Ungefroren H, Kruse ML, Trauzold A, Roeschmann S, Roeder C, Arlt A, Henne-Bruns D, Kalthoff H (2001) FAP-1 in pancreatic cancer cells: functional and mechanistic studies on its inhibitory role in CD95-mediated apoptosis. J Cell Sci 114(Pt 15):2735–2746
117. Ungefroren H, Voss M, Jansen M, Roeder C, Henne-Bruns D, Kremer B, Kalthoff H (1998) Human pancreatic adenocarcinomas express Fas and Fas ligand yet are resistant to Fas-mediated apoptosis. Cancer Res 58(8):1741–1749
118. Ivanov VN, Lopez Bergami P, Maulit G, Sato TA, Sassoon D, Ronai Z (2003) FAP-1 association with Fas (Apo-1) inhibits Fas expression on the cell surface. Mol Cell Biol 23(10):3623–3635
119. He RJ, Yu ZH, Zhang RY, Zhang ZY (2014) Protein tyrosine phosphatases as potential therapeutic targets. Acta Pharmacol Sin 35(10):1227–1246. doi:10.1038/aps.2014.80. aps201480 [pii]
120. Meinhold-Heerlein I, Stenner-Liewen F, Liewen H, Kitada S, Krajewska M, Krajewski S, Zapata JM, Monks A, Scudiero DA, Bauknecht T, Reed JC (2001) Expression and potential role of Fas-associated phosphatase-1 in ovarian cancer. Am J Pathol 158(4):1335–1344. doi:10.1016/S0002-9440(10)64084-9. S0002-9440(10)64084-9 [pii]
121. Yao H, Song E, Chen J, Hamar P (2004) Expression of FAP-1 by human colon adenocarcinoma: implication for resistance against Fas-mediated apoptosis in cancer. Br J Cancer 91(9):1718–1725
122. Wieckowski E, Atarashi Y, Stanson J, Sato TA, Whiteside TL (2007) FAP-1-mediated activation of NF-kappaB induces resistance of head and neck cancer to Fas-induced apoptosis. J Cell Biochem 100(1):16–28. doi:10.1002/jcb.20922
123. Lee SH, Shin MS, Lee HS, Bae JH, Lee HK, Kim HS, Kim SY, Jang JJ, Joo M, Kang YK, Park WS, Park JY, Oh RR, Han SY, Lee JH, Kim SH, Lee JY, Yoo NJ (2001) Expression of Fas and Fas-related molecules in human hepatocellular carcinoma. Hum Pathol 32(3):250–256. doi:10.1053/hupa.2001.22769. S0046-8177(01)06822-8 [pii]
124. Baer C, Nees M, Breit S, Selle B, Kulozik AE, Schaefer KL, Braun Y, Wai D, Poremba C (2004) Profiling and functional annotation of mRNA gene expression in pediatric rhabdomyosarcoma and Ewing's sarcoma. Int J Cancer 110(5):687–694. doi:10.1002/ijc.20171
125. Abaan OD, Levenson A, Khan O, Furth PA, Uren A, Toretsky JA (2005) PTPL1 is a direct transcriptional target of EWS-FLI1 and modulates Ewing's Sarcoma tumorigenesis. Oncogene 24(16):2715–2722. doi:10.1038/sj.onc.1208247. 1208247 [pii]
126. Xiao ZY, Wu W, Eagleton N, Chen HQ, Shao J, Teng H, Liu TH, Jiang ZM, Yao HR (2010) Silencing Fas-associated phosphatase 1 expression enhances efficiency of chemotherapy for colon carcinoma with oxaliplatin. World J Gastroenterol 16(1):112–118
127. Schickel R, Park SM, Murmann AE, Peter ME (2010) miR-200c regulates induction of apoptosis through CD95 by targeting FAP-1. Mol Cell 38(6):908–915. doi:10.1016/j.molcel.2010.05.018. S1097-2765(10)00380-1 [pii]
128. Ivanov VN, Ronai Z, Hei TK (2006) Opposite roles of FAP-1 and dynamin in the regulation of Fas (CD95) translocation to the cell surface and susceptibility to Fas ligand-mediated apoptosis. J Biol Chem 281(3):1840–1852

129. Foehr ED, Lorente G, Vincent V, Nikolich K, Urfer R (2005) FAS associated phosphatase (FAP-1) blocks apoptosis of astrocytomas through dephosphorylation of FAS. J Neurooncol 74(3):241–248
130. Gump JM, Staskiewicz L, Morgan MJ, Bamberg A, Riches DW, Thorburn A (2014) Autophagy variation within a cell population determines cell fate through selective degradation of Fap-1. Nat Cell Biol 16(1):47–54. doi:10.1038/ncb2886. ncb2886 [pii]
131. Gonzalez-Garcia A, R-Borlado L, Leonardo E, Merida I, Martinez AC, Carrera AC (1997) Lck is necessary and sufficient for Fas-ligand expression and apoptotic cell death in mature cycling T cells. J Immunol 158(9):4104–4112
132. Simon HU, Yousefi S, Dibbert B, Hebestreit H, Weber M, Branch DR, Blaser K, Levi-Schaffer F, Anderson GP (1998) Role for tyrosine phosphorylation and Lyn tyrosine kinase in fas receptor-mediated apoptosis in eosinophils. Blood 92(2):547–557
133. Yu XZ, Levin SD, Madrenas J, Anasetti C (2004) Lck is required for activation-induced T cell death after TCR ligation with partial agonists. J Immunol 172(3):1437–1443
134. Schneider TJ, Fischer GM, Donohoe TJ, Colarusso TP, Rothstein TL (1999) A novel gene coding for a Fas apoptosis inhibitory molecule (FAIM) isolated from inducibly Fas-resistant B lymphocytes. J Exp Med 189(6):949–956
135. Rothstein TL, Zhong X, Schram BR, Negm RS, Donohoe TJ, Cabral DS, Foote LC, Schneider TJ (2000) Receptor-specific regulation of B-cell susceptibility to Fas-mediated apoptosis and a novel Fas apoptosis inhibitory molecule. Immunol Rev 176:116–133
136. Rothstein TL (2000) Inducible resistance to Fas-mediated apoptosis in B cells. Cell Res 10(4):245–266. doi:10.1038/sj.cr.7290053
137. Zhong X, Schneider TJ, Cabral DS, Donohoe TJ, Rothstein TL (2001) An alternatively spliced long form of Fas apoptosis inhibitory molecule (FAIM) with tissue-specific expression in the brain. Mol Immunol 38(1):65–72
138. Huo J, Xu S, Lam KP (2010) Fas apoptosis inhibitory molecule regulates T cell receptor-mediated apoptosis of thymocytes by modulating Akt activation and Nur77 expression. J Biol Chem 285(16):11827–11835. doi:10.1074/jbc.M109.072744. M109.072744 [pii]
139. Huo J, Xu S, Guo K, Zeng Q, Lam KP (2009) Genetic deletion of faim reveals its role in modulating c-FLIP expression during CD95-mediated apoptosis of lymphocytes and hepatocytes. Cell Death Differ 16(7):1062–1070. doi:10.1038/cdd.2009.26. cdd200926 [pii]
140. Safa AR (2013) Roles of c-FLIP in apoptosis, necroptosis, and autophagy. J Carcinog Mutagen Suppl 6. doi:10.4172/2157-2518.S6-003
141. Ueffing N, Keil E, Freund C, Kuhne R, Schulze-Osthoff K, Schmitz I (2008) Mutational analyses of c-FLIPR, the only murine short FLIP isoform, reveal requirements for DISC recruitment. Cell Death Differ 15(4):773–782. doi:10.1038/sj.cdd.4402314. 4402314 [pii]
142. Planells-Ferrer L, Urresti J, Coccia E, Galenkamp KM, Calleja-Yague I, Lopez-Soriano J, Carriba P, Barneda-Zahonero B, Segura MF, Comella JX (2016) Fas apoptosis inhibitory molecules: more than death-receptor antagonists in the nervous system. J Neurochem 139(1):11–21. doi:10.1111/jnc.13729
143. Gentles AJ, Bratman SV, Lee LJ, Harris JP, Feng W, Nair RV, Shultz DB, Nair VS, Hoang CD, West RB, Plevritis SK, Alizadeh AA, Diehn M (2015) Integrating tumor and stromal gene expression signatures with clinical indices for survival stratification of early-stage non-small cell lung cancer. J Natl Cancer Inst 107(10). doi:10.1093/jnci/djv211. djv211 [pii]
144. Huo J, Xu S, Lin B, Chng WJ, Lam KP (2013) Fas apoptosis inhibitory molecule is upregulated by IGF-1 signaling and modulates Akt activation and IRF4 expression in multiple myeloma. Leukemia 27(5):1165–1171. doi:10.1038/leu.2012.326. leu2012326 [pii]
145. Patron JP, Fendler A, Bild M, Jung U, Muller H, Arntzen MO, Piso C, Stephan C, Thiede B, Mollenkopf HJ, Jung K, Kaufmann SH, Schreiber J (2012) MiR-133b targets antiapoptotic genes and enhances death receptor-induced apoptosis. PLoS One 7(4):e35345. doi:10.1371/journal.pone.0035345. PONE-D-11-20757 [pii]
146. Wise JF, Berkova Z, Mathur R, Zhu H, Braun FK, Tao RH, Sabichi AL, Ao X, Maeng H, Samaniego F (2013) Nucleolin inhibits Fas ligand binding and suppresses Fas-mediated

apoptosis in vivo via a surface nucleolin-Fas complex. Blood 121(23):4729–4739. doi:10.1182/blood-2012-12-471094. blood-2012-12-471094 [pii]
147. Srivastava M, Pollard HB (1999) Molecular dissection of nucleolin's role in growth and cell proliferation: new insights. FASEB J 13(14):1911–1922
148. Hovanessian AG, Puvion-Dutilleul F, Nisole S, Svab J, Perret E, Deng JS, Krust B (2000) The cell-surface-expressed nucleolin is associated with the actin cytoskeleton. Exp Cell Res 261(2):312–328. doi:10.1006/excr.2000.5071. S0014-4827(00)95071-7 [pii]
149. Chen CY, Gherzi R, Andersen JS, Gaietta G, Jurchott K, Royer HD, Mann M, Karin M (2000) Nucleolin and YB-1 are required for JNK-mediated interleukin-2 mRNA stabilization during T-cell activation. Genes Dev 14(10):1236–1248
150. Christian S, Pilch J, Akerman ME, Porkka K, Laakkonen P, Ruoslahti E (2003) Nucleolin expressed at the cell surface is a marker of endothelial cells in angiogenic blood vessels. J Cell Biol 163(4):871–878. doi:10.1083/jcb.200304132. jcb.200304132 [pii]
151. Otake Y, Soundararajan S, Sengupta TK, Kio EA, Smith JC, Pineda-Roman M, Stuart RK, Spicer EK, Fernandes DJ (2007) Overexpression of nucleolin in chronic lymphocytic leukemia cells induces stabilization of bcl2 mRNA. Blood 109(7):3069–3075. doi:10.1182/blood-2006-08-043257. blood-2006-08-043257 [pii]
152. Said EA, Courty J, Svab J, Delbe J, Krust B, Hovanessian AG (2005) Pleiotrophin inhibits HIV infection by binding the cell surface-expressed nucleolin. FEBS J 272(18):4646–4659. doi:10.1111/j.1742-4658.2005.04870.x. EJB4870 [pii]
153. Reyes-Reyes EM, Akiyama SK (2008) Cell-surface nucleolin is a signal transducing P-selectin binding protein for human colon carcinoma cells. Exp Cell Res 314(11–12):2212–2223. doi:10.1016/j.yexcr.2008.03.016. S0014-4827(08)00140-7 [pii]
154. Tate A, Isotani S, Bradley MJ, Sikes RA, Davis R, Chung LW, Edlund M (2006) Met-independent hepatocyte growth factor-mediated regulation of cell adhesion in human prostate cancer cells. BMC Cancer 6:197. doi:10.1186/1471-2407-6-197. 1471-2407-6-197 [pii]
155. Pasternack MS, Bleier KJ, McInerney TN (1991) Granzyme A binding to target cell proteins. Granzyme A binds to and cleaves nucleolin in vitro. J Biol Chem 266(22):14703–14708
156. Mi Y, Thomas SD, Xu X, Casson LK, Miller DM, Bates PJ (2003) Apoptosis in leukemia cells is accompanied by alterations in the levels and localization of nucleolin. J Biol Chem 278(10):8572–8579. doi:10.1074/jbc.M207637200. M207637200 [pii]
157. Bose S, Tholanikunnel TE, Reuben A, Tholanikunnel BG, Spicer EK (2016) Regulation of nucleolin expression by miR-194, miR-206, and HuR. Mol Cell Biochem 417(1–2):141–153. doi:10.1007/s11010-016-2721-2. 10.1007/s11010-016-2721-2 [pii]
158. Tominaga K, Srikantan S, Lee EK, Subaran SS, Martindale JL, Abdelmohsen K, Gorospe M (2011) Competitive regulation of nucleolin expression by HuR and miR-494. Mol Cell Biol 31(20):4219–4231. doi:10.1128/MCB.05955-11. MCB.05955-11 [pii]
159. Berkova Z, Wang S, Ao X, Wise JF, Braun FK, Rezaeian AH, Sehgal L, Goldenberg DM, Samaniego F (2014) CD74 interferes with the expression of fas receptor on the surface of lymphoma cells. J Exp Clin Cancer Res 33(1):80. doi:10.1186/PREACCEPT-1190264577137976. s13046-014-0080-y [pii]
160. Becker-Herman S, Arie G, Medvedovsky H, Kerem A, Shachar I (2005) CD74 is a member of the regulated intramembrane proteolysis-processed protein family. Mol Biol Cell 16(11):5061–5069. doi:10.1091/mbc.E05-04-0327. E05-04-0327 [pii]
161. Stein R, Mattes MJ, Cardillo TM, Hansen HJ, Chang CH, Burton J, Govindan S, Goldenberg DM (2007) CD74: a new candidate target for the immunotherapy of B-cell neoplasms. Clin Cancer Res 13(18 Pt 2):5556s–5563s. doi:10.1158/1078-0432.CCR-07-1167. 13/18/5556s [pii]
162. Shachar I, Haran M (2011) The secret second life of an innocent chaperone: the story of CD74 and B cell/chronic lymphocytic leukemia cell survival. Leuk Lymphoma 52(8):1446–1454. doi:10.3109/10428194.2011.565437
163. Berkova Z, Tao RH, Samaniego F (2010) Milatuzumab - a promising new immunotherapeutic agent. Expert Opin Investig Drugs 19(1):141–149. doi:10.1517/13543780903463854

164. Alinari L, Christian B, Baiocchi RA (2012) Novel targeted therapies for mantle cell lymphoma. Oncotarget 3(2):203–211. 426 [pii]
165. Kaufman JL, Niesvizky R, Stadtmauer EA, Chanan-Khan A, Siegel D, Horne H, Wegener WA, Goldenberg DM (2013) Phase I, multicentre, dose-escalation trial of monotherapy with milatuzumab (humanized anti-CD74 monoclonal antibody) in relapsed or refractory multiple myeloma. Br J Haematol 163(4):478–486. doi:10.1111/bjh.12565
166. Burton JD, Ely S, Reddy PK, Stein R, Gold DV, Cardillo TM, Goldenberg DM (2004) CD74 is expressed by multiple myeloma and is a promising target for therapy. Clin Cancer Res 10(19):6606–6611. doi:10.1158/1078-0432.CCR-04-0182. 10/19/6606 [pii]
167. Starlets D, Gore Y, Binsky I, Haran M, Harpaz N, Shvidel L, Becker-Herman S, Berrebi A, Shachar I (2006) Cell-surface CD74 initiates a signaling cascade leading to cell proliferation and survival. Blood 107(12):4807–4816. doi:10.1182/blood-2005-11-4334. 2005-11-4334 [pii]
168. Binsky I, Haran M, Starlets D, Gore Y, Lantner F, Harpaz N, Leng L, Goldenberg DM, Shvidel L, Berrebi A, Bucala R, Shachar I (2007) IL-8 secreted in a macrophage migration-inhibitory factor- and CD74-dependent manner regulates B cell chronic lymphocytic leukemia survival. Proc Natl Acad Sci U S A 104(33):13408–13413. doi:10.1073/pnas.0701553104. 0701553104 [pii]
169. Ohta S, Misawa A, Fukaya R, Inoue S, Kanemura Y, Okano H, Kawakami Y, Toda M (2012) Macrophage migration inhibitory factor (MIF) promotes cell survival and proliferation of neural stem/progenitor cells. J Cell Sci 125(Pt 13):3210–3220. doi:10.1242/jcs.102210. jcs.102210 [pii]
170. Leng L, Metz CN, Fang Y, Xu J, Donnelly S, Baugh J, Delohery T, Chen Y, Mitchell RA, Bucala R (2003) MIF signal transduction initiated by binding to CD74. J Exp Med 197(11):1467–1476. doi:10.1084/jem.20030286. jem.20030286 [pii]
171. Shi X, Leng L, Wang T, Wang W, Du X, Li J, McDonald C, Chen Z, Murphy JW, Lolis E, Noble P, Knudson W, Bucala R (2006) CD44 is the signaling component of the macrophage migration inhibitory factor-CD74 receptor complex. Immunity 25(4):595–606. doi:10.1016/j.immuni.2006.08.020. S1074-7613(06)00432-8 [pii]
172. Wang ZQ, Milne K, Webb JR, Watson PH (2016) CD74 and intratumoral immune response in breast cancer. Oncotarget. doi:10.18632/oncotarget.8610. 8610 [pii]
173. Ekmekcioglu S, Davies MA, Tanese K, Roszik J, Shin-Sim M, Bassett RL Jr, Milton DR, Woodman SE, Prieto VG, Gershenwald JE, Morton DL, Hoon DS, Grimm EA (2016) Inflammatory marker testing identifies CD74 expression in melanoma tumor cells, and its expression associates with favorable survival for stage III melanoma. Clin Cancer Res 22(12):3016–3024. doi:10.1158/1078-0432.CCR-15-2226. 1078-0432.CCR-15-2226 [pii]
174. Otterstrom C, Soltermann A, Opitz I, Felley-Bosco E, Weder W, Stahel RA, Triponez F, Robert JH, Serre-Beinier V (2014) CD74: a new prognostic factor for patients with malignant pleural mesothelioma. Br J Cancer 110(8):2040–2046. doi:10.1038/bjc.2014.117. bjc2014117 [pii]
175. Matza D, Lantner F, Bogoch Y, Flaishon L, Hershkoviz R, Shachar I (2002) Invariant chain induces B cell maturation in a process that is independent of its chaperonic activity. Proc Natl Acad Sci U S A 99(5):3018–3023. doi:10.1073/pnas.052703299. 052703299 [pii]
176. Lantner F, Starlets D, Gore Y, Flaishon L, Yamit-Hezi A, Dikstein R, Leng L, Bucala R, Machluf Y, Oren M, Shachar I (2007) CD74 induces TAp63 expression leading to B-cell survival. Blood 110(13):4303–4311. doi:10.1182/blood-2007-04-087486. blood-2007-04-087486 [pii]
177. Mark T, Martin P, Leonard JP, Niesvizky R (2009) Milatuzumab: a promising new agent for the treatment of lymphoid malignancies. Expert Opin Investig Drugs 18(1):99–104. doi:10.1517/13543780802636162
178. Stein R, Smith MR, Chen S, Zalath M, Goldenberg DM (2009) Combining milatuzumab with bortezomib, doxorubicin, or dexamethasone improves responses in multiple myeloma cell

lines. Clin Cancer Res 15(8):2808–2817. doi:10.1158/1078-0432.CCR-08-1953. 1078-0432.CCR-08-1953 [pii]
179. Hertlein E, Triantafillou G, Sass EJ, Hessler JD, Zhang X, Jarjoura D, Lucas DM, Muthusamy N, Goldenberg DM, Lee RJ, Byrd JC (2010) Milatuzumab immunoliposomes induce cell death in CLL by promoting accumulation of CD74 on the surface of B cells. Blood 116(14):2554–2558. doi:10.1182/blood-2009-11-253203. blood-2009-11-253203 [pii]
180. Alinari L, Yu B, Christian BA, Yan F, Shin J, Lapalombella R, Hertlein E, Lustberg ME, Quinion C, Zhang X, Lozanski G, Muthusamy N, Praetorius-Ibba M, O'Connor OA, Goldenberg DM, Byrd JC, Blum KA, Baiocchi RA (2011) Combination anti-CD74 (milatuzumab) and anti-CD20 (rituximab) monoclonal antibody therapy has in vitro and in vivo activity in mantle cell lymphoma. Blood 117(17):4530–4541. doi:10.1182/blood-2010-08-303354. blood-2010-08-303354 [pii]
181. Alinari L, Mahoney E, Patton J, Zhang X, Huynh L, Earl CT, Mani R, Mao Y, Yu B, Quinion C, Towns WH, Chen CS, Goldenberg DM, Blum KA, Byrd JC, Muthusamy N, Praetorius-Ibba M, Baiocchi RA (2011) FTY720 increases CD74 expression and sensitizes mantle cell lymphoma cells to milatuzumab-mediated cell death. Blood 118(26):6893–6903. doi:10.1182/blood-2011-06-363879. blood-2011-06-363879 [pii]
182. Alinari L, Baiocchi RA, Praetorius-Ibba M (2012) FTY720-induced blockage of autophagy enhances anticancer efficacy of milatuzumab in mantle cell lymphoma: is FTY720 the next autophagy-blocking agent in lymphoma treatment? Autophagy 8(3):416–417. doi:10.4161/auto.19050. 19050 [pii]
183. Gupta P, Goldenberg DM, Rossi EA, Cardillo TM, Byrd JC, Muthusamy N, Furman RR, Chang CH (2012) Dual-targeting immunotherapy of lymphoma: potent cytotoxicity of anti-CD20/CD74 bispecific antibodies in mantle cell and other lymphomas. Blood 119(16):3767–3778. doi:10.1182/blood-2011-09-381988. blood-2011-09-381988 [pii]
184. Mao Y, Triantafillou G, Hertlein E, Towns W, Stefanovski M, Mo X, Jarjoura D, Phelps M, Marcucci G, Lee LJ, Goldenberg DM, Lee RJ, Byrd JC, Muthusamy N (2013) Milatuzumab-conjugated liposomes as targeted dexamethasone carriers for therapeutic delivery in CD74+ B-cell malignancies. Clin Cancer Res 19(2):347–356. doi:10.1158/1078-0432.CCR-12-2046. 1078-0432.CCR-12-2046 [pii]
185. Gajate C, Mollinedo F (2007) Edelfosine and perifosine induce selective apoptosis in multiple myeloma by recruitment of death receptors and downstream signaling molecules into lipid rafts. Blood 109(2):711–719. doi:10.1182/blood-2006-04-016824. blood-2006-04-016824 [pii]
186. Mollinedo F, de la Iglesia-Vicente J, Gajate C, Estella-Hermoso de Mendoza A, Villa-Pulgarin JA, Campanero MA, Blanco-Prieto MJ (2010) Lipid raft-targeted therapy in multiple myeloma. Oncogene 29(26):3748–3757
187. Mollinedo F, de la Iglesia-Vicente J, Gajate C, Estella-Hermoso de Mendoza A, Villa-Pulgarin JA, de Frias M, Roue G, Gil J, Colomer D, Campanero MA, Blanco-Prieto MJ (2010) In vitro and In vivo selective antitumor activity of Edelfosine against mantle cell lymphoma and chronic lymphocytic leukemia involving lipid rafts. Clin Cancer Res 16(7):2046–2054
188. Gajate C, Del Canto-Janez E, Acuna AU, Amat-Guerri F, Geijo E, Santos-Beneit AM, Veldman RJ, Mollinedo F (2004) Intracellular triggering of Fas aggregation and recruitment of apoptotic molecules into Fas-enriched rafts in selective tumor cell apoptosis. J Exp Med 200(3):353–365
189. Gajate C, Fonteriz RI, Cabaner C, Alvarez-Noves G, Alvarez-Rodriguez Y, Modolell M, Mollinedo F (2000) Intracellular triggering of Fas, independently of FasL, as a new mechanism of antitumor ether lipid-induced apoptosis. Int J Cancer 85(5):674–682
190. Parlato S, Giammarioli AM, Logozzi M, Lozupone F, Matarrese P, Luciani F, Falchi M, Malorni W, Fais S (2000) CD95 (APO-1/Fas) linkage to the actin cytoskeleton through ezrin in human T lymphocytes: a novel regulatory mechanism of the CD95 apoptotic pathway. EMBO J 19(19):5123–5134. doi:10.1093/emboj/19.19.5123
191. Grassme H, Cremesti A, Kolesnick R, Gulbins E (2003) Ceramide-mediated clustering is required for CD95-DISC formation. Oncogene 22(35):5457–5470

192. Grassme H, Jekle A, Riehle A, Schwarz H, Berger J, Sandhoff K, Kolesnick R, Gulbins E (2001) CD95 signaling via ceramide-rich membrane rafts. J Biol Chem 276(23):20589–20596
193. Gajate C, Mollinedo F (2002) Biological activities, mechanisms of action and biomedical prospect of the antitumor ether phospholipid ET-18-OCH_3 (Edelfosine), a proapoptotic agent in tumor cells. Curr Drug Metab 3(5):491–525
194. Mollinedo F (2014) Editorial: antitumor alkylphospholipid analogs: a promising and growing family of synthetic cell membrane-targeting molecules for cancer treatment. Anticancer Agents Med Chem 14(4):495–498. doi:ACAMC-EPUB-59632 [pii]
195. Jaffres PA, Gajate C, Bouchet AM, Couthon-Gourves H, Chantome A, Potier-Cartereau M, Besson P, Bougnoux P, Mollinedo F, Vandier C (2016) Alkyl ether lipids, ion channels and lipid raft reorganization in cancer therapy. Pharmacol Ther 165:114–131. doi:10.1016/j.pharmthera.2016.06.003. S0163-7258(16)30093-6 [pii]
196. Hueber AO, Bernard AM, Herincs Z, Couzinet A, He HT (2002) An essential role for membrane rafts in the initiation of Fas/CD95-triggered cell death in mouse thymocytes. EMBO Rep 3(2):190–196
197. Nieto-Miguel T, Gajate C, Gonzalez-Camacho F, Mollinedo F (2008) Proapoptotic role of Hsp90 by its interaction with c-Jun N-terminal kinase in lipid rafts in edelfosine-mediated antileukemic therapy. Oncogene 27(12):1779–1787
198. Gajate C, Gonzalez-Camacho F, Mollinedo F (2009) Involvement of raft aggregates enriched in Fas/CD95 death-inducing signaling complex in the antileukemic action of edelfosine in Jurkat cells. PLoS One 4(4):e5044
199. Gajate C, Gonzalez-Camacho F, Mollinedo F (2009) Lipid raft connection between extrinsic and intrinsic apoptotic pathways. Biochem Biophys Res Commun 380(4):780–784
200. Reis-Sobreiro M, Gajate C, Mollinedo F (2009) Involvement of mitochondria and recruitment of Fas/CD95 signaling in lipid rafts in resveratrol-mediated antimyeloma and antileukemia actions. Oncogene 28(36):3221–3234
201. Lotocki G, Alonso OF, Dietrich WD, Keane RW (2004) Tumor necrosis factor receptor 1 and its signaling intermediates are recruited to lipid rafts in the traumatized brain. J Neurosci 24(49):11010–11016. doi:10.1523/JNEUROSCI.3823-04.2004. 24/49/11010 [pii]
202. Song JH, Tse MC, Bellail A, Phuphanich S, Khuri F, Kneteman NM, Hao C (2007) Lipid rafts and nonrafts mediate tumor necrosis factor related apoptosis-inducing ligand induced apoptotic and nonapoptotic signals in non small cell lung carcinoma cells. Cancer Res 67(14):6946–6955. doi:10.1158/0008-5472.CAN-06-3896. 67/14/6946 [pii]
203. Ouyang W, Yang C, Liu Y, Xiong J, Zhang J, Zhong Y, Zhang G, Zhou F, Zhou Y, Xie C (2011) Redistribution of DR4 and DR5 in lipid rafts accounts for the sensitivity to TRAIL in NSCLC cells. Int J Oncol 39(6):1577–1586. doi:10.3892/ijo.2011.1129
204. Ouyang W, Yang C, Zhang S, Liu Y, Yang B, Zhang J, Zhou F, Zhou Y, Xie C (2013) Absence of death receptor translocation into lipid rafts in acquired TRAIL-resistant NSCLC cells. Int J Oncol 42(2):699–711. doi:10.3892/ijo.2012.1748
205. Grassme H, Schwarz H, Gulbins E (2001) Molecular mechanisms of ceramide-mediated CD95 clustering. Biochem Biophys Res Commun 284(4):1016–1030
206. Paris F, Grassme H, Cremesti A, Zager J, Fong Y, Haimovitz-Friedman A, Fuks Z, Gulbins E, Kolesnick R (2001) Natural ceramide reverses Fas resistance of acid sphingomyelinase(-/-) hepatocytes. J Biol Chem 276(11):8297–8305
207. Cremesti A, Paris F, Grassme H, Holler N, Tschopp J, Fuks Z, Gulbins E, Kolesnick R (2001) Ceramide enables fas to cap and kill. J Biol Chem 276(26):23954–23961
208. Kolesnick R (2002) The therapeutic potential of modulating the ceramide/sphingomyelin pathway. J Clin Invest 110(1):3–8
209. Johnston I, Johnston LJ (2006) Ceramide promotes restructuring of model raft membranes. Langmuir 22(26):11284–11289
210. Ira JLJ (2008) Sphingomyelinase generation of ceramide promotes clustering of nanoscale domains in supported bilayer membranes. Biochim Biophys Acta 1778(1):185–197. doi:10.1016/j.bbamem.2007.09.021. S0005-2736(07)00379-3 [pii]

211. Prinetti A, Chigorno V, Prioni S, Loberto N, Marano N, Tettamanti G, Sonnino S (2001) Changes in the lipid turnover, composition, and organization, as sphingolipid-enriched membrane domains, in rat cerebellar granule cells developing in vitro. J Biol Chem 276(24):21136–21145
212. Cremesti AE, Goni FM, Kolesnick R (2002) Role of sphingomyelinase and ceramide in modulating rafts: do biophysical properties determine biologic outcome? FEBS Lett 531(1):47–53
213. Chiantia S, Ries J, Chwastek G, Carrer D, Li Z, Bittman R, Schwille P (2008) Role of ceramide in membrane protein organization investigated by combined AFM and FCS. Biochim Biophys Acta 1778(5):1356–1364. doi:10.1016/j.bbamem.2008.02.008. S0005-2736(08)00078-3 [pii]
214. Castro BM, de Almeida RF, Goormaghtigh E, Fedorov A, Prieto M (2011) Organization and dynamics of Fas transmembrane domain in raft membranes and modulation by ceramide. Biophys J 101(7):1632–1641. doi:10.1016/j.bpj.2011.08.022. S0006-3495(11)00968-4 [pii]
215. Silva LC, de Almeida RF, Castro BM, Fedorov A, Prieto M (2007) Ceramide-domain formation and collapse in lipid rafts: membrane reorganization by an apoptotic lipid. Biophys J 92(2):502–516. doi:10.1529/biophysj.106.091876. S0006-3495(07)70850-0 [pii]
216. Megha, London E (2004) Ceramide selectively displaces cholesterol from ordered lipid domains (rafts): implications for lipid raft structure and function. J Biol Chem 279(11):9997–10004
217. Yu C, Alterman M, Dobrowsky RT (2005) Ceramide displaces cholesterol from lipid rafts and decreases the association of the cholesterol binding protein caveolin-1. J Lipid Res 46(8):1678–1691
218. Staneva G, Chachaty C, Wolf C, Koumanov K, Quinn PJ (2008) The role of sphingomyelin in regulating phase coexistence in complex lipid model membranes: competition between ceramide and cholesterol. Biochim Biophys Acta 1778(12):2727–2739. doi:10.1016/j.bbamem.2008.07.025. S0005-2736(08)00232-0 [pii]
219. Chakrabandhu K, Herincs Z, Huault S, Dost B, Peng L, Conchonaud F, Marguet D, He HT, Hueber AO (2007) Palmitoylation is required for efficient Fas cell death signaling. EMBO J 26(1):209–220. doi:10.1038/sj.emboj.7601456. 7601456 [pii]
220. Feig C, Tchikov V, Schutze S, Peter ME (2007) Palmitoylation of CD95 facilitates formation of SDS-stable receptor aggregates that initiate apoptosis signaling. EMBO J 26(1):221–231. doi:10.1038/sj.emboj.7601460
221. Kamitani T, Nguyen HP, Yeh ET (1997) Activation-induced aggregation and processing of the human Fas antigen. Detection with cytoplasmic domain-specific antibodies. J Biol Chem 272(35):22307–22314
222. Hawash IY, Hu XE, Adal A, Cassady JM, Geahlen RL, Harrison ML (2002) The oxygen-substituted palmitic acid analogue, 13-oxypalmitic acid, inhibits Lck localization to lipid rafts and T cell signaling. Biochim Biophys Acta 1589(2):140–150. S0167488902001659 [pii]
223. Greaves J, Chamberlain LH (2007) Palmitoylation-dependent protein sorting. J Cell Biol 176(3):249–254. doi:10.1083/jcb.200610151. jcb.200610151 [pii]
224. Levental I, Lingwood D, Grzybek M, Coskun U, Simons K (2010) Palmitoylation regulates raft affinity for the majority of integral raft proteins. Proc Natl Acad Sci U S A 107(51):22050–22054. doi:10.1073/pnas.1016184107. 1016184107 [pii]
225. Aicart-Ramos C, Valero RA, Rodriguez-Crespo I (2011) Protein palmitoylation and subcellular trafficking. Biochim Biophys Acta 1808(12):2981–2994. doi:10.1016/j.bbamem.2011.07.009. S0005-2736(11)00214-8 [pii]
226. Rossin A, Durivault J, Chakhtoura-Feghali T, Lounnas N, Gagnoux-Palacios L, Hueber AO (2015) Fas palmitoylation by the palmitoyl acyltransferase DHHC7 regulates Fas stability. Cell Death Differ 22(4):643–653. doi:10.1038/cdd.2014.153
227. Leon-Bollotte L, Subramaniam S, Cauvard O, Plenchette-Colas S, Paul C, Godard C, Martinez-Ruiz A, Legembre P, Jeannin JF, Bettaieb A (2011) S-nitrosylation of the death receptor fas promotes fas ligand-mediated apoptosis in cancer cells. Gastroenterology 140(7):2009–2018, 2018 e2001–2004. doi:10.1053/j.gastro.2011.02.053

228. Rossin A, Kral R, Lounnas N, Chakrabandhu K, Mailfert S, Marguet D, Hueber AO (2010) Identification of a lysine-rich region of Fas as a raft nanodomain targeting signal necessary for Fas-mediated cell death. Exp Cell Res 316(9):1513–1522. doi:10.1016/j.yexcr.2010.03.002
229. Peter ME, Hellbardt S, Schwartz-Albiez R, Westendorp MO, Walczak H, Moldenhauer G, Grell M, Krammer PH (1995) Cell surface sialylation plays a role in modulating sensitivity towards APO-1-mediated apoptotic cell death. Cell Death Differ 2(3):163–171
230. Keppler OT, Peter ME, Hinderlich S, Moldenhauer G, Stehling P, Schmitz I, Schwartz-Albiez R, Reutter W, Pawlita M (1999) Differential sialylation of cell surface glycoconjugates in a human B lymphoma cell line regulates susceptibility for CD95 (APO-1/Fas)-mediated apoptosis and for infection by a lymphotropic virus. Glycobiology 9(6):557–569. cwc054 [pii]
231. Swindall AF, Bellis SL (2011) Sialylation of the Fas death receptor by ST6Gal-I provides protection against Fas-mediated apoptosis in colon carcinoma cells. J Biol Chem 286(26):22982–22990. doi:10.1074/jbc.M110.211375
232. Schultz MJ, Swindall AF, Bellis SL (2012) Regulation of the metastatic cell phenotype by sialylated glycans. Cancer Metastasis Rev 31(3–4):501–518. doi:10.1007/s10555-012-9359-7
233. Lee KH, Feig C, Tchikov V, Schickel R, Hallas C, Schutze S, Peter ME, Chan AC (2006) The role of receptor internalization in CD95 signaling. EMBO J 25(5):1009–1023
234. Schutze S, Tchikov V, Schneider-Brachert W (2008) Regulation of TNFR1 and CD95 signalling by receptor compartmentalization. Nat Rev Mol Cell Biol 9(8):655–662. doi:10.1038/nrm2430. nrm2430 [pii]
235. Schutze S, Schneider-Brachert W (2009) Impact of TNF-R1 and CD95 internalization on apoptotic and antiapoptotic signaling. Results Probl Cell Differ 49:63–85. doi:10.1007/400_2008_23
236. Tchikov V, Bertsch U, Fritsch J, Edelmann B, Schutze S (2011) Subcellular compartmentalization of TNF receptor-1 and CD95 signaling pathways. Eur J Cell Biol 90(6–7):467–475. doi:10.1016/j.ejcb.2010.11.002
237. Hanada M, Feng J, Hemmings BA (2004) Structure, regulation and function of PKB/AKT—a major therapeutic target. Biochim Biophys Acta 1697(1–2):3–16
238. Scheid MP, Marignani PA, Woodgett JR (2002) Multiple phosphoinositide 3-kinase-dependent steps in activation of protein kinase B. Mol Cell Biol 22(17):6247–6260
239. Scheid MP, Woodgett JR (2001) PKB/AKT: functional insights from genetic models. Nat Rev Mol Cell Biol 2(10):760–768
240. Scheid MP, Woodgett JR (2003) Unravelling the activation mechanisms of protein kinase B/Akt. FEBS Lett 546(1):108–112
241. Franke TF (2008) PI3K/Akt: getting it right matters. Oncogene 27(50):6473–6488
242. Duronio V (2008) The life of a cell: apoptosis regulation by the PI3K/PKB pathway. Biochem J 415(3):333–344
243. Zhuang L, Lin J, Lu ML, Solomon KR, Freeman MR (2002) Cholesterol-rich lipid rafts mediate akt-regulated survival in prostate cancer cells. Cancer Res 62(8):2227–2231
244. Hill MM, Feng J, Hemmings BA (2002) Identification of a plasma membrane Raft-associated PKB Ser473 kinase activity that is distinct from ILK and PDK1. Curr Biol 12(14):1251–1255
245. Adam RM, Mukhopadhyay NK, Kim J, Di Vizio D, Cinar B, Boucher K, Solomon KR, Freeman MR (2007) Cholesterol sensitivity of endogenous and myristoylated Akt. Cancer Res 67(13):6238–6246
246. Lasserre R, Guo XJ, Conchonaud F, Hamon Y, Hawchar O, Bernard AM, Soudja SM, Lenne PF, Rigneault H, Olive D, Bismuth G, Nunes JA, Payrastre B, Marguet D, He HT (2008) Raft nanodomains contribute to Akt/PKB plasma membrane recruitment and activation. Nat Chem Biol 4(9):538–547
247. Remijsen Q, Vanden Berghe T, Parthoens E, Asselbergh B, Vandenabeele P, Willems J (2009) Inhibition of spontaneous neutrophil apoptosis by parabutoporin acts independently of NADPH oxidase inhibition but by lipid raft-dependent stimulation of Akt. J Leukoc Biol 85(3):497–507
248. Calay D, Vind-Kezunovic D, Frankart A, Lambert S, Poumay Y, Gniadecki R (2010) Inhibition of Akt signaling by exclusion from lipid rafts in normal and transformed epidermal keratinocytes. J Invest Dermatol 130(4):1136–1145

249. Beneteau M, Pizon M, Chaigne-Delalande B, Daburon S, Moreau P, De Giorgi F, Ichas F, Rebillard A, Dimanche-Boitrel MT, Taupin JL, Moreau JF, Legembre P (2008) Localization of Fas/CD95 into the lipid rafts on down-modulation of the phosphatidylinositol 3-kinase signaling pathway. Mol Cancer Res 6(4):604–613
250. Reis-Sobreiro M, Roue G, Moros A, Gajate C, de la Iglesia-Vicente J, Colomer D, Mollinedo F (2013) Lipid raft-mediated Akt signaling as a therapeutic target in mantle cell lymphoma. Blood Cancer J 3:e118
251. Brazil DP, Hemmings BA (2001) Ten years of protein kinase B signalling: a hard Akt to follow. Trends Biochem Sci 26(11):657–664
252. Varadhachary AS, Edidin M, Hanlon AM, Peter ME, Krammer PH, Salgame P (2001) Phosphatidylinositol 3′-kinase blocks CD95 aggregation and caspase-8 cleavage at the death-inducing signaling complex by modulating lateral diffusion of CD95. J Immunol 166(11):6564–6569
253. Varadhachary AS, Peter ME, Perdow SN, Krammer PH, Salgame P (1999) Selective up-regulation of phosphatidylinositol 3′-kinase activity in Th2 cells inhibits caspase-8 cleavage at the death-inducing complex: a mechanism for Th2 resistance from Fas-mediated apoptosis. J Immunol 163(9):4772–4779
254. Chiarini F, Del Sole M, Mongiorgi S, Gaboardi GC, Cappellini A, Mantovani I, Follo MY, McCubrey JA, Martelli AM (2008) The novel Akt inhibitor, perifosine, induces caspase-dependent apoptosis and downregulates P-glycoprotein expression in multidrug-resistant human T-acute leukemia cells by a JNK-dependent mechanism. Leukemia 22(6):1106–1116
255. Moretti S, Procopio A, Lazzarini R, Rippo MR, Testa R, Marra M, Tamagnone L, Catalano A (2008) Semaphorin3A signaling controls Fas (CD95)-mediated apoptosis by promoting Fas translocation into lipid rafts. Blood 111(4):2290–2299
256. Dang P, Smythe E, Furley AJ (2012) TAG1 regulates the endocytic trafficking and signaling of the semaphorin3A receptor complex. J Neurosci 32(30):10370–10382. doi:10.1523/JNEUROSCI.5874-11.2012. 32/30/10370 [pii]
257. Cottin V, Doan JE, Riches DW (2002) Restricted localization of the TNF receptor CD120a to lipid rafts: a novel role for the death domain. J Immunol 168(8):4095–4102
258. Marconi M, Ascione B, Ciarlo L, Vona R, Garofalo T, Sorice M, Gianni AM, Locatelli SL, Carlo-Stella C, Malorni W, Matarrese P (2013) Constitutive localization of DR4 in lipid rafts is mandatory for TRAIL-induced apoptosis in B-cell hematologic malignancies. Cell Death Dis 4:e863. doi:10.1038/cddis.2013.389
259. Sorice M, Parolini I, Sansolini T, Garofalo T, Dolo V, Sargiacomo M, Tai T, Peschle C, Torrisi MR, Pavan A (1997) Evidence for the existence of ganglioside-enriched plasma membrane domains in human peripheral lymphocytes. J Lipid Res 38(5):969–980
260. Rajendran L, Simons K (2005) Lipid rafts and membrane dynamics. J Cell Sci 118(Pt 6):1099–1102. doi:10.1242/jcs.01681. 118/6/1099 [pii]
261. Fujita A, Cheng J, Hirakawa M, Furukawa K, Kusunoki S, Fujimoto T (2007) Gangliosides GM1 and GM3 in the living cell membrane form clusters susceptible to cholesterol depletion and chilling. Mol Biol Cell 18(6):2112–2122. doi:10.1091/mbc.E07-01-0071. E07-01-0071 [pii]
262. Janich P, Corbeil D (2007) GM1 and GM3 gangliosides highlight distinct lipid microdomains within the apical domain of epithelial cells. FEBS Lett 581(9):1783–1787. doi:10.1016/j.febslet.2007.03.065. S0014-5793(07)00341-9 [pii]
263. Lacour S, Hammann A, Grazide S, Lagadic-Gossmann D, Athias A, Sergent O, Laurent G, Gambert P, Solary E, Dimanche-Boitrel MT (2004) Cisplatin-induced CD95 redistribution into membrane lipid rafts of HT29 human colon cancer cells. Cancer Res 64(10):3593–3598
264. Rebillard A, Tekpli X, Meurette O, Sergent O, LeMoigne-Muller G, Vernhet L, Gorria M, Chevanne M, Christmann M, Kaina B, Counillon L, Gulbins E, Lagadic-Gossmann D, Dimanche-Boitrel MT (2007) Cisplatin-induced apoptosis involves membrane fluidification via inhibition of NHE1 in human colon cancer cells. Cancer Res 67 (16):7865-7874. doi:10.1158/0008-5472.CAN-07-0353. 67/16/7865 [pii]

265. Huang CR, Jin ZX, Dong L, Tong XP, Yue S, Kawanami T, Sawaki T, Sakai T, Miki M, Iwao H, Nakajima A, Masaki Y, Fukushima Y, Tanaka M, Fujita Y, Nakajima H, Okazaki T, Umehara H (2010) Cisplatin augments FAS-mediated apoptosis through lipid rafts. Anticancer Res 30(6):2065–2071. 30/6/2065 [pii]
266. Rebillard A, Jouan-Lanhouet S, Jouan E, Legembre P, Pizon M, Sergent O, Gilot D, Tekpli X, Lagadic-Gossmann D, Dimanche-Boitrel MT (2010) Cisplatin-induced apoptosis involves a Fas-ROCK-ezrin-dependent actin remodelling in human colon cancer cells. Eur J Cancer 46(8):1445–1455. doi:10.1016/j.ejca.2010.01.034. S0959-8049(10)00082-1 [pii]
267. Miyaji M, Jin ZX, Yamaoka S, Amakawa R, Fukuhara S, Sato SB, Kobayashi T, Domae N, Mimori T, Bloom ET, Okazaki T, Umehara H (2005) Role of membrane sphingomyelin and ceramide in platform formation for Fas-mediated apoptosis. J Exp Med 202(2):249–259
268. Micheau O, Solary E, Hammann A, Dimanche-Boitrel MT (1999) Fas ligand-independent, FADD-mediated activation of the Fas death pathway by anticancer drugs. J Biol Chem 274(12):7987–7992
269. Zhuang S, Kochevar IE (2003) Ultraviolet A radiation induces rapid apoptosis of human leukemia cells by Fas ligand-independent activation of the Fas death pathways. Photochem Photobiol 78(1):61–67
270. Mollinedo F, Fernandez-Luna JL, Gajate C, Martin-Martin B, Benito A, Martinez-Dalmau R, Modolell M (1997) Selective induction of apoptosis in cancer cells by the ether lipid ET-18-OCH_3 (Edelfosine): molecular structure requirements, cellular uptake, and protection by Bcl-2 and Bcl-X_L. Cancer Res 57(7):1320–1328
271. Watanabe S, Mukaida N, Ikeda N, Akiyama M, Harada A, Nakanishi I, Nariuchi H, Watanabe Y, Matsushima K (1995) Prevention of endotoxin shock by an antibody against leukocyte integrin beta 2 through inhibiting production and action of TNF. Int Immunol 7(7):1037–1046
272. Ogasawara J, Watanabe-Fukunaga R, Adachi M, Matsuzawa A, Kasugai T, Kitamura Y, Itoh N, Suda T, Nagata S (1993) Lethal effect of the anti-Fas antibody in mice. Nature 364(6440):806–809
273. Costelli P, Aoki P, Zingaro B, Carbo N, Reffo P, Lopez-Soriano FJ, Bonelli G, Argiles JM, Baccino FM (2003) Mice lacking TNFalpha receptors 1 and 2 are resistant to death and fulminant liver injury induced by agonistic anti-Fas antibody. Cell Death Differ 10(9):997–1004. doi:10.1038/sj.cdd.4401281. 4401281 [pii]
274. Gerspach J, Pfizenmaier K, Wajant H (2011) Therapeutic targeting of CD95 and the TRAIL death receptors. Recent Pat Anticancer Drug Discov 6(3):294–310. BSP/PRA/EPUB/00043 [pii]
275. Wajant H, Gerspach J, Pfizenmaier K (2013) Engineering death receptor ligands for cancer therapy. Cancer Lett 332(2):163–174. doi:10.1016/j.canlet.2010.12.019
276. Micheau O, Shirley S, Dufour F (2013) Death receptors as targets in cancer. Br J Pharmacol 169(8):1723–1744. doi:10.1111/bph.12238
277. Walczak H, Miller RE, Ariail K, Gliniak B, Griffith TS, Kubin M, Chin W, Jones J, Woodward A, Le T, Smith C, Smolak P, Goodwin RG, Rauch CT, Schuh JC, Lynch DH (1999) Tumoricidal activity of tumor necrosis factor-related apoptosis-inducing ligand in vivo. Nat Med 5(2):157–163
278. Ashkenazi A, Pai RC, Fong S, Leung S, Lawrence DA, Marsters SA, Blackie C, Chang L, McMurtrey AE, Hebert A, DeForge L, Koumenis IL, Lewis D, Harris L, Bussiere J, Koeppen H, Shahrokh Z, Schwall RH (1999) Safety and antitumor activity of recombinant soluble Apo2 ligand. J Clin Invest 104(2):155–162
279. Nesterov A, Nikrad M, Johnson T, Kraft AS (2004) Oncogenic Ras sensitizes normal human cells to tumor necrosis factor-alpha-related apoptosis-inducing ligand-induced apoptosis. Cancer Res 64(11):3922–3927
280. Merino D, Lalaoui N, Morizot A, Solary E, Micheau O (2007) TRAIL in cancer therapy: present and future challenges. Expert Opin Ther Targets 11(10):1299–1314. doi:10.1517/14728222.11.10.1299

281. Ashkenazi A, Holland P, Eckhardt SG (2008) Ligand-based targeting of apoptosis in cancer: the potential of recombinant human apoptosis ligand 2/Tumor necrosis factor-related apoptosis-inducing ligand (rhApo2L/TRAIL). J Clin Oncol 26(21):3621–3630. doi:10.1200/JCO.2007.15.7198. 26/21/3621 [pii]
282. Jo M, Kim TH, Seol DW, Esplen JE, Dorko K, Billiar TR, Strom SC (2000) Apoptosis induced in normal human hepatocytes by tumor necrosis factor-related apoptosis-inducing ligand. Nat Med 6(5):564–567
283. Mollinedo F, Gajate C, Morales AI, del Canto-Janez E, Justies N, Collia F, Rivas JV, Modolell M, Iglesias A (2009) Novel anti-inflammatory action of edelfosine lacking toxicity with protective effect in experimental colitis. J Pharmacol Exp Ther 329(2):439–449
284. Lim SC, Parajuli KR, Han SI (2016) The alkyllysophospholipid edelfosine enhances TRAIL-mediated apoptosis in gastric cancer cells through death receptor 5 and the mitochondrial pathway. Tumour Biol 37(5):6205–6216. doi:10.1007/s13277-015-4485-9. 10.1007/s13277-015-4485-9 [pii]
285. Rao-Bindal K, Zhou Z, Kleinerman ES (2012) MS-275 sensitizes osteosarcoma cells to Fas ligand-induced cell death by increasing the localization of Fas in membrane lipid rafts. Cell Death Dis 3:e369
286. Pizon M, Rampanarivo H, Tauzin S, Chaigne-Delalande B, Daburon S, Castroviejo M, Moreau P, Moreau JF, Legembre P (2011) Actin-independent exclusion of CD95 by PI3K/AKT signalling: implications for apoptosis. Eur J Immunol 41(8):2368–2378
287. DeMorrow S, Glaser S, Francis H, Venter J, Vaculin B, Vaculin S, Alpini G (2007) Opposing actions of endocannabinoids on cholangiocarcinoma growth: recruitment of Fas and Fas ligand to lipid rafts. J Biol Chem 282(17):13098–13113
288. Xu ZX, Ding T, Haridas V, Connolly F, Gutterman JU (2009) Avicin D, a plant triterpenoid, induces cell apoptosis by recruitment of Fas and downstream signaling molecules into lipid rafts. PLoS One 4(12):e8532
289. Yan S, Qu X, Xu L, Che X, Ma Y, Zhang L, Teng Y, Zou H, Liu Y (2014) Bufalin enhances TRAIL-induced apoptosis by redistributing death receptors in lipid rafts in breast cancer cells. Anticancer Drugs 25(6):683–689. doi:10.1097/CAD.0000000000000095
290. Barua S, Linton RS, Gamboa J, Banerjee I, Yarmush ML, Rege K (2010) Lytic peptide-mediated sensitization of TRAIL-resistant prostate cancer cells to death receptor agonists. Cancer Lett 293(2):240–253. doi:10.1016/j.canlet.2010.01.012
291. Vondalova Blanarova O, Jelinkova I, Szoor A, Skender B, Soucek K, Horvath V, Vaculova A, Andera L, Sova P, Szollosi J, Hofmanova J, Vereb G, Kozubik A (2011) Cisplatin and a potent platinum(IV) complex-mediated enhancement of TRAIL-induced cancer cells killing is associated with modulation of upstream events in the extrinsic apoptotic pathway. Carcinogenesis 32(1):42–51. doi:10.1093/carcin/bgq220. bgq220 [pii]
292. Chen YC, Kung FL, Tsai IL, Chou TH, Chen IS, Guh JH (2010) Cryptocaryone, a natural dihydrochalcone, induces apoptosis in human androgen independent prostate cancer cells by death receptor clustering in lipid raft and nonraft compartments. J Urol 183(6):2409–2418. doi:10.1016/j.juro.2010.01.065
293. Vanoosten RL, Moore JM, Ludwig AT, Griffith TS (2005) Depsipeptide (FR901228) enhances the cytotoxic activity of TRAIL by redistributing TRAIL receptor to membrane lipid rafts. Mol Ther 11(4):542–552. doi:10.1016/j.ymthe.2004.12.008. S1525-0016(04)01574-6 [pii]
294. Aroui S, Brahim S, Hamelin J, De Waard M, Breard J, Kenani A (2009) Conjugation of doxorubicin to cell penetrating peptides sensitizes human breast MDA-MB 231 cancer cells to endogenous TRAIL-induced apoptosis. Apoptosis 14(11):1352–1365. doi:10.1007/s10495-009-0397-8
295. Xu L, Qu X, Luo Y, Zhang Y, Liu J, Qu J, Zhang L, Liu Y (2011) Epirubicin enhances TRAIL-induced apoptosis in gastric cancer cells by promoting death receptor clustering in lipid rafts. Mol Med Rep 4(3):407–411. doi:10.3892/mmr.2011.439
296. Xu L, Qu X, Zhang Y, Hu X, Yang X, Hou K, Teng Y, Zhang J, Sada K, Liu Y (2009) Oxaliplatin enhances TRAIL-induced apoptosis in gastric cancer cells by CBL-regulated

death receptor redistribution in lipid rafts. FEBS Lett 583(5):943–948. doi:10.1016/j.febslet.2009.02.014. S0014-5793(09)00113-6 [pii]
297. Psahoulia FH, Drosopoulos KG, Doubravska L, Andera L, Pintzas A (2007) Quercetin enhances TRAIL-mediated apoptosis in colon cancer cells by inducing the accumulation of death receptors in lipid rafts. Mol Cancer Ther 6(9):2591–2599. doi:10.1158/1535-7163.MCT-07-0001. 6/9/2591 [pii]
298. Delmas D, Rebe C, Micheau O, Athias A, Gambert P, Grazide S, Laurent G, Latruffe N, Solary E (2004) Redistribution of CD95, DR4 and DR5 in rafts accounts for the synergistic toxicity of resveratrol and death receptor ligands in colon carcinoma cells. Oncogene 23(55):8979–8986
299. Delmas D, Rebe C, Lacour S, Filomenko R, Athias A, Gambert P, Cherkaoui-Malki M, Jannin B, Dubrez-Daloz L, Latruffe N, Solary E (2003) Resveratrol-induced apoptosis is associated with Fas redistribution in the rafts and the formation of a death-inducing signaling complex in colon cancer cells. J Biol Chem 278(42):41482–41490
300. Stel AJ, Ten Cate B, Jacobs S, Kok JW, Spierings DC, Dondorff M, Helfrich W, Kluin-Nelemans HC, de Leij LF, Withoff S, Kroesen BJ (2007) Fas receptor clustering and involvement of the death receptor pathway in rituximab-mediated apoptosis with concomitant sensitization of lymphoma B cells to fas-induced apoptosis. J Immunol 178(4):2287–2295
301. Yun SH, Park ES, Shin SW, Ju MH, Han JY, Jeong JS, Kim SH, Stonik VA, Kwak JY, Park JI (2015) By activating Fas/ceramide synthase 6/p38 kinase in lipid rafts, stichoposide D inhibits growth of leukemia xenografts. Oncotarget 6(29):27596–27612. doi:10.18632/oncotarget.4820. 4820 [pii]
302. Lin ML, Chen SS, Wu TS (2015) Synthetic bichalcone TSWU-BR23 induces apoptosis of human colon cancer HT-29 cells by p53-mediated mitochondrial oligomerization of BAX/BAK and lipid raft localization of CD95/FADD. Anticancer Res 35(10):5407–5416. 35/10/5407 [pii]
303. Elyassaki W, Wu S (2006) Lipid rafts mediate ultraviolet light-induced Fas aggregation in M624 melanoma cells. Photochem Photobiol 82(3):787–792
304. Lim SC, Duong HQ, Choi JE, Lee TB, Kang JH, SH O, Han SI (2011) Lipid raft-dependent death receptor 5 (DR5) expression and activation are critical for ursodeoxycholic acid-induced apoptosis in gastric cancer cells. Carcinogenesis 32(5):723–731. doi:10.1093/carcin/bgr038
305. Lim SC, Han SI (2015) Ursodeoxycholic acid effectively kills drug-resistant gastric cancer cells through induction of autophagic death. Oncol Rep 34(3):1261–1268. doi:10.3892/or.2015.4076

Chapter 10
Role of Sphingolipids in Death Receptor Signalling

Fatima Bilal, Michaël Pérès, Nathalie Andrieu-Abadie, Thierry Levade, Bassam Badran, Ahmad Daher, and Bruno Ségui

Abstract Sphingolipids (SLs) are sphingoid base-containing lipids, which are enriched in plasma membrane microdomains. Some SLs behave as bioactive molecules, modulating cell signalling in various pathophysiological contexts. Whereas ceramide triggers apoptosis and impairs cell migration, sphingosine-1-phosphate (S1P) induces the opposite effects. CD95/Fas, TRAIL-R1 (DR4), and TRAIL-R2 (DR5) are death receptors (DRs) and members of the TNF-R1 superfamily. DRs

F. Bilal
INSERM UMR 1037, CRCT, 31037 Toulouse, France

Equipe Labellisée Ligue Contre Le Cancer, 31037 Toulouse, France

Université Libanaise, Ecole Doctorale de Sciences et Technologies, Campus Universitaire de Rafic Hariri, Hadath, Lebanon

Université Toulouse III—Paul Sabatier, 118 route de Narbonne, 31062 Toulouse, France

M. Pérès • N. Andrieu-Abadie
INSERM UMR 1037, CRCT, 31037 Toulouse, France

Equipe Labellisée Ligue Contre Le Cancer, 31037 Toulouse, France

T. Levade
INSERM UMR 1037, CRCT, 31037 Toulouse, France

Equipe Labellisée Ligue Contre Le Cancer, 31037 Toulouse, France

Université Toulouse III—Paul Sabatier, 118 route de Narbonne, 31062 Toulouse, France

Laboratoire de Biochimie, Institut Fédératif de Biologie, CHU Purpan, 31059 Toulouse, France

B. Badran • A. Daher
Université Libanaise, Ecole Doctorale de Sciences et Technologies, Campus Universitaire de Rafic Hariri, Hadath, Lebanon

B. Ségui (✉)
INSERM UMR 1037, CRCT, 31037 Toulouse, France

Equipe Labellisée Ligue Contre Le Cancer, 31037 Toulouse, France

Université Toulouse III—Paul Sabatier, 118 route de Narbonne, 31062 Toulouse, France
e-mail: bruno.segui@inserm.fr

O. Micheau (ed.), *TRAIL, Fas Ligand, TNF and TLR3 in Cancer*, Resistance to Targeted Anti-Cancer Therapeutics, DOI 10.1007/978-3-319-56805-8_10

trigger apoptosis of various cell types, including cancer cells. Over the last two decades, a growing body of evidence indicates that SLs modulate DR signalling. DR stimulation triggers the generation of SLs, including ceramide, sphingosine, and gangliosides. Ceramide has been reported to facilitate DR clustering into lipid rafts upon pro-apoptotic DR agonists. Moreover, ceramide and its metabolites likely contribute to the mitochondrial route of apoptosis. More recently, SLs have been shown to modulate CD95-mediated cell migration of triple negative breast cancer cell lines and Th17 lymphoid cells in response to a nonapoptotic form of CD95L. Herein, we review the role of SLs in DR signalling, including apoptotic and migration pathways.

Keywords Death receptors • CD95 • Sphingolipids • Apoptosis • Migration

10.1 Sphingolipid Metabolism at a Glance

Sphingolipids (SLs) are one of the most complex and structurally diverse classes of lipids. They are defined by an aliphatic amino alcohol sphingoid backbone called sphingosine. Modification of this core results in the formation of a multitude of SLs that play important roles in membrane biology and signal transduction.

SL metabolism begins with the "de novo" biosynthesis pathway of ceramide. This reaction occurs on the cytosolic surface of the endoplasmic reticulum (ER) membrane, via the condensation of L-serine and palmitoyl coenzyme A (palmitoyl-CoA) into 3-ketodihydrosphingosine (3-KDS), catalyzed by the enzyme serine palmitoyltransferase (SPT) [1]. 3-KDS is subsequently reduced to form dihydrosphingosine (sphinganine), which is then N-acylated to generate dihydroceramide (dhCer) by the action of six mammalian dhCer synthases [also known as LASS or ceramide synthases (CerS)], *each* of which synthesizes dhCer with a specific chain length fatty acyl CoA. dhCer desaturase next desaturates dhCer to give ceramide, the central molecule in SL metabolism [2] (Fig. 10.1).

Following transport to the Golgi apparatus, ceramide can then serve as a precursor for the biosynthesis of sphingomyelin (SM) and glycosphingolipids (GSLs), by the addition of various polar head groups. SM synthases (SMS) 1 and 2 transfer a phosphocholine headgroup from phosphatidylcholine to ceramide, thereby generating SM and diacylglycerol (DAG) [3]. On the other hand glucosylceramide synthase (GCS) attaches glucose to ceramide, thus generating glucosylceramide (GlcCer). Ceramide can also be glycosylated by galactosylceramide synthase (GalCerS) to galactosylceramide (GalCer) at the ER. GlcCer and GalCer are the precursors of the hundreds of the most complex GSLs including gangliosides, which are with SM the major plasma membrane lipid raft components. There, SM can be hydrolyzed by acid sphingomyelinase (aSMase) (on the outer leaflet) and neutral sphingomyelinases (nSMase) (on the inner leaflet) to produce ceramide. SM

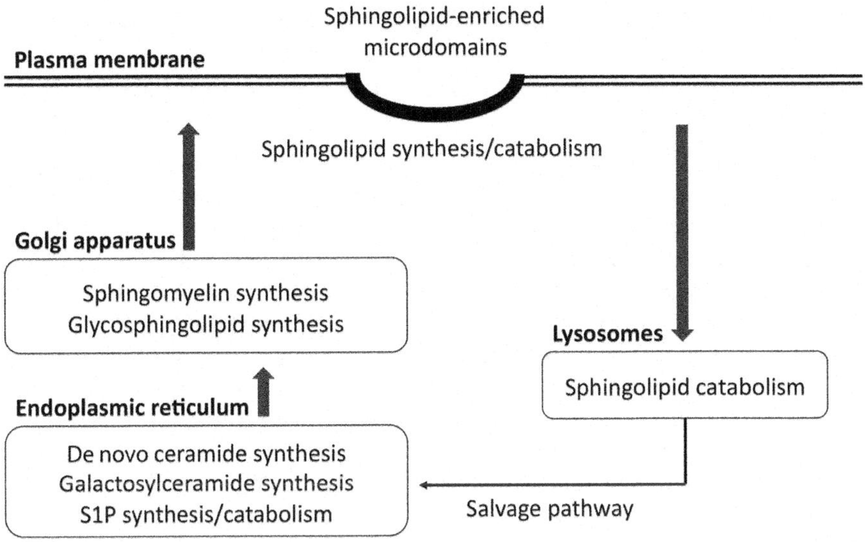

Fig. 10.1 Subcellular compartmentalization of sphingolipid metabolism. Whereas most of the sphingolipid synthesis occurs in the endoplasmic reticulum and Golgi apparatus, most of the sphingolipid catabolism takes place in the lysosomes. Sphingolipid metabolism also occurs at the plasma membrane

can be also catabolized to ceramide in the lysosomal compartment by aSMase. Another important source of ceramide is provided by the hydrolysis of GSLs by specific β-glucosidases and galactosidases [4] (Fig. 10.1).

By the action of ceramide kinase, ceramide can be phosphorylated to form ceramide-1-phosphate (C1P), which in turn can be recycled by a C1P phosphatase [5]. Ceramide can be also deacylated by ceramidases to sphingosine, which in turn can be phosphorylated to sphingosine-1-phosphate (S1P) by sphingosine kinases 1 and 2 [6]. Ceramidases are also distinguished according to their optimum pH and subcellular localization. Neutral ceramidase is located at the plasma membrane, acid ceramidase is lysosomal, and the alkaline ceramidase is located at the ER and Golgi apparatus. Ceramidase has been shown to be also present in the mitochondria [7].

Various alterations of SL catabolism due to gene mutations lead to lysosomal storage diseases. For instance, aSMase deficiency is responsible for type A and B Niemann-Pick diseases (NPD), the type A being the most severe form associated with the strongest loss of aSMase enzyme activity and lysosomal accumulation of SM [8]. Moreover, human genetic disorders of SL biosynthesis have been recently described in patients [9].

10.2 Role of Sphingolipids in CD95-Mediated Cell Apoptosis

10.2.1 Ceramide-Mediated CD95 Clustering in Lipid Rafts

The cell membrane of eukaryotic cells consists of a lipid bilayer containing predominantly SLs, cholesterol and glycerophospholipids with embedded proteins. Hydrophilic interactions between the polar head groups of SLs on one hand, and interactions between SLs and cholesterol on the other hand, result in the separation of cholesterol and SLs from the other lipids within the bilayer of the cell membrane and the formation of distinct microdomains named lipid rafts [10]. These small domains can float freely within the cellular membrane bilayer or assemble together to form large ordered platforms that play a central role in many cellular processes, including CD95-mediated apoptosis [11]. An important early event at the plasma membrane following the initiation of CD95-mediated apoptosis involves the clustering of CD95 in these lipid rafts for efficient and rapid transmembrane signalling [12] (Fig. 10.2). One should note, however, that CD95 constitutively resides or not in lipid rafts depending on the cell type. Indeed, CD95 was located in lipid rafts in type I cells but not in type II cells [13]. Whereas disruption of lipid rafts impaired CD95-induced apoptosis in type I cells [13], forced distribution of CD95 in rafts

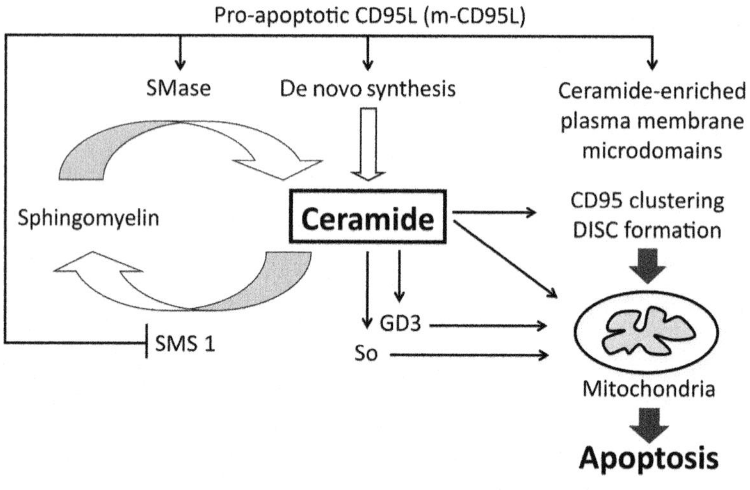

Fig. 10.2 Sphingolipids in CD95L-induced apoptosis. Binding of Membrane-bound CD95L (m-CD95L) to its cognate receptor CD95 leads to the activation of sphingomyelinase (SMase). SMase catalyzes the hydrolysis of membrane sphingomyelin to ceramide, thus forming ceramide-enriched plasma membrane platforms that facilitate CD95 clustering in lipid rafts and DISC formation. m-CD95L/CD95 interaction rises also the intracellular ceramide level through different pathways. Whereas it enhances ceramide synthesis by the de novo pathway, it inhibits the metabolism of ceramide to sphingomyelin by inactivating sphingomyelin synthase 1 (SMS 1). Ceramide, sphingosine (So), and ganglioside 3 (GD3) activate the mitochondrial pathway leading to apoptosis

enhances type II cell death [14], arguing that CD95 location in lipid rafts is important for potent apoptosis signalling initiation.

CD95 engagement triggers a rapid translocation of the aSMase from intracellular stores to the plasma membrane outer surface. ASMase is one of the enzymes expressed by the mammalian cells that are responsible for catalyzing the hydrolysis of SM to phosphocholine and ceramide. The SMases are characterized by their optimal pH: acid, neutral, or alkaline [15]. Of these enzymes, the aSMase is rapidly activated, within a few seconds to minutes, upon stimulation via CD95 [12]. ASMase showed strong activity with an optimum pH of 5.0, however, it can be active even at a neutral or slightly acidic pH. Indeed, an increase of the pH lowers the enzyme's affinity for its substrate, while the activity of the enzyme remains unaffected. Since SM is essentially, but not exclusively, located in the anti-cytosolic leaflet of biological membranes, translocated aSMase, which localizes to SL-rich rafts, catalyzes the breakdown of SM to ceramide at the cell surface. Extracellularly orientated ceramides self-associate with each other and, therefore, induce the transformation of small existing rafts into large active signalling platforms called ceramide-enriched membrane domains that mediate selective clustering of CD95 and transmit the apoptotic stimulus from outside into the cell [12].

The formation of ceramide-enriched membrane platforms has been demonstrated in vitro by the treatment of SM-containing liposomes with immobilized SMase onto micro-beads [16] and *in cellulo* by the use of confocal microscopy employing anti-ceramide antibodies [17]. One should note, however, that the specificity of the anti-ceramide antibodies has not been firmly established, and the possibility that antibodies cross-react with complex SLs cannot be ruled out. The significance of these membrane platforms for CD95 signalling was indicated by the finding that the disruption of rafts using *methyl-β-cyclodextrin*, a compound that extracts cholesterol from the cell membrane, the neutralization of surface ceramides by treatment with anti-ceramide antibody or aSMase deficiency, prevented CD95 clustering and apoptosis. Moreover, providing cells with natural exogenous ceramide rescued aSMase-deficient cells and restored CD95 clustering and apoptosis [12]. Another interesting observation further argues that SLs in rafts play a critical role in CD95 pro-apoptotic signalling pathway activation. Indeed, SMS deficiency in murine leukemia cells, which altered plasma membrane composition and properties through SM depletion, impaired CD95 location into lipid rafts and conferred partial resistance to CD95-mediated apoptosis [18]. It is tempting to speculate that SM depletion impairs apoptosis because of the lack of substrate for aSMase-dependent ceramide generation in response to CD95 engagement.

The molecular mechanisms leading to aSMase activation and translocation to the cell surface upon CD95 stimulation have been investigated. FADD and caspase-8 are both required for CD95-induced aSMase activation [19] and overexpression of FADD (Fas-associated protein with death domain) or caspase-8 triggers ceramide production [20]. Upon CD95/CD95L interaction, the adaptor protein FADD is recruited to the CD95 death domain. Next, FADD activates a limited pool of caspase-8, which would be sufficient for the activation of aSMase and the mobilization of intracellular aSMase-containing vesicles to fuse with the cell membrane, resulting in the secretion or the exposure of the enzyme on the extracellular leaflet [21]. It was demonstrated that aSMase inactive mutants still translocate to the cell surface, indicating that aSMase cell surface exposure is independent on the enzyme activation [22]. This translocation is mediated by an exocytosis phenomenon implicating the t-SNARE protein Syntaxin 4 and requires an intact cytoskeleton [23, 24]. Following SM breakdown to ceramide, CD95 clustering, which results in a very high receptor density in the cell membrane, may stabilize the death-inducing signalling complex (DISC), leading to potent FADD-dependent caspase-8 activation and amplifying CD95-mediated cell death signalling [25].

Several studies have documented the significance of aSMase as a general requisite for the induction of CD95-mediated apoptosis. ASMase knockout mice were partially, yet significantly, resistant to fulminant hepatitis induced by the injection of anti-CD95, as compared to their wild-type counterparts [26]. Exogenous natural ceramide overcame resistance of aSMase-deficient hepatocytes towards CD95 agonist [27]. Furthermore, genetic studies employing lymphoblastoid cell lines (LCL) from NPD patients, which suffer from an in-born defect of aSMase, showed LCL resistance to apoptosis induced by an anti-CD95 agonist, while aSMase-positive control cells rapidly underwent programmed cell death. CD95-induced apoptosis was restored in aSMase-deficient cells by the addition of exogenous ceramide or aSMase [28]. However, others and we have questioned the role of aSMase in CD95-mediated cell death. Indeed, thymocytes, activated T and B cells derived from both aSMase-deficient and wild-type mice were equally sensitive to anti-CD95 or CD95L [26]. Moreover, LCL as well as SV40-transformed human fibroblasts deficient for aSMase died upon CD95 stimulation. Caspase-3 activation as well as ceramide production occurred to a similar extent in aSMase-deficient and -proficient cells in response to CD95 engagement [29, 30]. Thus, aSMase is not essential for the induction of CD95-induced apoptosis and ceramide increase. In this context, ceramide can be generated by different pathways including ceramide de novo synthesis [31], activation of nSMase [30], and inhibition of SM synthesis [32, 33].

10.2.2 Relationship Between Ceramide and Caspases in CD95-Induced Apoptosis

The molecular connection between ceramide and caspases in CD95 signalling has been essentially documented in type II Jurkat leukemia T cells, in which CD95 stimulation triggers ceramide accumulation concomitantly to apoptosis induction [33–36]. Ceramide increase was prevented by the broad-spectrum caspase inhibitor zVAD-fmk [34, 36], arguing that CD95-mediated ceramide accumulation occurs in a caspase-dependent manner. One should note, however, that the effector caspase inhibitor DEVD-CHO, which completely prevented CD95-mediated apoptosis, failed to block ceramide increase. Thus, whereas CD95-induced ceramide increase is caspase-dependent, it occurs upstream of effector caspase activation and is unlikely a mere consequence of apoptosis induction [37]. Rather, ceramide may be instrumental in

CD95 pro-apoptotic signalling pathway since exogenous short-chain ceramides potently activate caspase-3 and trigger apoptosis in Jurkat T cells [36–38].

The role of initiator caspases in ceramide generation upon CD95 stimulation has been investigated by diverse groups. Caspase-8 deficiency abolished anti-CD95-induced ceramide increase [35]. Moreover, caspase-8 and caspase-10 doubly deficiency totally abolished ceramide production in response to CD95L [38], further arguing that apical caspases are required for ceramide generation in CD95 signalling. In contrast, neither the caspase-9 inhibitor zLEHD-fmk [34] nor caspase-9 deficiency [38] impaired CD95-induced ceramide production. Accordingly, Bcl-xL overexpression, which impairs cytochrome c release from the mitochondria, did not impair CD95-induced ceramide production [36]. Thus, CD95-induced ceramide increase likely occurs in between the activation of apical caspases-8/-10 and mitochondrial events leading to cytochrome c release, which is required for caspase-9 activation.

10.2.3 Sphingolipids in CD95-Induced Intrinsic Pathway Activation

A growing body of evidence in the literature indicates that ceramide is instrumental in the activation of the intrinsic pathway, which involves cytochrome c release from the mitochondria and subsequent caspase-9 activation (Fig. 10.2). Cuvillier and coworkers have documented that treatment of Jurkat cells with exogenous ceramide and sphingosine led to cytochrome c release from the mitochondria and caspase-9 activation [36]. More recently, we have shown that exogenous ceramide-induced apoptosis of Jurkat cells occurred in a caspase-9-dependent manner [38]. Indeed, caspase-9-deficient Jurkat cells, which potently resisted CD95-mediated apoptosis [39], were also resistant towards C2- and C16-ceramides. Our data are in good agreement with the resistance of neuronal cells towards C2-ceramide conferred by caspase-9 pharmacological inhibition or overexpression of a dominant negative form of caspase-9 [40]. Of note, caspase-9 inhibition did not compromise exogenous ceramide-induced apoptosis in K562 leukemia cells [41], indicating that the role of caspase-9 might be dependent on the cell type or the experimental conditions. As a matter of fact, we observed that caspase-9 deficiency failed to confer resistance of Jurkat cells upon incubation with a high C2-ceramide concentration (i.e., 20 μM), which triggered necrosis rather than apoptosis [38]. We have also illustrated the role of endogenous ceramide in CD95L-induced caspase-9 activation in Jurkat cells. Indeed, SMS1 knockdown not only facilitated ceramide accumulation due to the reduced conversion of ceramide to SM but also enhanced cytochrome c release from the mitochondria and caspase-9 activation upon CD95L [38]. Moreover, the tricyclodecan-9-yl-xanthogenate D609, which inhibited SM synthesis and, albeit to a lesser extent, GlcCer synthesis in Jurkat T cells and in PHA-activated human T cells, increased endogenous ceramide levels and significantly enhanced caspase activation and apoptosis in response to CD95L. Interestingly, D609 not only overcame zVAD-fmk-conferred resistance to CD95L but also bypassed RIP deficiency. Mitochondrial events were likely involved, since Bcl-xL overexpression abolished D609 effects. Thus, the inhibition of ceramide conversion to SM enhanced CD95L-induced both caspase-dependent and -independent cell death in T cells [42].

The molecular mechanisms by which ceramide enhances CD95-induced mitochondrial pathway activation are not yet completely elucidated. Exogenous ceramides triggered mitochondrial outer-membrane permeabilization (MOMP) on purified mitochondria, most likely via ceramide channel formation. Moreover, SLs likely cooperated with canonical pathways, which involve pro-apoptotic Bcl-2 family members (Bid, Bax, Bad). Indeed, the cleavage of Bid by apical caspases-8 and -10 in response to CD95L [43] triggers cytochrome c release from the mitochondria in a Bax/Bak-dependent manner. Exogenous ceramides synergistically cooperated with Bax to induce the MOMP on purified mitochondria [44]. Moreover, the ceramide catabolites, S1P and hexadecenal, a product of S1P degradation by sphingosine-1-phosphate lyase, cooperated with Bak and Bax, respectively, to enhance tBid-induced MOMP on purified mitochondria [45]. Moreover, ceramide, which inhibits the PI3K/Akt pathway, likely facilitates the activation of Bad, another pro-apoptotic member of the Bcl-2 family involved in MOMP [46]. Finally, another interesting hypothesis is to consider that ceramide triggers an alternative splicing of the mRNA encoding caspase-9 and Bcl-xL, leading to pro-apoptotic caspase-9 and Bcl-x(s) expression [47].

Testi and coworkers have provided evidence that CD95 engagement led to GD3 ganglioside production, which disrupted mitochondrial transmembrane potential in hematopoietic cells. Pharmacological and epigenetic approaches inhibiting GD3 synthesis, impaired CD95-induced apoptosis [48]. The mechanism of GD3 production upon CD95 engagement remains a matter of debate. Whereas aSMase has been initially described as required for GD3 production in CD95 signalling [28], others did not confirm aSMase involvement [49]. Alternatively, GD3 production is due to an enhanced GD3 synthase gene expression as a consequence of NF-κB activation following CD95 engagement [50]. An intriguing point to consider is how a raft component (i.e., GD3) migrates to mitochondria upon CD95 stimulation. Interaction between GD3 and microtubules via CLIPR-59, a CLIP-170-related protein, has been shown to facilitate the redistribution of GD3 from rafts to mitochondria [51, 52]. GD3 is unlikely the only ganglioside produced in CD95 signalling. Moreover, the role of gangliosides in CD95-induced cell death has been challenged by the observation that inhibiting glucosylceramide synthase, which critically contributes to ganglioside production, did not abrogate the apoptotic process [49].

10.3 Role of Sphingolipids in cl-CD95L-Mediated Cell Motility

Even though to date CD95/CD95L is one of the best characterized apoptosis-inducing receptor–ligand system, it can also trigger, in different pathophysiological contexts, nonapoptotic signalling [53]. Such signalling ranges from inflammation to carcinogenesis and even increased cell motility, which, in case of breast cancer, enables cancer cells to migrate and form metastatic tumors. In this context, it was shown that the level of the soluble form of CD95L is higher in the blood of patients with triple negative breast cancer (TNBC) than that of patients affected with other breast cancer subtypes, and was associated with increased risk of developing distant metastases [54].

CD95L is a transmembrane member of the TNFα superfamily whose extracellular domain can be cleaved by metalloproteases or cathepsins, to produce a soluble ligand released into the connective tissue and the bloodstream [55]. This soluble form was initially described as an inert ligand competing with its membrane-bound and pro-apoptotic counterpart (m-CD95L) for binding to CD95, thus acting as an antagonist of the death signal [56, 57]. More recent studies have shown that, unlike m-CD95L, the metalloprotease-cleaved CD95L (cl-CD95L) fails to trigger apoptosis, but instead may exert nonapoptotic functions by promoting the survival and motility of cancer cells, and can also aggravate inflammation in chronic inflammatory disorders [54, 58].

From a molecular standpoint, binding of m-CD95L to CD95 leads to receptor clustering, which is crucial to promote the formation of DISC [59]. In contrast, cl-CD95L fails to induce DISC formation and instead promotes the formation of an atypical pro-migratory CD95-containing complex called motility-inducing signalling complex (MISC), which is devoid of both FADD and caspase-8/-10 but contains the src kinase c-yes [60]. TNBC cells exposed to metalloprotease-cleaved CD95L showed enhanced cell migration demonstrated by using the Boyden chamber assay. In these cells, MISC formation induces Nox3 (nicotinamide adenine dinucleotide phosphate oxidase 3)-driven reactive oxygen species (ROS) generation. ROS activate Src kinase c-yes, which in turn implement Orai1-mediated increase of intracellular calcium levels and recruits and activates EGF receptor (EGFR) in an EGF-independent manner, leading to PI3K signalling [61]. Moreover, in a very recent study it was shown that cl-CD95L activates NHE1, the Na^+/H^+ plasma membrane transporter whose main function is to regulate intracellular pH and cell volume, which thereby enhances cell spreading and migration [62].

Together with Legembre et al. and Micheau et al., we have shown, using electron paramagnetic resonance, that cl-CD95L treatment induced plasma membrane fluidity increase in TNBC cells and this phenomenon is impaired by C16-ceramide [63]. Our findings raise the possibility of an instrumental role played by some SLs in CD95-mediated pro-migratory signalling pathway owing to their role as essential plasma membrane components and/or bioactive molecules (Fig. 10.3).

At the plasma membrane, in contrary to SM and GSLs, ceramide is not the major component. It can be generated via hydrolysis of SM by SMases or via ceramide synthase (CerS)-mediated de novo ceramide biosynthesis. The latter pathway involves acylation of sphinganine with fatty acyl-CoAs of chain lengths ranging from C14 to C26 to produce dihydroceramide. Alternatively, CerS can synthesize ceramide by the salvage pathway through direct acylation of sphingosine, which is derived from sphingolipid catabolism [64]. Ceramide synthesis is orchestrated by six mammalian CerS proteins, each of which produces ceramides with restricted

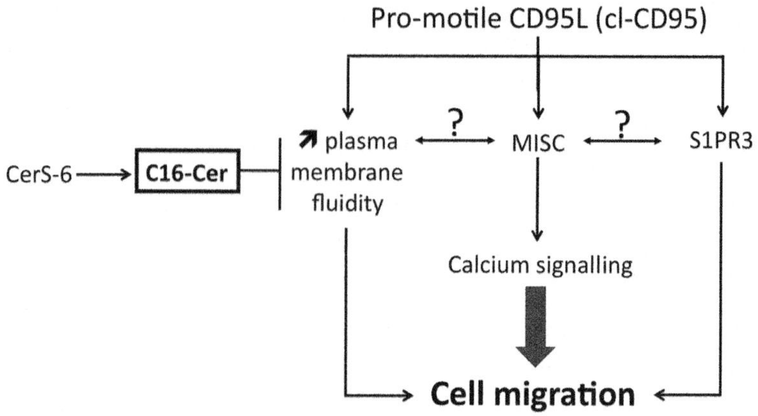

Fig. 10.3 Modulation of CD95L-induced cell motility by sphingolipids. Binding of cleaved CD95L (cl-CD95L) to CD95 promotes MISC (motility inducing signalling complex) formation, plasma membrane fluidity increase and calcium signalling, which triggers cell migration. Whereas sphingosine-1-phosphate receptor 3 (S1PR3) signalling is involved in cell migration triggered by cl-CD95L, the interconnection between plasma membrane fluidity increase, S1PR3 signalling and MISC remains to be evaluated. Cl-CD95L-triggered cell motility is blocked by C16:0 Ceramide (C16-Cer), which is produced by ceramide synthase 6 (CerS6) and increases plasma membrane rigidity

acyl chain lengths [65]. Accumulation of ceramides, with *N*-acyl chain longer than C12, rigidifies the plasma membrane [66]. Accordingly, incubation of TNBC with exogenous C16-ceramide increases plasma membrane rigidity [63]. Furthermore, an increased membrane fluidity was observed in CerS2-null mice which was directly associated with changes in SL composition [67].

The epithelial–mesenchymal transition (EMT) allows epithelial cells to acquire features of mesenchymal cells, increasing cell motility and invasiveness properties. EMT is associated with changes in SL metabolism, and SL metabolites, such as gangliosides, modulate EMT [68]. In this context, an integrative analysis of gene expression in National Cancer Institute (NCI) tumor cell lines revealed that the expression of CerS6 decreased during EMT. As a matter of fact, CerS6 expression was lower in cancer cell lines, which exhibit a mesenchymal gene signature such as TNBC cell lines, than in cancer cells having an epithelial gene signature. In epithelial cells, TGFβ-induced EMT was associated with a significant reduction of CerS6 transcript levels [63]. We next established that downregulation of CerS6 expression during EMT is instrumental in increasing plasma membrane fluidity and cell motility in response to cl-CD95L. Indeed, pharmacological and epigenetic approaches aiming at inhibiting CerS6 expression/activity in breast cancer cells with epithelial gene signature not only reduced the level of C16-ceramide but also increased plasma membrane fluidity and cell motility in response to cl-CD95L. Conversely, overexpression of CerS6 in TNBC cell lines, which exhibit mesenchymal-like gene signature, increased C16-ceramide levels, rigidified plasma membrane, and impaired cl-CD95L-induced cell motility [63]. Thus, we identified *CERS6* as a novel EMT-regulated gene, which impairs cell migration in response to cl-CD95L.

More recently, Legembre and coworkers have demonstrated the involvement of the S1P receptor 3 (S1PR3) in cl-CD95L-induced T-cell helper 17 (Th17) endothelial transmigration [69] (Fig. 10.3). In this study, cl-CD95L likely facilitated the secretion of S1P, which stimulated S1PR3, thereby increasing migration properties of Th17 cells and contributing to autoimmune disorders in a CD95-driven lupus mouse model. Future studies are needed to decipher the molecular mechanisms by which cl-CD95L triggers S1P production. Considering that EGFR, which is part of the MISC complex, is known to activate both sphingosine kinase 1 and 2 [70], it is tempting to speculate that cl-CD95L-induced S1P production occurs in an EGFR-dependent manner. Moreover, it would be of interest to determine whether the S1P pathway is involved in the motility of cancer cells in response to cl-CD95L. The latter tenet gets further credence considering that sphingosine kinases 1 and 2 are both involved in breast cancer cell motility [70, 71].

10.4 Role of Sphingolipids in TRAIL Signalling

Tumor-necrosis-factor related apoptosis-inducing ligand (TRAIL) belongs to the tumor necrosis factor (TNF) superfamily. Also known as Apo2L, TRAIL plays an important role in multiple cellular processes including proliferation, differentiation, and apoptosis. A growing body of evidence in the literature indicates that TRAIL has a remarkable property: it is able to trigger apoptosis in a broad range of cancer cell types, while having no or little cytotoxicity to most of the normal cells and tissues [72]. Clinical trials indicate that TRAIL may serve as a potent anti-cancer molecule [72]. However, different molecular events impair TRAIL-induced apoptosis in cancer cells [73–75], thereby limiting the use of TRAIL or TRAIL analogs in oncology.

TRAIL is a type II transmembrane protein, which is expressed at the cell surface of different leukocyte populations, including T lymphocytes and natural killers [76, 77]. TRAIL can be secreted as a consequence of a proteolytic cleavage, leading to the generation of a soluble form [77]. Five TRAIL receptors have been identified so far [78]. Three receptors are type I transmembrane proteins, two of them being agonistic receptors [TRAIL-R1 (DR4) and TRAIL-R2 (DR5)] with a functional intracellular death domain, similar in structure to that of CD95. The third one, TRAIL-R4 (dcR2), contains a truncated and nonfunctional death domain, which is unable to trigger apoptotic signalling, and thus behaves as a decoy receptor [79, 80]. Another decoy receptor, TRAIL-R3 (dcR1), is associated to the plasma membrane via a glycosyl phosphatidyl inositol (GPI) anchor. Finally, osteoprotegerin is a soluble TRAIL receptor known to neutralize TRAIL.

TRAIL triggers apoptosis through interacting with its receptors on the cell surface of target cells. Once bound to agonistic receptors (DR4 and DR5), TRAIL induces receptor oligomerization followed by the formation of the DISC, leading to intrinsic and extrinsic apoptotic signalling pathway activation [81].

SLs are also putative biologically active molecules in TRAIL signalling [8, 82, 83]. Cellular levels of ceramide and its metabolites are highly regulated by several SL-metabolizing enzymes (see Sect. 10.1) that may participate in regulating apoptotic responses to TRAIL [79]. For instance, aSMase, as for CD95L signalling pathway (see Sect. 10.2.1), plays a key role in TRAIL-induced apoptosis, through its ability to hydrolyze SM into ceramide. Upon TRAIL, aSMase translocates onto the cell surface via lysosome trafficking and fusion, enabling ceramide-enriched membrane platforms that contain DR4 and DR5 clusters. This process was impaired in aSMase-deficient splenocytes and coronary arterial endothelial cells (CAECs) isolated from aSMase knockout mice [79, 80].

Taking into account the various alterations of SL metabolism in cancer cells [84], it is tempting to speculate that some SL changes contribute to resistance of cancer cells to TRAIL-induced apoptosis. For instance, acid ceramidase, which is frequently overexpressed in cancer, catabolizes ceramide and prevents TRAIL-induced cytotoxicity in the murine fibrosarcoma L929 cell line [85]. One should note that TRAIL-induced L929 cell death is associated with necrosis features rather than apoptosis, indicating that ceramide is likely involved in TRAIL-induced necroptosis in this cell type. Furthermore, CerS6 is weakly expressed in SW620 colon cancer cells, which are resistant to TRAIL, and expressed at high levels in SW480 colon cancer cells, which are sensitive to TRAIL [86]. Whereas downregulation of CerS6 by siRNA in SW480 conferred resistance to TRAIL-induced apoptosis, the overexpression of this enzyme in SW620 had the opposite effect [86]. More recently, subtoxic doses of docosahexaenoic acid (DHA), a fish oil fatty acid, which enhanced C16-ceramide intracellular contents, sensitized SW620 metastatic colon cancer cells to TRAIL. This effect was reduced by fumonisin B1, which prevented de novo ceramide synthesis [87]. One should note however that CerS6 knock-down or overexpression in breast cancer cell lines failed to modulate DR-mediated cell death [63], indicating that CerS6 function in DR apoptotic signalling cannot be generalized to all cancer subtypes.

Other studies argue that targeting sphingolipid metabolism sensitizes cancer cells to TRAIL. For instance, incubation of cells with exogenous ceramides enhanced TRAIL-induced apoptosis in different cell lines and restored sensitivity of resistant cancer cells to TRAIL [79, 88]. More recently, sphingosine kinase 2 was reported to be overexpressed in TRAIL resistant non-small cell lung cancer cell lines (NSCLC). Targeting sphingosine kinase 2 with the selective inhibitor ABC294640 or by siRNA strategy is associated with a significant sensitization of NSCLC cancer cell lines to TRAIL. This phenomenon is associated with an increase of DR4 and/or DR5 expression at the cell surface via unknown mechanisms [89]. Similar findings have been reported upon treatment of cancer cells with FTY720, a sphingosine analog used in the clinic to treat multiple sclerosis. FTY720 potently synergizes with TRAIL to trigger apoptosis in various cancer cell lines (renal, breast, and colon carcinoma) [90]. Mechanistically, FTY720 downregulates the anti-apoptotic Bcl-2 family member Mcl-1 and upregulates DR5. Moreover, renal carcinoma tumor growth in nude mice is abolished with FTY720 and TRAIL association [90]. Whereas the combination of FTY720 with TRAIL in cancer patients seems to be a promising therapeutic strategy, FTY720 is a potent immunosuppressor, which prevents lymphocyte egress from thymus and lymph nodes. Thus, FTY720-based therapy should be adapted with caution to avoid tumor progression due to immunosuppression.

10.5 Concluding Remarks

The role of SLs in CD95L- and TRAIL-mediated apoptosis has been intensively investigated during the last two decades. CD95L and TRAIL trigger the activation of different metabolic pathways, including SMase activation, ceramide de novo synthesis increase, and SMS inhibition. Early ceramide production likely facilitates DR redistribution in lipid rafts and DISC formation. A growing body of evidence indicates that ceramide and possibly its metabolites contribute to the DR-mediated intrinsic signalling pathway. More recently, SLs have emerged as being involved in the modulation of CD95-induced cell migration. Deciphering the molecular mechanisms by which SLs modulate DR-driven cell motility and cell death may help better clarifying the role of SLs in cancer and autoimmune diseases. Interfering with SL metabolism may represent an interesting therapeutic strategy to limit cell motility and stimulate apoptosis triggered by DR.

Acknowledgements This work was supported by Ligue nationale contre le cancer, Institut National du Cancer (INCa), INSERM and Paul Sabatier University (Toulouse III). FB is a recipient of a grant from Association de Spécialisation et d'Orientation Scientifique.

References

1. Hanada K (2003) Serine palmitoyltransferase, a key enzyme of sphingolipid metabolism. Biochim Biophys Acta 1632:16–30
2. Levy M, Futerman AH (2010) Mammalian ceramide synthases. IUBMB Life 62:347–356. doi:10.1002/iub.319
3. Tafesse FG, Ternes P, Holthuis JCM (2006) The multigenic sphingomyelin synthase family. J Biol Chem 281:29421–29425. doi:10.1074/jbc.R600021200
4. Lahiri S, Futerman AH (2007) The metabolism and function of sphingolipids and glycosphingolipids. Cell Mol Life Sci CMLS 64:2270–2284. doi:10.1007/s00018-007-7076-0
5. Van Overloop H, Gijsbers S, Van Veldhoven PP (2006) Further characterization of mammalian ceramide kinase: substrate delivery and (stereo)specificity, tissue distribution, and subcellular localization studies. J Lipid Res 47:268–283. doi:10.1194/JLR.M500321-JLR200
6. Hait NC, Oskeritzian CA, Paugh SW et al (2006) Sphingosine kinases, sphingosine 1-phosphate, apoptosis and diseases. Biochim Biophys Acta 1758:2016–2026. doi:10.1016/j.Bbamem.2006.08.007
7. Mao C, Obeid LM (2008) Ceramidases: regulators of cellular responses mediated by ceramide, sphingosine, and sphingosine-1-phosphate. Biochim Biophys Acta 1781:424–434. doi:10.1016/j.Bbalip.2008.06.002
8. Sabourdy F, Kedjouar B, Sorli SC et al (2008) Functions of sphingolipid metabolism in mammals—lessons from genetic defects. Biochim Biophys Acta 1781:145–183. doi:10.1016/j.Bbalip.2008.01.004
9. Astudillo L, Sabourdy F, Therville N et al (2015) Human genetic disorders of sphingolipid biosynthesis. J Inherit Metab Dis 38:65–76. doi:10.1007/s10545-014-9736-1

10. Simons K, Ikonen E (1997) Functional rafts in cell membranes. Nature 387:569–572. doi:10.1038/42408
11. Simons K, Ehehalt R (2002) Cholesterol, lipid rafts, and disease. J Clin Invest 110:597–603. doi:10.1172/JCI16390
12. Grassme H, Jekle A, Riehle A et al (2001) CD95 signaling via ceramide-rich membrane rafts. J Biol Chem 276:20589–20596. doi:10.1074/jbc.M101207200
13. Muppidi JR, Siegel RM (2004) Ligand-independent redistribution of Fas (CD95) into lipid rafts mediates clonotypic T cell death. Nat Immunol 5:182–189. doi:10.1038/ni1024
14. Legembre P, Daburon S, Moreau P et al (2005) Amplification of Fas-mediated apoptosis in type II cells via microdomain recruitment. Mol Cell Biol 25:6811–6820. doi:10.1128/MCB.25.15.6811-6820.2005
15. Gault CR, Obeid LM, Hannun YA (2010) An overview of sphingolipid metabolism: from synthesis to breakdown. Adv Exp Med Biol 688:1–23
16. Nurminen TA, Holopainen JM, Zhao H, Kinnunen PKJ (2002) Observation of topical catalysis by sphingomyelinase coupled to microspheres. J Am Chem Soc 124:12129–12134
17. Grassmé H, Schwarz H, Gulbins E (2001) Molecular mechanisms of ceramide-mediated CD95 clustering. Biochem Biophys Res Commun 284:1016–1030. doi:10.1006/bbrc.2001.5045
18. Miyaji M, Jin Z-X, Yamaoka S et al (2005) Role of membrane sphingomyelin and ceramide in platform formation for Fas-mediated apoptosis. J Exp Med 202:249–259. doi:10.1084/jem.20041685
19. Brenner B, Ferlinz K, Grassmé H et al (1998) Fas/CD95/Apo-I activates the acidic sphingomyelinase via caspases. Cell Death Differ 5:29–37. doi:10.1038/sj.Cdd.4400307
20. Grullich C, Sullards MC, Fuks Z et al (2000) CD95(Fas/APO-1) signals ceramide generation independent of the effector stage of apoptosis. J Biol Chem 275:8650–8656
21. Grassmé H, Cremesti A, Kolesnick R, Gulbins E (2003) Ceramide-mediated clustering is required for CD95-DISC formation. Oncogene 22:5457–5470. doi:10.1038/sj.Onc.1206540
22. Gulbins E, Kolesnick R (2000) Measurement of sphingomyelinase activity. Methods Enzymol 322:382–388
23. Perrotta C, Bizzozero L, Cazzato D et al (2010) Syntaxin 4 is required for acid sphingomyelinase activity and apoptotic function. J Biol Chem 285:40240–40251. doi:10.1074/jbc.M110.139287
24. Grassmé H, Bock J, Kun J, Gulbins E (2002) Clustering of CD40 ligand is required to form a functional contact with CD40. J Biol Chem 277:30289–30299. doi:10.1074/jbc.M200494200
25. Grassmé H, Riethmüller J, Gulbins E (2007) Biological aspects of ceramide-enriched membrane domains. Prog Lipid Res 46:161–170. doi:10.1016/j.Plipres.2007.03.002
26. Lin T, Genestier L, Pinkoski MJ et al (2000) Role of acidic sphingomyelinase in Fas/CD95-mediated cell death. J Biol Chem 275:8657–8663
27. Paris F, Grassmé H, Cremesti A et al (2001) Natural ceramide reverses Fas resistance of acid sphingomyelinase(−/−) hepatocytes. J Biol Chem 276:8297–8305. doi:10.1074/jbc.M008732200
28. De Maria R, Rippo MR, Schuchman EH, Testi R (1998) Acidic sphingomyelinase (ASM) is necessary for fas-induced GD3 ganglioside accumulation and efficient apoptosis of lymphoid cells. J Exp Med 187:897–902
29. Cock JG, Tepper AD, de Vries E et al (1998) CD95 (Fas/APO-1) induces ceramide formation and apoptosis in the absence of a functional acid sphingomyelinase. J Biol Chem 273:7560–7565
30. Bezombes C, Ségui B, Cuvillier O et al (2001) Lysosomal sphingomyelinase is not solicited for apoptosis signaling. FASEB J 15:297–299. doi:10.1096/fj.00-0466fje
31. Chalfant CE, Ogretmen B, Galadari S et al (2001) FAS activation induces dephosphorylation of SR proteins; dependence on the de novo generation of ceramide and activation of protein phosphatase 1. J Biol Chem 276:44848–44855. doi:10.1074/jbc.M106291200
32. Watanabe M, Kitano T, Kondo T et al (2004) Increase of nuclear ceramide through caspase-3-dependent regulation of the "sphingomyelin cycle" in Fas-induced apoptosis. Cancer Res 64:1000–1007

33. Lafont E, Milhas D, Carpentier S et al (2010) Caspase-mediated inhibition of sphingomyelin synthesis is involved in FasL-triggered cell death. Cell Death Differ 17:642–654. doi:10.1038/cdd.2009.130
34. Tepper AD, de Vries E, van Blitterswijk WJ, Borst J (1999) Ordering of ceramide formation, caspase activation, and mitochondrial changes during CD95- and DNA damage-induced apoptosis. J Clin Invest 103:971–978. doi:10.1172/JCI5457
35. Juo P, Woo MS, Kuo CJ et al (1999) FADD is required for multiple signaling events downstream of the receptor Fas. Cell Growth Differ 10:797–804
36. Cuvillier O, Edsall L, Spiegel S (2000) Involvement of sphingosine in mitochondria-dependent Fas-induced apoptosis of type II Jurkat T cells. J Biol Chem 275:15691–15700. doi:10.1074/jbc.M000280200
37. Tepper AD, Cock JG, de Vries E et al (1997) CD95/Fas-induced ceramide formation proceeds with slow kinetics and is not blocked by caspase-3/CPP32 inhibition. J Biol Chem 272:24308–24312
38. Lafont E, Dupont R, Andrieu-Abadie N et al (2012) Ordering of ceramide formation and caspase-9 activation in CD95L-induced Jurkat leukemia T cell apoptosis. Biochim Biophys Acta 1821:684–693. doi:10.1016/j.Bbalip.2012.01.012
39. Samraj AK, Keil E, Ueffing N et al (2006) Loss of caspase-9 provides genetic evidence for the type I/II concept of CD95-mediated apoptosis. J Biol Chem 281:29652–29659. doi:10.1074/jbc.M603487200
40. Movsesyan VA, Yakovlev AG, Dabaghyan EA et al (2002) Ceramide induces neuronal apoptosis through the caspase-9/caspase-3 pathway. Biochem Biophys Res Commun 299:201–207
41. Nica AF, Tsao CC, Watt JC et al (2008) Ceramide promotes apoptosis in chronic myelogenous leukemia-derived K562 cells by a mechanism involving caspase-8 and JNK. Cell Cycle 7:3362–3370. doi:10.4161/cc.7.21.6894
42. Milhas D, Andrieu-Abadie N, Levade T et al (2012) The tricyclodecan-9-yl-xanthogenate D609 triggers ceramide increase and enhances FasL-induced caspase-dependent and -independent cell death in T lymphocytes. Int J Mol Sci 13:8834–8852. doi:10.3390/ijms13078834
43. Milhas D, Cuvillier O, Therville N et al (2005) Caspase-10 triggers Bid cleavage and caspase cascade activation in FasL-induced apoptosis. J Biol Chem 280:19836–19842. doi:10.1074/jbc.M414358200
44. Ganesan V, Perera MN, Colombini D et al (2010) Ceramide and activated Bax act synergistically to permeabilize the mitochondrial outer membrane. Apoptosis 15:553–562. doi:10.1007/s10495-009-0449-0
45. Chipuk JE, McStay GP, Bharti A et al (2012) Sphingolipid metabolism cooperates with BAK and BAX to promote the mitochondrial pathway of apoptosis. Cell 148:988–1000. doi:10.1016/j.Cell.2012.01.038
46. Zundel W, Giaccia A (1998) Inhibition of the anti-apoptotic PI(3)K/Akt/Bad pathway by stress. Genes Dev 12:1941–1946
47. Chalfant CE, Rathman K, Pinkerman RL et al (2002) De novo ceramide regulates the alternative splicing of caspase 9 and Bcl-x in A549 lung adenocarcinoma cells. Dependence on protein phosphatase-1. J Biol Chem 277:12587–12595. doi:10.1074/jbc.M112010200
48. De Maria R, Lenti L, Malisan F et al (1997) Requirement for GD3 ganglioside in CD95- and ceramide-induced apoptosis. Science 277:1652–1655
49. Popa I, Therville N, Carpentier S et al (2011) Production of multiple brain-like ganglioside species is dispensable for fas-induced apoptosis of lymphoid cells. PLoS One 6:e19974. doi:10.1371/journal.Pone.0019974
50. Kang N-Y, Kang Y, Kang S-K et al (2006) Transcriptional regulation of the human GD3 synthase gene expression in Fas-induced Jurkat T cells: a critical role of transcription factor NF-kappaB in regulated expression. Glycobiology 16:375–389. doi:10.1093/glycob/cwj087
51. Sorice M, Matarrese P, Tinari A et al (2009) Raft component GD3 associates with tubulin following CD95/Fas ligation. FASEB J 23:3298–3308. doi:10.1096/fj.08-128140
52. Sorice M, Matarrese P, Manganelli V et al (2010) Role of GD3-CLIPR-59 association in lymphoblastoid T cell apoptosis triggered by CD95/Fas. PLoS One 5:e8567. doi:10.1371/journal.Pone.0008567

53. Peter ME, Hadji A, Murmann AE et al (2015) The role of CD95 and CD95 ligand in cancer. Cell Death Differ 22:549–559. doi:10.1038/cdd.2015.3
54. Malleter M, Tauzin S, Bessede A et al (2013) CD95L cell surface cleavage triggers a prometastatic signaling pathway in triple-negative breast cancer. Cancer Res 73:6711–6721. doi:10.1158/0008-5472.CAN-13-1794
55. Fouqué A, Debure L, Legembre P (2014) The CD95/CD95L signaling pathway: a role in carcinogenesis. Biochim Biophys Acta 1846:130–141. doi:10.1016/j.Bbcan.2014.04.007
56. Suda T, Hashimoto H, Tanaka M et al (1997) Membrane Fas ligand kills human peripheral blood T lymphocytes, and soluble Fas ligand blocks the killing. J Exp Med 186:2045–2050
57. Schneider P, Holler N, Bodmer JL et al (1998) Conversion of membrane-bound Fas(CD95) ligand to its soluble form is associated with downregulation of its proapoptotic activity and loss of liver toxicity. J Exp Med 187:1205–1213
58. O'Reilly LA, Tai L, Lee L et al (2009) Membrane-bound Fas ligand only is essential for Fas-induced apoptosis. Nature 461:659–663. doi:10.1038/nature08402
59. Kischkel FC, Hellbardt S, Behrmann I et al (1995) Cytotoxicity-dependent APO-1 (Fas/CD95)-associated proteins form a death-inducing signaling complex (DISC) with the receptor. EMBO J 14:5579–5588
60. Tauzin S, Chaigne-Delalande B, Selva E et al (2011) The naturally processed CD95L elicits a c-yes/calcium/PI3K-driven cell migration pathway. PLoS Biol 9:e1001090. doi:10.1371/journal.Pbio.1001090
61. Khadra N, Bresson-Bepoldin L, Penna A et al (2011) CD95 triggers Orai1-mediated localized Ca^{2+} entry, regulates recruitment of protein kinase C (PKC) β2, and prevents death-inducing signaling complex formation. Proc Natl Acad Sci U S A 108:19072–19077. doi:10.1073/pnas.1116946108
62. Monet M, Poët M, Tauzin S et al (2016) The cleaved FAS ligand activates the Na(+)/H(+) exchanger NHE1 through Akt/ROCK1 to stimulate cell motility. Sci Rep 6:28008. doi:10.1038/srep28008
63. Edmond V, Dufour F, Poiroux G et al (2015) Downregulation of ceramide synthase-6 during epithelial-to-mesenchymal transition reduces plasma membrane fluidity and cancer cell motility. Oncogene 34:996–1005. doi:10.1038/onc.2014.55
64. Hannun YA, Obeid LM (2008) Principles of bioactive lipid signalling: lessons from sphingolipids. Nat Rev Mol Cell Biol 9:139–150. doi:10.1038/nrm2329
65. Mullen TD, Hannun YA, Obeid LM (2012) Ceramide synthases at the centre of sphingolipid metabolism and biology. Biochem J 441:789–802. doi:10.1042/BJ20111626
66. Goñi FM, Alonso A (2009) Effects of ceramide and other simple sphingolipids on membrane lateral structure. Biochim Biophys Acta 1788:169–177. doi:10.1016/j.Bbamem.2008.09.002
67. Pewzner-Jung Y, Park H, Laviad EL et al (2010) A critical role for ceramide synthase 2 in liver homeostasis: I. Alterations in lipid metabolic pathways. J Biol Chem 285:10902–10910. doi:10.1074/jbc.M109.077594
68. Levade T, Andrieu-Abadie N, Micheau O et al (2015) Sphingolipids modulate the epithelial–mesenchymal transition in cancer. Cell Death Discov 1:15001. doi:10.1038/cddiscovery.2015.1
69. Poissonnier A, Sanséau D, Le Gallo M et al (2016) CD95-mediated calcium signaling promotes T helper 17 trafficking to inflamed organs in lupus-prone mice. Immunity 45:209–223. doi:10.1016/j.Immuni.2016.06.028
70. Hait NC, Sarkar S, Le Stunff H et al (2005) Role of sphingosine kinase 2 in cell migration toward epidermal growth factor. J Biol Chem 280:29462–29469. doi:10.1074/jbc.M502922200
71. Sarkar S, Maceyka M, Hait NC et al (2005) Sphingosine kinase 1 is required for migration, proliferation and survival of MCF-7 human breast cancer cells. FEBS Lett 579:5313–5317. doi:10.1016/j.Febslet.2005.08.055
72. Ashkenazi A, Holland P, Eckhardt SG (2008) Ligand-based targeting of apoptosis in cancer: the potential of recombinant human apoptosis ligand 2/tumor necrosis factor-related apoptosis-inducing ligand (rhApo2L/TRAIL). J Clin Oncol 26:3621–3630. doi:10.1200/JCO.2007.15.7198

73. LeBlanc H, Lawrence D, Varfolomeev E et al (2002) Tumor-cell resistance to death receptor—induced apoptosis through mutational inactivation of the proapoptotic Bcl-2 homolog Bax. Nat Med 8:274–281. doi:10.1038/nm0302-274
74. Ndozangue-Touriguine O, Sebbagh M, Mérino D et al (2008) A mitochondrial block and expression of XIAP lead to resistance to TRAIL-induced apoptosis during progression to metastasis of a colon carcinoma. Oncogene 27:6012–6022. doi:10.1038/onc.2008.197
75. Micheau O, Shirley S, Dufour F (2013) Death receptors as targets in cancer. Br J Pharmacol 169:1723–1744. doi:10.1111/bph.12238
76. Wiley SR, Schooley K, Smolak PJ et al (1995) Identification and characterization of a new member of the TNF family that induces apoptosis. Immunity 3:673–682
77. Almasan A, Ashkenazi A (2003) Apo2L/TRAIL: apoptosis signaling, biology, and potential for cancer therapy. Cytokine Growth Factor Rev 14:337–348
78. Mérino D, Lalaoui N, Morizot A et al (2007) TRAIL in cancer therapy: present and future challenges. Expert Opin Ther Targets 11:1299–1314. doi:10.1517/14728222.11.10.1299
79. Dumitru CA, Gulbins E (2006) TRAIL activates acid sphingomyelinase via a redox mechanism and releases ceramide to trigger apoptosis. Oncogene 25:5612–5625. doi:10.1038/sj.Onc.1209568
80. Xiang H, Reyes AE, Eppler S et al (2013) Death receptor 5 agonistic antibody PRO95780: preclinical pharmacokinetics and concentration-effect relationship support clinical dose and regimen selection. Cancer Chemother Pharmacol 72:405–415. doi:10.1007/s00280-013-2200-3
81. Walczak H, Krammer PH (2000) The CD95 (APO-1/Fas) and the TRAIL (APO-2L) apoptosis systems. Exp Cell Res 256:58–66. doi:10.1006/excr.2000.4840
82. Pettus BJ, Chalfant CE, Hannun YA (2002) Ceramide in apoptosis: an overview and current perspectives. Biochim Biophys Acta 1585:114–125
83. Ségui B, Andrieu-Abadie N, Jaffrézou J-P et al (2006) Sphingolipids as modulators of cancer cell death: potential therapeutic targets. Biochim Biophys Acta 1758:2104–2120. doi:10.1016/j.Bbamem.2006.05.024
84. Truman J-P, García-Barros M, Obeid LM, Hannun YA (2014) Evolving concepts in cancer therapy through targeting sphingolipid metabolism. Biochim Biophys Acta 1841:1174–1188. doi:10.1016/j.Bbalip.2013.12.013
85. Thon L, Mathieu S, Kabelitz D, Adam D (2006) The murine TRAIL receptor signals caspase-independent cell death through ceramide. Exp Cell Res 312:3808–3821. doi:10.1016/j.Yexcr.2006.08.017
86. White-Gilbertson S, Mullen T, Senkal C et al (2009) Ceramide synthase 6 modulates TRAIL sensitivity and nuclear translocation of active caspase-3 in colon cancer cells. Oncogene 28:1132–1141. doi:10.1038/onc.2008.468
87. Skender B, Hofmanová J, Slavík J et al (2014) DHA-mediated enhancement of TRAIL-induced apoptosis in colon cancer cells is associated with engagement of mitochondria and specific alterations in sphingolipid metabolism. Biochim Biophys Acta 1841:1308–1317. doi:10.1016/j.Bbalip.2014.06.005
88. Voelkel-Johnson C, Hannun YA, El-Zawahry A (2005) Resistance to TRAIL is associated with defects in ceramide signaling that can be overcome by exogenous C6-ceramide without requiring down-regulation of cellular FLICE inhibitory protein. Mol Cancer Ther 4:1320–1327. doi:10.1158/1535-7163.MCT-05-0086
89. Yang J, Yang C, Zhang S et al (2015) ABC294640, a sphingosine kinase 2 inhibitor, enhances the antitumor effects of TRAIL in non-small cell lung cancer. Cancer Biol Ther 16:1194–1204. doi:10.1080/15384047.2015.1056944
90. Woo SM, Seo BR, Min K, Kwon TK (2015) FTY720 enhances TRAIL-mediated apoptosis by up-regulating DR5 and down-regulating Mcl-1 in cancer cells. Oncotarget 6:11614–11626. doi:10.18632/oncotarget.3426

Chapter 11
Posttranslational Modifications and Death Receptor Signalling

Olivier Micheau

Abstract Members of the TNF family are key players of the immune system. Their ability to trigger a wide variety of signalling pathways leading, but not limited, to inflammation, survival, differentiation, or cell death, makes them effective host defense tools to control and eradicate pathogens or unwanted malignant cells. Binding of these ligands to their cognate receptors induces the formation of a macromolecular complex, through protein–protein interactions, enabling the activation of a myriad of signalling pathways. The molecular and regulatory events activated downstream of most of these receptors are fairly understood. However, the impact of posttranslational modifications (PTMs) on the early events, including glycosylations or proteolytic cleavage of these receptors and ligands, is less known. This book chapter aims at providing an overview of the main PTMs and their importance in the regulation of apoptosis by TNF receptors.

Keywords TNF family • Receptors • Glycosylation • Apoptosis • Signalling • Posttranslational modifications

O. Micheau (✉)
Université de Bourgogne Franche-Comté, LNC UMR1231, 21079 Dijon, France

Institut National de la Santé et de la Recherche Médicale (INSERM), LNC UMR1231, 21079 Dijon, France

FCS Bourgogne Franche-Comté, Laboratoire d'Excellence LipSTIC, 21079 Dijon, France

UFR Science de santé, Inserm LNC UMR1231,
7 Boulevard Jeanne d'Arc, 21079 Dijon, cedex, France
e-mail: omicheau@u-bourgogne.fr

O. Micheau (ed.), *TRAIL, Fas Ligand, TNF and TLR3 in Cancer*, Resistance to Targeted Anti-Cancer Therapeutics, DOI 10.1007/978-3-319-56805-8_11

11.1 Introduction

11.1.1 TNF Family

11.1.1.1 TNFSF

Ligands of the tumor necrosis factor superfamily (TNFSF) transduce a plethora of signalling pathways leading to cell growth, cell survival, differentiation, inflammation, or cell death [1–6]. Members of this family were originally identified owing to their homology with the carboxy-terminal domain of TNF [7]. TNFSF ligands are type II transmembrane glycoproteins [8] whose expression is mostly restricted to immune cells [9–12]. EDA-A1 and TL1A are probably the sole exceptions, as these ligands are expressed in epithelial cells during embryonic skin development and endothelial cells, respectively [13, 14]. TNFSF is composed of 19 ligands (Fig. 11.1), many of which play a central role during acquired or innate immunity [15–17]. Dysregulation of their expression or mutation events targeting the ligands themselves, their cognate receptors or downstream signalling partners can result in autoimmune and autoinflammatory diseases [18–21], dysplasias [22, 23], as well as cancers [24–31].

11.1.1.2 TNFRSF

TNFSF ligands have the ability to bind to cognate TNF receptors (TNFRSF). Among the 29 receptors identified (Table 11.1), so far, all TNFRSF receptors, but DcR3 and OPG which are secreted, are expressed at the cell surface (Fig. 11.1). With the exception of DcR1, these receptors are bound to the cell surface owing to

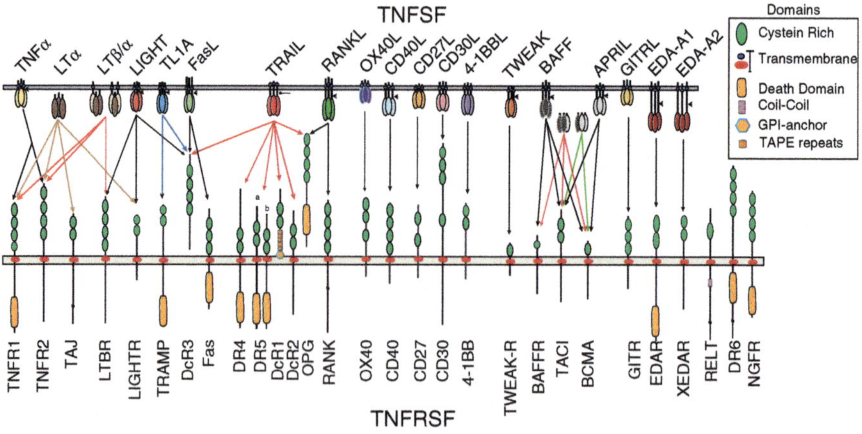

Fig. 11.1 Schematic representation of ligands and receptors of the TNF superfamily. *Arrows* indicate ligand–receptor interactions. Main structural domains are described in the *inset*

Table 11.1 TNFRSF and corresponding ligands

TNFRSF	Usual name	Aliases	Reference (TNFRSF)	TNFSF ligand	Reference (TNFSF)	Exogenous ligand	Reference (other)
1A	TNFR1 (*TNFRSF1A*, P19438)	CD120a, p55TNFR, TNFAR, TNF-R55	[42–44]	Lymphotoxin-α (*lta*, p01374)tumor necrosis factor membrane form (*tnf*, p01375)tumor necrosis factor shed form (*tnf*, p01375)	[45, 46]		
1B	TNFR2 (*TNFRSF1B*, P20333)	Tumor necrosis factor receptor superfamily, member 1B, CD120b, p75 TNFR, TNFalpha-R2, TNF-R75, TNFRII	[44, 47, 48]	Lymphotoxin-α (*LTA*, P01374)tumor necrosis factor membrane form (*TNF*, P01375)	[45]		
3	*LTBR* (P36941)	Lymphotoxin beta receptor, CD18, TNFCR, TNFR III, TNFR2-RP, LT-beta receptor, LTbetaR, TNF receptor-related protein	[49]	Lymphotoxin β2α1 heterotrimer (*LTA*, *LTB*, Q06643, P01374) LIGHT	[50, 51]		
4	OX40 (*TNFRSF4*, P43489)	Activated glycoprotein 1, tumor necrosis factor (ligand) superfamily, member 4, ACT35, CD134, TXGP1L, MRC OX40, OX40L receptor, Tax-transcriptionally	[52]	OX-40 ligand (*TNFSF4*, P23510)			
5	*CD40* (P25942)	TNF receptor superfamily member 5, TNFRSF5	[53]	CD40 ligand (*CD40LG*, P29965)	[54]		
6A	*FAS* (P25445)	*DR2*, APO-1, CD95, apoptosis-mediating surface antigen FAS, FAS1, Fas receptor, FASLG receptor, Fas cell surface death receptor, FAS1, TNFRSF6A	[55]	Fas ligand (*FASLG*, P48023)	[56]		

(continued)

Table 11.1 (continued)

TNFRSF	Usual name	Aliases	Reference (TNFRSF)	TNFSF ligand	Reference (TNFSF)	Exogenous ligand	Reference (other)
6B	decoy receptor 3 (*TNFRSF6B*, O95407)	*DcR3*, decoy receptor for Fas ligand, tumor necrosis factor receptor superfamily, member 6b, decoy	[57]	LIGHT (*TNFSF14*, O43557)	[2, 13, 57–61]		
				TL1A (*TNFSF15*, O95150)			
				Fas ligand (*FASLG*, P48023)			
				TRAIL (TNFSF10, P50591)			
7	*CD27* (P26842)	CD antigen 27, Tp55	[62]	CD70 (*CD70*, P32970)	[63]		
8	CD30 (*TNFRSF8*, P28908)	CD30L receptor, tumor necrosis factor receptor superfamily, member 8	[64]	CD30 ligand (*TNFSF8*, P32971)	[65]		
9	4-1BB (*TNFRSF9*, Q07011)	ILA, CD137, Ly63, tumor necrosis factor receptor superfamily, member 9	[66]	4-1BB ligand (*TNFSF9*, P41273)	[67]		
10A	TRAIL-R1 (TNFRSF10A, O00220)	*DR4*, tumor necrosis factor receptor superfamily, member 10a, CD261, Apo2, TNF-related apoptosis-inducing ligand receptor 1, TRAILR-1	[68]	TRAIL (*TNFSF10*, P50591)	[2]	Emilin2 (Q9BXX0)	[69]
10B	TRAIL-R2 (TNFRSF10B, O14763)	*DR5*, tumor necrosis factor receptor superfamily, member 10b, CD262, Killer/Ly98, TNF-related apoptosis-inducing ligand receptor 2, TRICK2A, TRICKB	[70–72]	TRAIL (*TNFSF10*, P50591)	[2]	UL141 (HCMV viral protein)	[73, 74]

TNFRSF	Usual name	Aliases	Reference (TNFRSF)	TNFSF ligand	Reference (TNFSF)	Exogenous ligand	Reference (other)
10C	TRAIL-R3 (TNFRSF10C, O14798)	*DcR1*, antagonist decoy receptor for TRAIL/Apo-2L, lymphocyte inhibitor of TRAIL, TNF-related apoptosis-inducing ligand receptor 3, TRAIL receptor 3, tumor necrosis factor receptor superfamily member 10C, CD263,LIT, tumor necrosis factor receptor superfamily, member 10c, decoy without an intracellular domain	[33, 70, 75, 76]	TRAIL (*TNFSF10*, P50591)	[2]		
10D	TRAIL-R4 (TNFRSF10D, Q9UBN6)	*DcR2*, TNF-related apoptosis-inducing ligand receptor 4, TRAIL receptor 4, TRAILR4, TRUNDD, tumor necrosis factor receptor superfamily member 10D, CD264, tumor necrosis factor receptor superfamily, member 10d, decoy with truncated death domain	[77, 78]	TRAIL (*TNFSF10*, P50591)	[2]		
11A	RANK (TNFRSF11A, Q9Y6Q6)	*Receptor activator of NF-kappa B*, CD265, ODFR, osteoclast differentiation factor receptor, TRANCE-R, tumor necrosis factor receptor superfamily, member 11a, NFKB activator, tumor necrosis factor receptor superfamily, member 11a	[79]	RANK ligand (*TNFSF11*, O14788)	[80]		
11B	OPG (TNFRSF11B, O00300)	*Osteoprotegerin*, osteoclastogenesis inhibitory factor, TR1, tumor necrosis factor receptor superfamily, member 11b	[81]	RANK ligand (*TNFSF11*, O14788) TRAIL (*TNFSF10*, P50591).	[80]		

(continued)

Table 11.1 (continued)

TNFRSF	Usual name	Aliases	Reference (TNFRSF)	TNFSF ligand	Reference (TNFSF)	Exogenous ligand	Reference (other)
12A	TWEAK-R (TNFRSF12A, Q9NP84)	Fn14, tumor necrosis factor receptor superfamily, member 12a, CD266, FGF-inducible 14, TweakR, tumor necrosis factor receptor superfamily, member 12A	[82]	TWEAK (*TNFSF12*, O43508)	[83]		
13B	TACI (TNFRSF13B, O14836)	CD267, tumor necrosis factor receptor superfamily, member 13B, Transmembrane activator and CAML interactor	[84]	APRIL (*TNFSF13*, O75888)	[85, 86]		
				BAFF (*TNFSF13B*, Q9Y275)			
13C	BAFFR (TNFRSF13C, Q96RJ3)	B cell-activating factor receptor, tumor necrosis factor receptor superfamily, member 13c, BAFFR, Bcmd1, CD268, tumor necrosis factor receptor superfamily, member 13C	[87]	BAFF (*TNFSF13B*, Q9Y275)	[86, 88, 89]		
14	LIGHTR (*TNFRSF14*, Q92956)	ATAR, Herpesvirus entry mediator A, HVEA, HVEM, TR2, tumor necrosis factor receptor superfamily, member 14, CD270	[90]	Lymphotoxin-α (*LTA*, P01374)	[45, 46, 58]	B and T lymphocyte attenuator (*BTLA*, Q7Z6A9)	[91, 92]
				LIGHT (*TNFSF14*, O43557)			
16	NGFR (*NGFR*, P08138)	CD271, NGF receptor, p75NTR, Low affinity nerve growth factor receptor, nerve growth factor receptor (TNFR superfamily, member 16), LNGFR	[93]			NGF (*NGF*, P01138)	[94–97]
						BDNF (*BDNF*, P23560)	
						Neurotrophin-3 (*NTF3*, P20783)	
						Neurotrophin-4 (*NTF4*, P34130)	

TNFRSF	Usual name	Aliases	Reference (TNFRSF)	TNFSF ligand	Reference (TNFSF)	Exogenous ligand	Reference (other)
17	BCMA (*TNFRSF17*, Q02223)	Tumor necrosis factor receptor superfamily, member 17, BCM, CD269, TNFRSF13a	[98]	APRIL (*TNFSF13*, O75888)	[85, 86]		
				BAFF (*TNFSF13B*, Q9Y275)			
18	GITR (*TNFRSF18*, Q9Y5U5)	Activation-inducible TNFR family receptor, AITR, Glucocorticoid-induced TNFR-related protein, tumor necrosis factor receptor superfamily, member 18, CD357	[99]	TL6 (*TNFSF18*, Q9UNG2)	[100]		
19	TAJ (*TNFRSF19*, Q9NS68)	TRADE, TROY, tumor necrosis factor receptor superfamily, member 19, TAJ-alpha	[101]	Lymphotoxin-α (*LTA*, P01374)	[45, 46]		
19L	RELT (Q969Z4)	Receptor expressed in lymphoid tissues, tumor necrosis factor receptor superfamily, member 19-like, RELT tumor necrosis factor receptor, TNFRSF19L	[102]				
21	DR6 (*TNFRSF21*, O75509)	Tumor necrosis factor receptor superfamily, member 21, CD358	[103]			APP (P05067)	[40]
25	TRAMP (*TNFRSF25*, Q93038)	Apoptosis-mediating receptor DR3, apoptosis-mediating receptor TRAMP, death domain receptor 3, WSL-1, WSL-LR, tumor necrosis factor receptor superfamily, member 25, APO-3, DDR3, TNFRSF12, TR3	[104]	TL1A (*TNFSF15*, VEGI, O95150)	[13]		

(continued)

Table 11.1 (continued)

TNFRSF	Usual name	Aliases	Reference (TNFRSF)	TNFSF ligand	Reference (TNFSF)	Exogenous ligand	Reference (other)
27	XEDAR (*EDA2R*, Q9HAV5)	*Ectodysplasin A2 isoform receptor*, tumor necrosis factor receptor superfamily member 27, EDA-A2 receptor, TNFRSF27, XEDAR, X-linked ectodysplasin-A2 receptor	[105]	Ectodysplasin A2 (*EDA*, Q92838)	[106]		
	EDAR (Q9UNE0)	Ectodermal dysplasia receptor, ectodysplasin-A receptor, DL, ED1R, ED5, EDA3, ectodysplasin A receptor	[105]	Ectodysplasin A1 (*EDA*, Q92838)	[106]		

a hydrophobic transmembrane-spanning domain. DcR1 sits in the outer leaflet of the lipid bilayer and faces the extracellular environment thanks to its anchored glycosylphosphatidylinositol (GPI) carboxyl terminus [32, 33]. Their expression is generally less restricted than their cognate ligands [34, 35]. TNFSFs and TNFRSFs display a complex set of interactions. Except RELT, DR6 and NFGR, all receptors of the family are able to interact with at least one TNFSF ligands [36]. Some TNFSF ligands bind a single cognate receptor while others bind 2–6 distinct receptors (Fig. 11.1). On the other hand, DR6 and NGFR interact with several non-TNFSF ligands (Fig. 11.2a). NGFR binds low affinity ligands of the neurotrophin family (NGF, BDNF and neurotrophins) and transduces cell death as well as survival pathways in neuronal cells [37–39]. The binding of beta-amyloid precursor protein (APP) to DR6 also induces neuronal cell death [40], while the binding of S5a in monocytes induces NF-κB activation and their differentiation to macrophages [41].

In addition to their cognate ligands, other receptors of the family have also been found to interact with unrelated TNFSF ligands (Fig. 11.2b). Binding of B and T lymphocyte attenuator (BTLA) to LIGHTR, for example, represses both antigen-driven T cell activation [92] and proliferation of dendritic cells [107]. Moreover, some viruses are able to thwart the immune system, or enter the host cells by targeting TNFRSF receptors. Early on, it was found that LIGHTR, also coined HVEM or HveA for herpesvirus entry mediator or herpesvirus entry mediator A, respectively,

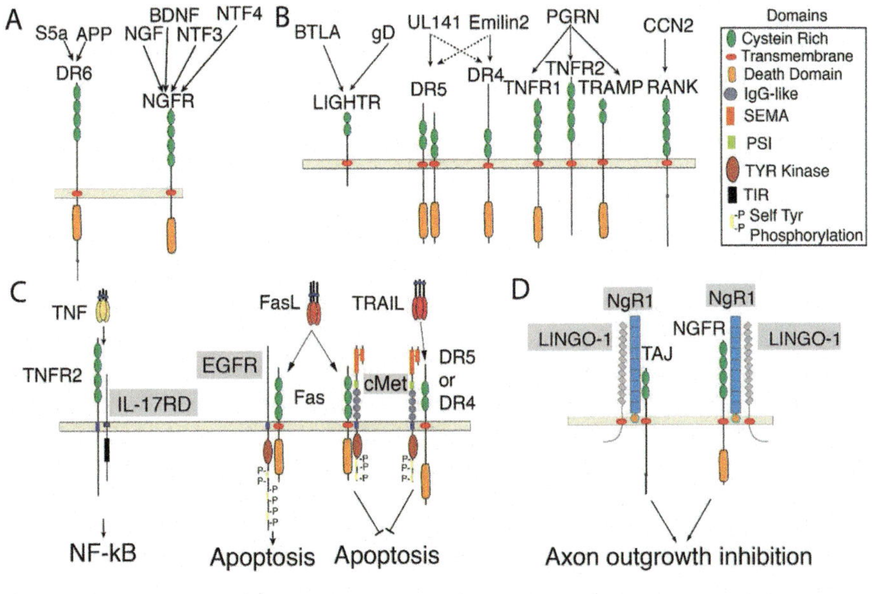

Fig. 11.2 Schematic representation of non-conventional TNFSF/TNFRS ligands and receptors interactions. Nonconventional ligands binding (**a**) TNFSF orphan DR6 and NGFR receptors and (**b**) TNFRSF the non-orphan receptors LIGHTR, DR5, DR4, TNFR1, TNFR2, TRAMP, and RANK. Heteromeric interactions of TNFRSF receptors with non-TNFRSF receptors induced by (**c**) TNFSF ligands or (**d**) non-TNFSF ligands. Main structural domains are described in the *inset*

is able to bind herpes simplex virus glycoprotein D (gD), acting as a co-receptor for virus entry [108, 109]. Human cytomegalovirus (HCMV) was next found to avoid death receptor mediated immune clearance not only because it can inhibit TNFRSF downstream signalling events during infection but also because it can induce the loss of TNFR1 [110], Fas [111], DR4 and DR5 [74] from the cell surface of the host cells. Interestingly enough, the HCMV glycoprotein UL141, which is responsible for the sequestration of DR5 in the intracellular compartments of the host cell, was found to be able to bind to DR4 and DR5 directly with high affinity [73, 74]. Similar to LIGHTR and the herpes simplex virus glycoprotein D [112], binding of UL141 to DR4 and DR5 is believed to be due to its "immunoglobulin-like" fold [113]. Other nonconventional bindings have been described. Likewise, Emilin2, an extracellular matrix glycoprotein, is also able to interact with DR4, and to a lesser extent with DR5 [69]. Contrary to UL141, though, binding of Emilin2 to DR4 and DR5 was found to trigger apoptosis in several cancer cell lines [69]. In other situations nonconventional TNFRSF binding partners were shown to enhance or inhibit TNFSF ligand's function. Henceforth, CCN2, a connective tissue growth factor, was found to bind RANK and to enhance osteoclast differentiation induced by RANKL [114]. Binding of the growth factor progranulin (PGRN) with TNFR1, TNFR2 or TRAMP, on the other hand, prevents signalling induced by TNF [115] or TL1A [116], respectively.

TNFSF ligands usually bind their cognate receptors as homotrimers, but heteromers have also been described to dictate receptor binding and signal transduction, including LTβ/α or BAFF/APRIL [117–119]. Conversely, heteromers of TNFRSF receptors can also contribute to the fine-tuning of signalling pathways, as evidenced with TRAIL [120–124]. Likewise, DR4 and DR5 are able to form homomers or heteromers upon TRAIL stimulation and trigger apoptosis in tumor cells [123, 125]. DR4 and DR5 can also form heteromers with DcR2 [123, 122]. But since DcR2 is devoid of DD, its interaction with DR4 and DR5 limits caspase-8 recruitment and thus apoptosis (see also Pollack and collaborators, Chap. 2).

In a limited number of studies, several TNFRSF receptors have also been demonstrated to be able to interact with unrelated receptors (Fig. 11.2c). Likewise, it has been demonstrated that heteromerization of IL-17RD with TNFR2 is required for TNF-induced NF-κB activation in renal epithelial cells [126]. These findings were proposed to explain the contribution of TNFR2 in renal dysfunction [127]. Similarly, co-recruitment of EGFR with Fas has been found to be required for Fas-ligand induced cell death [128–130]. Conversely, heteromerization of Fas, and DR4 or DR5 with cMET was found to inhibit apoptosis induced by FasL and TRAIL, respectively [131–133]. Last but not least some receptors of the TNFRSF heteromerize with unrelated TNFRSF receptors and contribute to TNFSF-independent signalling pathways (Fig. 11.2d). Likewise, recruitment of TAJ and NGFR with NgR1 and LINGO-1 in the Nogo-receptor complex has been demonstrated to contribute to RhoA-mediated inhibition of axonal regeneration [134, 135].

11.2 Signal Transduction of Death-Containing Receptors

With the exception of OPG, DcR1, and DcR3, all TNFRSF receptors are able to trigger the canonical NF-kB pathway, to a variable extent, but only 12 of these receptors (LTbetaR, p75TNFR, OX40, CD40, CD30, CD27, 4-1BB, RANK, LIGHTR, BCMA, TACI, and GITR) trigger the noncanonical NF-κB pathway [136]. Several TNF family receptors harbor a peculiar intracellular motif, sufficient and necessary to trigger cell death [137–139]. This domain, coined death domain (DD) is composed of six amphipathic α helices [140–142]. Receptors harboring a DD include TNFR1 [137], Fas or CD95 [55], TRAIL-R1 [68], TRAIL-R2 [32, 70–72], TRAMP [143–145], DR6 [103], NGFR [93], and EDAR [105]. The DD allows homotypic protein–protein interactions with the adaptor protein FADD [146, 147] and leads to the formation of the so-called DISC (Death-Inducing Signalling Complex) after Fas ligand or TRAIL stimulation (Fig. 11.3a and [148–150]). Provided that the activation of the caspase-8 is sufficient, apoptosis can occur directly through cleavage of the effector caspase-3 (Fig. 11.3b). In so-called type II cells, however, caspase-8 activation is weaker, but apoptosis can still occur thanks to an amplification loop involving Bid cleavage by the caspase-8 [151]. Cleavage of this BH3-only protein leads to the activation of Bax/Bak, mitochondrial permeabilization, release of the cytochrome c [152] and to the formation of the apoptosome [153], a soluble receptor platform allowing activation of caspase-9 (Fig. 11.3b). Similar to the initiator caspase-9 [154], activation of procaspase-8, within the DISC, is triggered by proximity-induced dimerization [155, 156]. Its activation is also tightly dependent on receptor aggregation and caspase-8 chain formation ((Fig. 11.3c) and [157–162]).

While TNFR1 also harbors a DD, its engagement by TNF primarily induces NF-κB activation and survival [163]. TNFR1 can nonetheless induce apoptosis provided that protein synthesis is inhibited [164] or that NF-κB signalling is defective [163]. Resistance induced by NF-kB activation is mainly due to an early transcriptional regulation of the caspase-8 inhibitor c-FLIP [165, 166]. However, and contrary to Fas or TRAIL receptors, despite the fact that FADD was known to be required for TNF-induced apoptosis, since the late 90s [167], TNFR1 is unable to recruit FADD and caspase-8 directly to the plasma membrane ([168, 169], Fig. 11.4). Binding of TNF to TNFR1 primarily induces the recruitment of the adaptor protein TRADD, RIPK1, and TRAF2 as well as other proteins such as cIAP-1 and cIAP2, and IKKs (see also Dubrez and Fulda, Chap. 3 for a detailed description). TNF triggers within seconds NF-κB activation from this membrane-bound complex [168–174]. This primary complex, coined complex I (Fig. 11.4) was found to give rise to a soluble complex, coined complex II, within which FADD and caspase-8 are recruited, allowing triggering of apoptosis [169]. How complex II arises after TNF stimulation has remained an open question until McCarthy and collaborators found out that the transition from complex I to complex II involves extensive posttranslational modifications of TNFR1. Likewise, it was found that the formation of complex II required shedding of the TNFR1 extracellular domain by TACE (TNF-Alpha

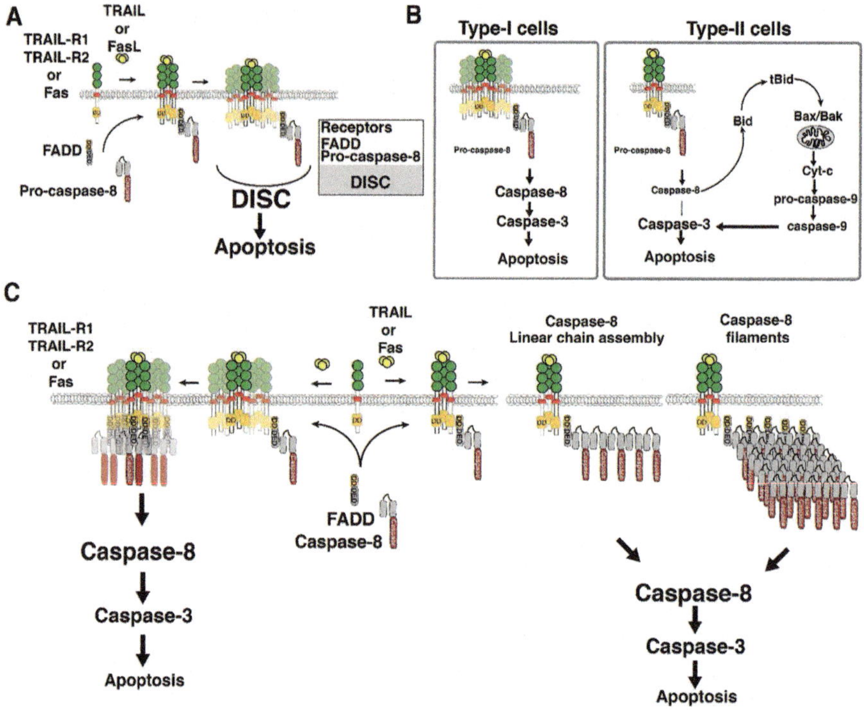

Fig. 11.3 Schematic representation of FasL- and TRAIL-induced apoptosis. (**a**) Binding of FasL or TRAIL to their cognate pro-apoptotic receptors induces receptor multimerization, recruitment of the adaptor protein FADD and initiator caspases-8 and -10, through death domain (DD) or death effector domain (DED) homotypic interactions, respectively, leading to the formation of the Death-Inducing Signalling Complex (DISC), which triggers apoptosis. (**b**) From the DISC, apoptosis is directly induced by caspase-8, in type I cells but requires an amplification loop in type II cells, owing to the fact that caspase-8 is not sufficiently activated. Amplification of the signal in these cells is mediated by a caspase-8-dependent cleavage of the BH3-only pro-apoptotic Bcl-2 member Bid. The resulting product (tBid) in turn translocates to mitochondria, allowing Bax/Bak activation, permeabilization of the mitochondrial outer plasma membrane, release of cytochrome c, and formation of a second macromolecular scaffold coined apoptosome (see also Eberle et al., Chap. 4 for a detailed description). The latter enables activation of the pro-caspase-9, another initiator caspase, which like caspase-8, cleaves the effector caspase-3. (**c**) Schematic representation of events leading to efficient caspase-8 activation after FasL or TRAIL stimulation (see text for details). Main signalling components and domains are described in the *inset*

Converting Enzyme) also known as ADAM17, internalization of complex I through a clathrin-dependent mechanism and post-processing of the receptor by the γ-secretase to release the intracellular domain of TNFR1 bound to TRADD, TRAF2, and RIPK1, among others proteins ([175], see also Fig. 11.4). The release of complex I to the cytosol subsequently allows recruitment of FADD and caspase-8 [175], leading to the formation of complex II [169], from which apoptosis can be initiated, provided that c-FLIP is not fueled by NF-κB activation [163, 165, 166].

TRAMP also primarily triggers NF-κB activation ([104, 143] and (Fig. 11.5)) via the recruitment of TRADD/RIP/TRAF2 after TL1A stimulation [176]. However,

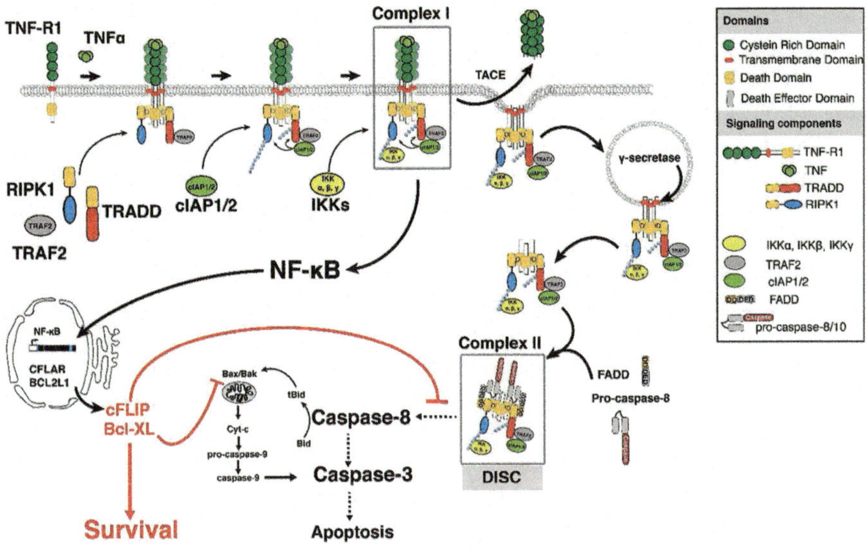

Fig. 11.4 Schematic representation of TNFR1-induced signal transduction. See text for details

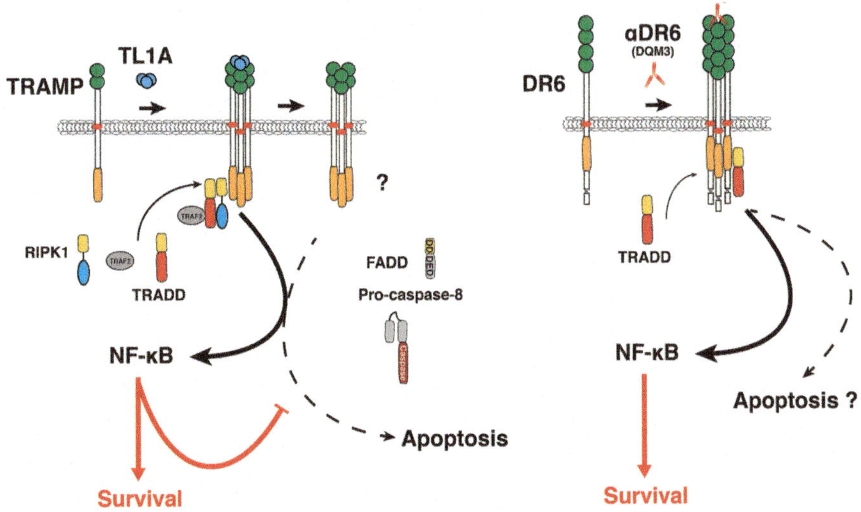

Fig. 11.5 Schematic representation of TRAMP- and DR6-induced signal transduction. See text for details

contrary to TNFR1 [177], recruitment of TRADD to TRAMP requires prior association of TRAF2 and RIP [178]. While it still remains unknown how TRAMP induces apoptosis [143], it has early on been demonstrated that a deficiency in FADD [167] or the overexpression of c-FLIP [179] would impair its triggering, suggesting that TRAMP-mediated apoptosis might be closely related to TNFR1-induced cell death

(Fig. 11.5). In the same vein, DR6 was first evidenced to induce NF-κB activation, to recruit TRADD and to trigger apoptosis [103, 104, 180]. However, contrary to TRAMP or TNFR1, DR6 may trigger apoptosis regardless of FADD or caspase-8 (Fig. 11.5), since neither a deficiency in Bid nor caspase-8 impairs cell death induced by DR6 [181]. In the same line, although antibodies targeting the extracellular domain of the low affinity NGFR have been shown to mediate apoptosis in cultured sympathetic neurons [182], the precise underlying signalling cascades have been difficult to dissect. Despite the fact that it also contains a DD, NGFR was suggested by an earlier study, using the yeast two hybrid approach, to be unable to interact with any DD-containing adaptor proteins known to contribute to TNFSF signalling, such as FADD or TRADD [183]. Consistently, cell death induced by NGFR in striatal neurons was shown to occur regardless of FADD, TRADD or caspase-8 [184]. Yet in this study, the authors also found that the viral homolog of c-FLIP, E8, could rescue cell death induced by NGFR [184]. More recently, however, TRADD was found to be recruited to NGFR and to be required for NGF-induced NF-κB activation in the breast cancer cell line MCF7 [185], suggesting that it might nonetheless be able to recruit TRADD. Moreover, beta-amyloid peptides as well as prion protein fragment PrP (106–126) were shown to bind NGFR and to trigger apoptosis in neuroblastoma cells [186]. Apoptosis induced by NGFR in these cells was found to require NGFR's DD and was also closely correlated with caspase-8 activation [186], suggesting again that the molecular mechanisms leading to NGFR-mediated cell death are likely to resemble those involved after TNF stimulation.

While the molecular mechanisms governing apoptosis-induced by DR6 and NGFR remain uncertain, EDAR is the sole receptor of the family with a DD, whose inability to trigger apoptosis is the less controversial. This receptor is involved during the development in hair follicle, nails, teeth, and sweat gland morphogenesis [187, 188]. Although it possesses a DD, EDAR is unable to recruit FADD or TRADD upon EDA binding [189]. Instead EDAR recruits another adaptor protein coined EDARADD [190] through which it transduces NF-kB activation via TRAF6, TAB2, and TAK1 [191].

Besides NF-κB and apoptosis, several DD-containing TNFRSF receptors, such as TNFR1, Fas, or TRAIL receptors, are also able to transduce necroptosis [192–196], a programmed form of necrosis orchestrated by RIPK1 and/or RIPK3, whose execution involves disruption of lysosomal, plasma and mitochondrial membranes [197–201].

Activation of apoptosis or necrosis by DD-containing receptors is tightly controlled by a limited number of adaptor proteins, most of which are shared among TNFRSF receptors, as described above. The outcome of the signal and its transduction, though, also rely on the metabolic and cellular environment of the target cell that affect inherent sensitivity to apoptosis [196, 202–205], but also on posttranslational modifications (PTMs) of components of the core machinery, including Bid and caspase-8 [206–209], or ligands and receptors themselves [210–215].

11.3 Posttranslational Modifications

In addition to the metabolic and cellular environment, pathogens and cancer cells are able to subvert TNFSF/TNFRSF signalling pathways. Almost all ligands and receptors of the TNFSF/TNFRSF family may be targeted. Since most of them contribute to innate or adaptive immunity, alteration of their signalling pathways is mandatory skill for viruses and cancer cells to thwart the immune system [216]. Early studies demonstrated that viral proteins could directly interfere with apoptosis-induced by DD-containing receptors [217]. These include viral homologs of the caspase-8 inhibitor c-FLIP, found in herpes viruses (HHV-8, EHV-2, BHV-4), the Kaposi sarcoma-associated herpes virus (KSHV), as well as in the molluscum contagiosum virus (MCV) [179, 218]. Like c-FLIP, these viral proteins harbor a Death-Effector-Domain (DED) and are either devoid of the caspase-like domain or contain a domain that lacks the catalytic cysteine that confers caspase's proteolytic activity. Their recruitment within the DISC interferes with caspase-8 cleavage and prevents apoptosis [219]. Additional interactions and regulations have been described to challenge DD-containing receptor signalling, most of which are nicely reviewed in the following reviews [220, 221]. More recently, however, even smarter subversive approaches have been described to contribute to pathogen virulence or cancer progression that include posttranslational modifications of TNFRSF receptors, or downstream signalling partners leading to inactivation of TNF receptor pro-apoptotic potential and immune escape.

11.3.1 Proteolytic Cleavage of TNFSF and TNFRSF

11.3.1.1 Cleavage of TNFSF

TNFSF are naturally found as trimers [222–224], and with the exception of lymphotoxin-alpha (LTα), which is naturally secreted [51, 225], TNFSF are expressed at the cell surface as anchored transmembrane proteins (Fig. 11.1). Most of these ligands can be, however, proteolytically processed from the cell surface to yield soluble bioactive or inactive oligomers [188, 226–229]. Soluble TNF was first evidenced in 1986 in the peritoneal fluid of mice injected with Picibanil, also coined OK-432 [230], a streptococcal preparation used in the treatment of head and neck lymphangiomas in pediatric patients [231]. The metalloproteinase found to exert this activity was latter coined TACE (TNF-a converting enzyme) [227]. This protease belongs to a family of disintegrin and metalloproteases and has been renamed ADAM17 [232]. Other ligands of the family are also prone to proteolytic cleavage and release from the cell surface (Fig. 11.6), such as FasL [233, 234], TRAIL [235], CD40L [236], EDA-A1 and EDA-A2 [228], 4-1BBL [237], BAFF [89], APRIL [238], LIGHT [239], TWEAK [240–242], RANKL [243], and TL1A [244]. TNFSF ligand shedding can be induced by metalloproteases of the ADAM family [237, 239, 245, 246], cathepsins [247], or furins [89, 248].

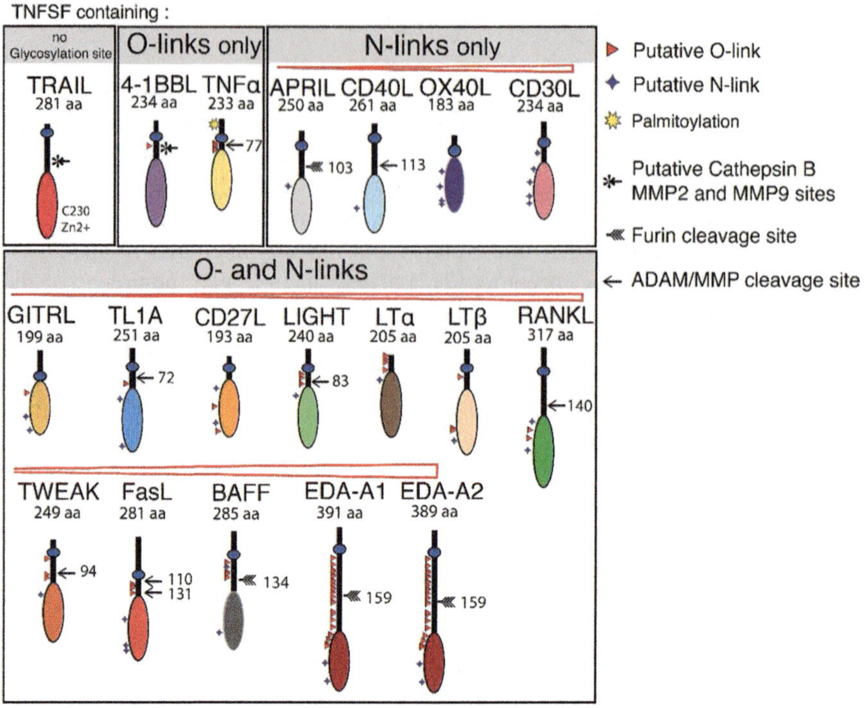

Fig. 11.6 Schematic representation of TNFSF ligands posttranslational modifications. TNFSF ligands are depicted and ranked based on their putative O- and/or N-linked glycosylation number. Palmitoylation and putative or effective cleavage sites are shown, see associated legend. Numbers shown on the right-hand side of each ligand correspond to the precise amino acid position of ADAM/MMP or Furin cleavage sites

11.3.1.2 Cleavage of TNFRSF

Like TNFSF, many receptors of the family are prone to shedding by ADAM17. These include TNFR1 and TNFR2, respectively [249], DR4 [250], CD30 [251], CD40 [252, 253], and 4-1BB [254]. In addition to this metalloprotease, other proteases of the family such as ADAM8, ADAM10, MMP7, or MMP8 are known to cleave the extracellular domain of TNFR1 [255, 256], CD27 [257], CD30 [258], or Fas [259], respectively. The ectodomain of XEDAR has also been found to be proteolytically cleaved by an unknown metalloprotease [260]. Apart from metalloproteases, some members of the TNFRSF are cleaved by γ-secretase, an intramembrane multi-subunit protease complex that cleaves transmembrane proteins at residues within the transmembrane domain. This protease cleaves TNFR1 [175], NGFR [261], and BCMA [262]. Finally, RANK ectodomain was proposed to be cleaved by an enteropeptidase [263].

11.3.1.3 Significance

Although the biological functions associated with TNFSF/TNFRSF cleavage and/or shedding remain poorly studied, several examples are well documented in the literature. For instance, EDA-A1-mediated morphogenesis of ectodermal structures requires shedding of the ligand from the cell surface by furin, allowing paracrine NF-κB signalling activation on distant target cells during development. Mutations of EDA-A1 furin cleavage site lead to X-linked hypohidrotic ectodermal dysplasia (XLHED), a human disorder characterized by impaired development of hair, sweat glands, and teeth [23]. Albeit less documented, TWEAK has been proposed to induce mammary epithelial branching morphogenesis [264]. Interestingly, elevations of soluble cleaved TWEAK have been correlated with mammary gland involution [241], suggesting that cleavage of membrane-bound TWEAK may work as a physiological negative feedback loop. Since cleavage of TWEAK [241] changes its binding and signalling capabilities [265], it has been proposed that inhibition of mammary epithelial morphogenesis may be due to its weakest ability to transduce NF-kB [266]. In keeping with these findings that proteases can affect the biological properties of TNFSF and TNFRSF, it has long been known that membrane-bound TNF binds to and transduce signalling through both TNFR1 and TNFR2 while soluble TNF solely binds TNFR1 [267, 268]. Albeit soluble TNF remains as efficient as membrane-bound TNF in inducing TNFR1-mediated NF-κB or cell death in tumor cells [169, 269], only membrane-bound TNF is able to bind to and transduce signalling through TNFR2 [270]. TNFR1 is also subject to extensive proteolytic cleavage. Apoptosis-induced by TNFR1 requires sequential cleavage of the receptor by ADAM17 and a γ-secretase [175] to allow complex II formation [169] and apoptosis (Fig. 11.4).

Shedding of these ligands or receptors can also occur in pathological conditions and contribute to disease progression. For example, cleavage RANK ectodomain by the enteropeptidase inhibits RANKL-induced signalling and therefore is likely to inhibit bone remodelling [263]. As regards DD-containing receptors, early findings unveiled in the mid-90s that soluble Fas, owing to its ability to inhibit apoptosis induced by FasL could contribute to autoimmune diseases such as systemic lupus erythematosus (SLE) [271]. More recently it was found that soluble FasL-mediated Th17 cell transmigration is likely to contribute to SLE in mice [272] (see Poissonnier et al., Chap. 7 for more details). Conversion of membrane-bound TRAIL or FasL to their soluble cleaved trimers by metalloproteases [246] or cathepsins [247] inhibits their pro-apoptotic potential [269]. Accumulating evidence suggests that soluble TNFSF ligands such as FasL or TRAIL can induce non-apoptotic signalling and promote tumorigenesis. The earliest studies indicating that Fas may induce direct, non-apoptotic, tumorigenic-like activity in vitro and in vivo, demonstrated that FasL could promote motility and invasiveness of tumor cells refractory to FasL-mediated killing [273–275]. It is worth noting not only that serum levels of soluble FasL are higher in patients with triple-negative breast cancer (TNBC) than any other breast cancer patients but that sFasL is alone sufficient to promote cell motility of TNBC cells in vitro [276, 277].

Although TRAIL was initially found to contribute to cancer immune surveillance of metastatic cancer cells in vivo [278–280], it has next been found to promote cell migration and invasion in resistant tumor cells in vitro [281], as well as metastasis in vivo [282, 283]. Invasion and metastatic TRAIL signalling capabilities were more recently assigned to TRAIL-R2 [284, 285]. While it remains to be determined whether soluble TRAIL trimers (sTRAIL) can be found in the serum of patients with advanced metastatic disease and whether it can alone promote cell migration and invasion, it is clear from these examples that cleavage of TNFSF ligands or TNFRSF receptors can dramatically alter their physiological functions, the result of which is likely to contribute to the pathogenesis of cancer or autoimmune diseases. Noteworthy, with the exception of TRAMP, GITRL, LTβ, CD27L, and OX40L, all other membrane-anchored TNFSF ligands or TNFRSF receptors harbor putative ADAM/MMP-, furin-, enteropeptidase-, or γ-secretase-protease cleavage sites (Figs. 11.6 and 11.7). Their cleavage is thus likely to occur, either during physiological or pathological conditions and have biological consequences.

11.3.2 Palmitoylation

Some members of the TNFSF/TNFRSF family, including TNF [286], Fas [287], DR4 [288], DR6 [211], and NGFR [289] have been reported to undergo particular PTM, namely palmitoylation (Figs. 11.6 and 11.7). This posttranslational

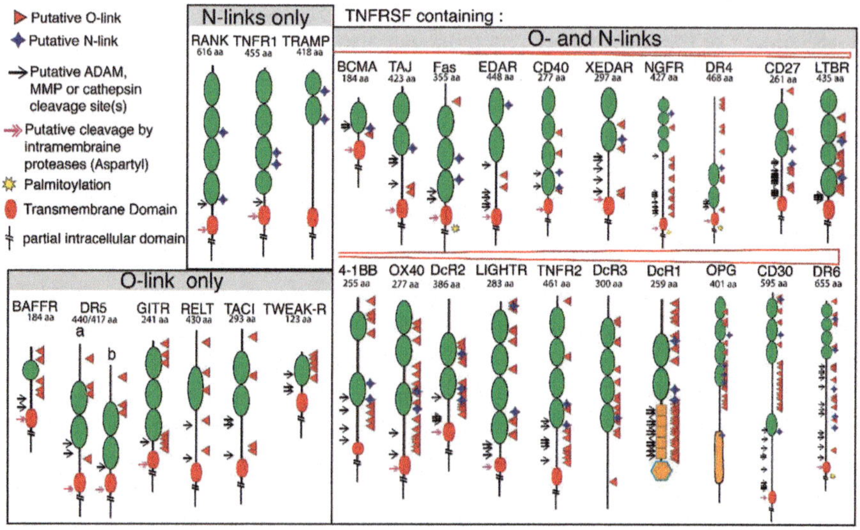

Fig. 11.7 Schematic representation of TNFSF ligands posttranslational modifications. TNFRSF receptors are depicted and ranked based on their putative O- and/or N-linked glycosylation number. Palmitoylation and putative or effective cleavage sites are shown, see associated legend

modification leads to the covalent attachment of a 16-carbon fatty acid, palmitate, to sulfhydryl groups of cysteine residues. The first study describing palmitoylation of a member of the TNF/TNFR super family, reported that TNF could undergo fatty acylation on the cysteine 30 [286]. However, myristyl acylation or myristoylation of lysines 19 and 20 has also been described for TNF [290]. Palmitoylation of TNF is not required for its shedding from the cell surface by ADAM17, but has been proposed to be required for its partitioning into lipid rafts [291]. It has been found more recently that lysine fatty acylation of TNF induces its retention to the lysosomal compartment [292], but that its deacetylation by SIRT6, a deacetylase of the mammalian sirtuin family, promotes its secretion [293]. The best example of TNFRSF receptor undergoing palmitoylation, so far, is Fas. This receptor can undergo S-palmitoylation of its cysteine 199 (C199), located within the Fas membrane proximal intracellular domain ([294] and Fig. 11.1). Fas palmitoylation contributes to its translocation into lipid rafts, aggregation, internalization, DISC formation and to apoptosis triggering [287, 294, 295]. The palmitoyl transferase responsible for Fas palmitoylation, DHHC7, has recently been characterized [296]. Similar to Fas, palmitoylation of DR4 on C336 was found to increase its pro-apoptotic potential, allowing DR4 partitioning to lipid rafts and increasing DR4 oligomerization upon TRAIL stimulation [288]. On the other hand, albeit cell death was not assessed in these studies, palmitoylation was not associated with translocation of DR6 into lipid-rich membrane subcellular compartments [211]. In an early study demonstrating NGFR palmitoylation, this PTM was not found to alter NGFR signalling [297]. However, it was found later on that palmitoylation of NGFR could affect not only its signalling capabilities but also its cleavage by gamma-secretase, suggesting that dysregulation of this PTM may somehow concur to neurogenerative diseases such as Alzheimer [289]. Although TNFR1, TRAMP, DR5, EDAR contain cysteine residues as well, in their membrane-proximal intracellular region, as potential sites for lipid modification, palmitoylation has, so far, only been detected on DR4, Fas, DR6, and NGFR [211, 288, 289].

11.3.3 S-Nitrosylation

Along the line, Fas and DR4 may also undergo S-nitrosylation at C199, C304 and C336, respectively [298, 299]. This PTM consists in the attachment of an NO (nitric oxide) radical to a thiol group of a cysteine residue [300]. The first study describing S-nitrosylation of a member of TNFR family reported that the NO donor nitrosylcobalamin (NO-Cbl), an analog of vitamin B12 that delivers NO, induced S-nitrosylation of DR4 but not DR5 at C336 [299]. S-nitrosylation of DR4 correlated with the potent antiproliferative activity of NO-Cbl in several human cell lines from different origins (melanoma, renal, and ovarian carcinomas). In the same vein, Fas was also found to undergo S-nitrosylation at cysteines 199 and 304. However, the biological effects of S-nitrosylation on Fas pro-apoptotic signalling were solely associated with PTM of C304, not C199. S-nitrosylation of C304 was found to increase Fas targeting to raft nanodomains as well as its aggregation, enhancing thus its pro-apoptotic potential [298].

11.3.4 Arginine N-GlcNAcylation

Arginine N-GlcNAcylation is a rather unusual posttranslational modification (PTM) that has been identified in several DD-containing proteins and associated with enteropathogenic Escherichia coli (EPEC) virulence. These gram-negative bacterial pathogens display a type III virulence secretion system (T3SS) that manipulates host's signalling pathways, allowing bacteria to thwart immune defenses. Remarkably, one of its secreted proteins, NleB, exhibits a N-acetylglucosamine (GlcNAc) transferase activity and induces GlcNAcylation of TNFR1, Fas, TRADD, FADD, and RIPK1 DD, as demonstrated by extensive mass spectrometry analysis [301, 302]. GlcNAcylation of these DD-containing proteins during infection, owing to its ability to impair DD homotypic interactions (Fig. 11.8), was found to be sufficient to inhibit both TNF-induced NF-κB activation and FADD-mediated cell death signalling after TNF, FasL, or TRAIL stimulation [301, 302].

11.3.5 O- and N-Glycosylation

Protein glycosylation is a complex process involving hundreds of distinct genes. It is estimated that more than 50% of the human proteome is glycosylated [303]. Protein N-linked and O-linked glycosylation of asparagine (Asn) [304] and serine (Ser) or threonine (Thr) amino acids, respectively, are the most abundant forms [305]. All TNFSF and TNFRSF members, but TRAIL, harbor putative N- and/or

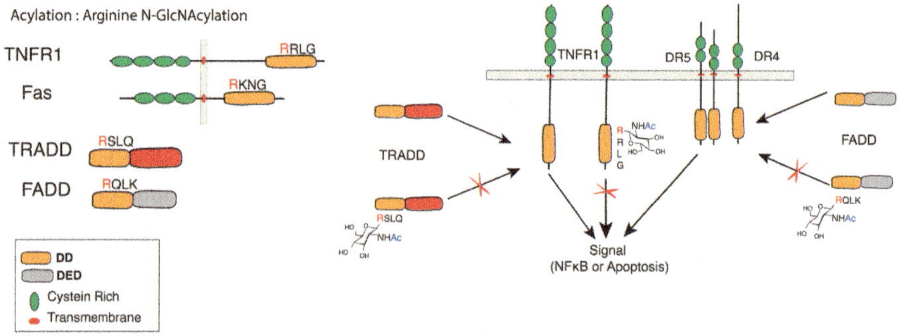

Fig. 11.8 Schematic representation of the impact of TNFR1, Fas, TRADD, and FADD arginine N-GlcNAcylation on NF-kB or apoptosis triggering. Arginine acylation of Fas, TNFR1, FADD, or TRADD impairs recruitment of the adaptor proteins FADD or TRADD to Fas, DR4, DR5, or TNFR1 and inhibits signal transduction of apoptosis and NF-kB (see text for details)

O-link glycosylation sites, as predicted using the bioinformatic tool GlycoEP [306] (Figs. 11.6 and 11.7). In the mid-80s and 90s, several TNFSF ligands and TNFRSF receptors were found to be glycosylated, including TNF [307], LTβ [212, 308, 309], TNFR1 [310], TNFR2 [311], and Fas [312]. While most of these ligands and receptors contain both type of glycosylation sites, or harbor only N- or O-link putative glycosylation sites (Figs. 11.6 and 11.7), little is known of the biological significance of these PTMs. Le Bivic and collaborators provided the first demonstration that O-glycosylation of NGFR stalk region is required for apical sorting of the receptor [313, 314]. Zunino et al. demonstrated, at the same time, that N-link glycosylation of Fas was not necessarily associated with receptor trafficking but related to its pro-apoptotic function ([210] and Fig. 11.9). Lavrik and collaborators next found out that mutation of two Fas N-link sites altered caspase-8 activation within the DISC [315]. In line with these findings, a seminal work by Ashkenazi and collaborators demonstrated that O-link glycosylation of DR5, one of the two TRAIL agonist receptors, contributes to DR5 pro-apoptotic potential [215]. More recently, we have demonstrated that the pro-apoptotic signalling of DR4 is, on the other hand, positively regulated by N-glycosylation [316]. Of importance, albeit most O- or N-glycosylation sites are found within the cysteine rich domains of TNFRSF receptors (Figs. 11.6 and 11.7), glycosylation of DR4 and DR5 within this domain neither increases nor inhibits TRAIL binding to its cognate receptors. Rather glycosylation of DR4 and DR5 promoted receptor aggregation, increasing TRAIL DISC formation and caspase-8 activation [215, 316]. N-link glycosylation of TNFR1, on the other hand, was found to be required for TNF binding and transduction of NF-kB [214]. Like Fas, TNFR1 and DR6 were shown to be N-glycosylated [211, 214, 317]. The biological significance of these PTMs remains, however, to be determined for these receptors.

Along this line, it is worth noting that glycan-modifying enzymes and glycan-binding lectins can regulate signalling properties of TNFSF/TNFRSF members, including cell death induced by DD-containing receptors [318]. Likewise, Krammer and collaborators found, early on, that Fas could be sialylated to a variable extent in B and T cell lymphoma cell lines and that removal of sialic acids in these cell lines using a neuraminidase would increase Fas-induced cell death, as well as apoptosis triggered by TNF ([319, 320], see also Fig. 11.9). In agreement with these findings it has been found more recently that the glycosyltransferase, ST6Gal-I, which adds sialic acid in α-2,6 to N-glycans, induces Fas sialylation and inhibits apoptosis-induced by this receptor [321]. The same team also showed that TNFR1, which is also subject to N-glycosylation [310], can be modified by ST6Gal-I and that its sialylation impairs its pro-apoptotic potential [322]. Conversely, fucosylation, another oligosaccharide modification, was found to contribute to apoptosis induced by TRAIL [323]. Miyoshi and collaborators discovered that a deficiency in GDP-mannose-4,6-dehydratase (GMDS), a GDP-mannose converting enzyme essential for de novo fucosylation, can confer colorectal cancer cell resistance to TRAIL [323]. They could demonstrate that fucosylation of DR4, but not DR5, would restore sensitivity to apoptosis-induced by TRAIL [324]. They also provided evidence that fucosylation of Fas could restore sensitivity to FasL-induced apoptosis (Fig. 11.9).

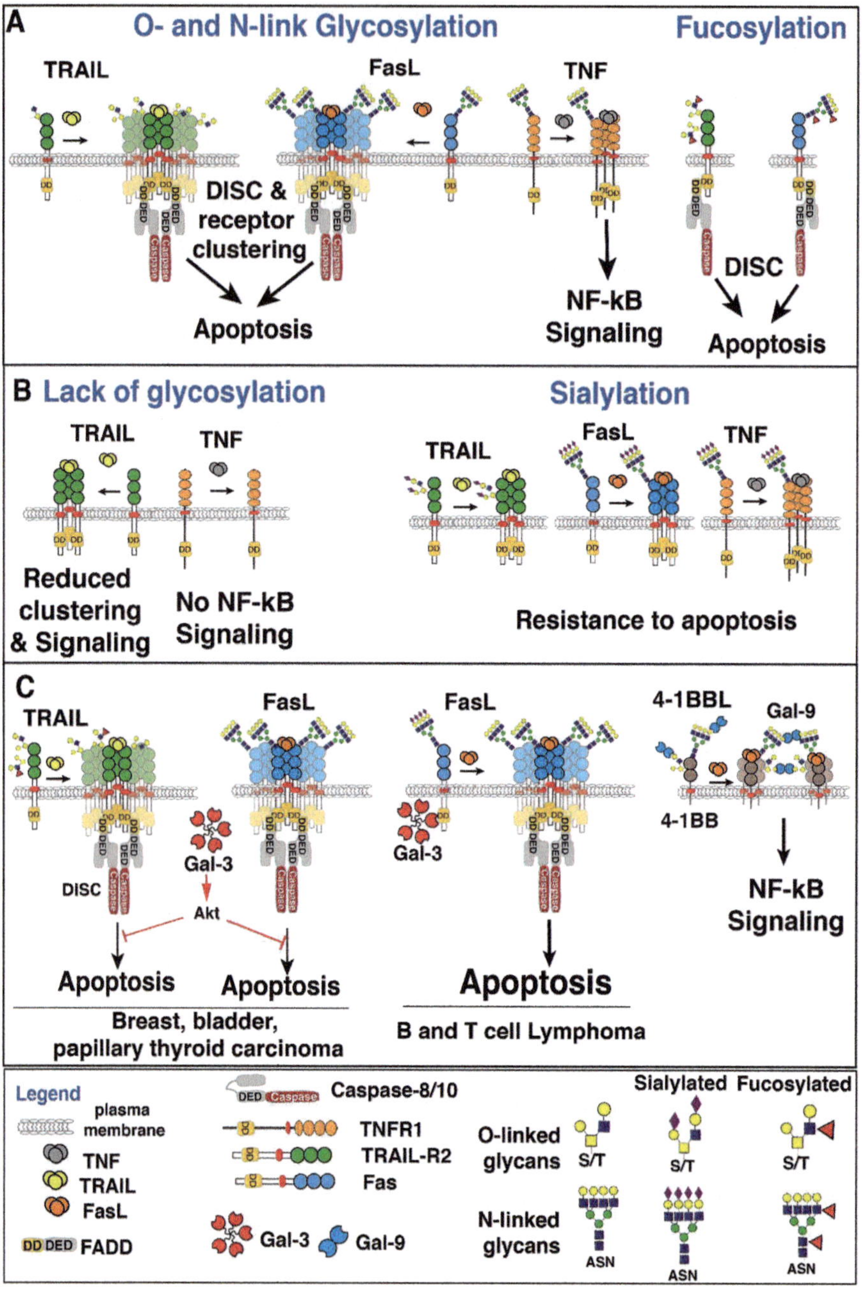

Fig. 11.9 Schematic representation of the impact of TNFRSF receptor glycosylation on signal transduction. (**a**) O-link and N-link glycosylation as well as fucosylation of DR5, Fas, or TNFR1 enhances receptor clustering and signal transduction after TRAIL, FasL, or TNF stimulation, while (**b**) a deficiency in glycosylation or sialylation of the corresponding receptors reduce receptor clustering after stimulation and prevents signalling. (**c**) glycan-binding proteins such as galectin-3 or galectin-9 can contribute to TNFRSF signal transduction regulation directly or indirectly (see text for details)

Consistent with these PTMs, glycan-binding proteins, including galectins have been demonstrated to interfere with, or to contribute to, TNFSF/TNFRSF signalling. Henceforth, it was found that galectin-3-mediated activation of AKT could inhibit TRAIL-induced apoptosis in the human breast carcinoma cell line BT459 [325]. Likewise, ectopic expression of galectin-3 in the human bladder carcinoma cell line J82, or in papillary thyroid cancer cells was found to inhibit TRAIL-induced cell death, owing galectin-3's ability to induce phosphorylation of Akt on serine 473 [326, 327]. In B and T lymphoma cell lines, by contrast, galectin-3 was not only found to be required for FasL-induced apoptosis but also associated with type I cells, characterized by their propensity to induce strong activation of the caspase-8 [328]. Noteworthy, galectin-3 was found in this study to interact with Fas, even in the absence of FasL [328]. Using the galectin-3-deficient cell line BT459, Mazurek and collaborators demonstrated that restoration of TRAIL-induced cell death by galectin-3 required its phosphorylation on serine-6 [329] and that TRAIL sensitivity may be influenced by a sequence polymorphism commonly found in galectin-3 coding for Pro64/His64, associated with breast cancer incidence [330]. This team also found out that the generation of a stable TRAIL-resistant clone, derived from the metastatic human colon cancer cell line LS-LiM6, by repeated exposure to TRAIL was associated with an increase in galectin-3 at the cell surface [331]. Interestingly, the authors also discovered that cell surface expressed galectin-3 could interact with both DR4 and DR5, and that inhibitors of glycosylation could restore TRAIL sensitivity in this resistant clone (Fig. 11.9).

In line with these findings that galectins are likely to regulate TNFSF/TNFRSF signalling through direct interaction with TNFRSF receptors, it has been demonstrated by Wazel and collaborators in two human leukemic T cell lines, namely Jurkat and CEM, that apoptosis induced by galectin-1 involved direct binding of the lectin to Fas and activation of caspase-8 [332]. More recently, a seminal work published by Croft and collaborators demonstrates that galectin-9 is not only able to interact with 4-1BB but is required for receptor aggregation and signalling [333].

Galectins are carbohydrate-binding proteins displaying high affinity for beta-galactoside containing glycoproteins. They are potentially able to bind to a large spectrum of glycosylated proteins and to behave differentially on a given signalling pathway depending on the cellular context [334] or their ability to bind to their interaction partners [335]. Binding of galectin-3 to galactoside moieties, for example, is severely compromised when its carbohydrate-binding partner is sialylated [336]. Moreover, as highlighted by Bresalier and collaborators, localization of these lectins, either intracellular or secreted, is also likely to determine their ability to interfere directly or not with a given target. Albeit these issues are scarcely evaluated altogether in most studies, galectins as well as TNFSFs and/or TNFRSFs glycosylation status are likely to play important regulatory functions.

11.4 Conclusion

It is becoming increasingly clear that TNFSF/TNFRSF ligand/receptor signalling is not only regulated by protein–protein interactions but also regulated by posttranslational modifications. Proteolytic cleavage, palmitoylation, and glycosylation events, occurring on a growing number of ligands and receptors of this family, have been found to change their signal transduction capabilities. Given that most of them harbor putative PTM sites and that PTMs are subject to major qualitative changes by metabolic flux [337], inflammation [338, 339], or diseases [340] such as cancer [341], understanding to what extent the family is concerned with these PTMs is likely to open novel clinical therapeutic opportunities, not only for autoimmune diseases or inflammation but also for cancer therapy.

Acknowledgments I apologize to the many authors whose excellent works could not be cited because of space limitations. Research in OM laboratory is supported by grants from the program "Investissements d'Avenir" with reference ANR-11-LABX-0021-01-LipSTIC Labex, the Conseil Regional de Bourgogne, la Ligue Nationale Contre le Cancer and the ANR (Agence Nationale de la Recherche, SphingoDR).

References

1. Stuber E, Neurath M, Calderhead D, Fell HP, Strober W (1995) Cross-linking of OX40 ligand, a member of the TNF/NGF cytokine family, induces proliferation and differentiation in murine splenic B cells. Immunity 2(5):507–521
2. Wiley SR, Schooley K, Smolak PJ, Din WS, Huang CP, Nicholl JK, Sutherland GR, Smith TD, Rauch C, Smith CA (1995) Identification and characterization of a new member of the TNF family that induces apoptosis. Immunity 3(6):673–682
3. Kowalczyk-Quintas C, Schneider P (2014) Ectodysplasin A (EDA) - EDA receptor signalling and its pharmacological modulation. Cytokine Growth Factor Rev 25(2):195–203. doi:10.1016/j.cytogfr.2014.01.004
4. Croft M (2014) The TNF family in T cell differentiation and function--unanswered questions and future directions. Semin Immunol 26(3):183–190. doi:10.1016/j.smim.2014.02.005
5. Blaser H, Dostert C, Mak TW, Brenner D (2016) TNF and ROS crosstalk in inflammation. Trends Cell Biol 26(4):249–261. doi:10.1016/j.tcb.2015.12.002
6. MacEwan DJ (2002) TNF ligands and receptors--a matter of life and death. Br J Pharmacol 135(4):855–875. doi:10.1038/sj.bjp.0704549
7. Bodmer JL, Schneider P, Tschopp J (2002) The molecular architecture of the TNF superfamily. Trends Biochem Sci 27(1):19–26. S0968000401019958 [pii]
8. Armitage RJ (1994) Tumor necrosis factor receptor superfamily members and their ligands. Curr Opin Immunol 6(3):407–413
9. Croft M (2009) The role of TNF superfamily members in T-cell function and diseases. Nat Rev Immunol 9(4):271–285. doi:10.1038/nri2526
10. So T, Lee SW, Croft M (2006) Tumor necrosis factor/tumor necrosis factor receptor family members that positively regulate immunity. Int J Hematol 83(1):1–11. doi:10.1532/IJH97.05120
11. Mirandola P, Ponti C, Gobbi G, Sponzilli I, Vaccarezza M, Cocco L, Zauli G, Secchiero P, Manzoli FA, Vitale M (2004) Activated human NK and CD8+ T cells express both TNF-

related apoptosis-inducing ligand (TRAIL) and TRAIL receptors but are resistant to TRAIL-mediated cytotoxicity. Blood 104(8):2418–2424
12. Kashii Y, Giorda R, Herberman RB, Whiteside TL, Vujanovic NL (1999) Constitutive expression and role of the TNF family ligands in apoptotic killing of tumor cells by human NK cells. J Immunol 163(10):5358–5366
13. Zhai Y, Ni J, Jiang GW, Lu J, Xing L, Lincoln C, Carter KC, Janat F, Kozak D, Xu S, Rojas L, Aggarwal BB, Ruben S, Li LY, Gentz R, GL Y (1999) VEGI, a novel cytokine of the tumor necrosis factor family, is an angiogenesis inhibitor that suppresses the growth of colon carcinomas in vivo. FASEB J 13(1):181–189
14. Laurikkala J, Pispa J, Jung HS, Nieminen P, Mikkola M, Wang X, Saarialho-Kere U, Galceran J, Grosschedl R, Thesleff I (2002) Regulation of hair follicle development by the TNF signal ectodysplasin and its receptor Edar. Development 129(10):2541–2553
15. Collette Y, Gilles A, Pontarotti P, Olive D (2003) A co-evolution perspective of the TNFSF and TNFRSF families in the immune system. Trends Immunol 24(7):387–394
16. Sedy J, Bekiaris V, Ware CF (2015) Tumor necrosis factor superfamily in innate immunity and inflammation. Cold Spring Harb Perspect Biol 7(4):a016279. doi:10.1101/cshperspect.a016279
17. Sonar S, Lal G (2015) Role of tumor necrosis factor superfamily in neuroinflammation and autoimmunity. Front Immunol 6:364. doi:10.3389/fimmu.2015.00364
18. Brenner D, Blaser H, Mak TW (2015) Regulation of tumour necrosis factor signalling: live or let die. Nat Rev Immunol 15(6):362–374. doi:10.1038/nri3834
19. Aganna E, Aksentijevich I, Hitman GA, Kastner DL, Hoepelman AI, Posma FD, Zweers EJ, McDermott MF (2001) Tumor necrosis factor receptor-associated periodic syndrome (TRAPS) in a Dutch family: evidence for a TNFRSF1A mutation with reduced penetrance. Eur J Hum Genet 9(1):63–66. doi:10.1038/sj.ejhg.5200573
20. McDermott MF, Aksentijevich I, Galon J, McDermott EM, Ogunkolade BW, Centola M, Mansfield E, Gadina M, Karenko L, Pettersson T, McCarthy J, Frucht DM, Aringer M, Torosyan Y, Teppo AM, Wilson M, Karaarslan HM, Wan Y, Todd I, Wood G, Schlimgen R, Kumarajeewa TR, Cooper SM, Vella JP, Amos CI, Mulley J, Quane KA, Molloy MG, Ranki A, Powell RJ, Hitman GA, O'Shea JJ, Kastner DL (1999) Germline mutations in the extracellular domains of the 55 kDa TNF receptor, TNFR1, define a family of dominantly inherited autoinflammatory syndromes. Cell 97(1):133–144
21. WD X, Zhao Y, Liu Y (2016) Role of the TWEAK/Fn14 pathway in autoimmune diseases. Immunol Res 64(1):44–50. doi:10.1007/s12026-015-8761-y
22. Chauhan M, Bombell S, McGuire W (2009) Tumour necrosis factor (--308A) polymorphism in very preterm infants with bronchopulmonary dysplasia: a meta-analysis. Arch Dis Child Fetal Neonatal Ed 94(4):F257–F259. doi:10.1136/adc.2008.153122
23. Schneider P, Street SL, Gaide O, Hertig S, Tardivel A, Tschopp J, Runkel L, Alevizopoulos K, Ferguson BM, Zonana J (2001) Mutations leading to X-linked hypohidrotic ectodermal dysplasia affect three major functional domains in the tumor necrosis factor family member ectodysplasin-A. J Biol Chem 276(22):18819–18827. doi:10.1074/jbc.M101280200
24. Miyamoto Y, Hanna DL, Zhang W, Baba H, Lenz HJ (2016) Molecular pathways: cachexia signaling-a targeted approach to cancer treatment. Clin Cancer Res. doi:10.1158/1078-0432.CCR-16-0495
25. Bell RB, Leidner RS, Crittenden MR, Curti BD, Feng Z, Montler R, Gough MJ, Fox BA, Weinberg AD, Urba WJ (2016) OX40 signaling in head and neck squamous cell carcinoma: overcoming immunosuppression in the tumor microenvironment. Oral Oncol 52:1–10. doi:10.1016/j.oraloncology.2015.11.009
26. van de Ven K, Borst J (2015) Targeting the T-cell co-stimulatory CD27/CD70 pathway in cancer immunotherapy: rationale and potential. Immunotherapy 7(6):655–667. doi:10.2217/imt.15.32
27. Richard AC, Ferdinand JR, Meylan F, Hayes ET, Gabay O, Siegel RM (2015) The TNF-family cytokine TL1A: from lymphocyte costimulator to disease co-conspirator. J Leukoc Biol 98(3):333–345. doi:10.1189/jlb.3RI0315-095R

28. Cullen SP, Martin SJ (2015) Fas and TRAIL 'death receptors' as initiators of inflammation: Implications for cancer. Semin Cell Dev Biol 39:26–34. doi:10.1016/j.semcdb.2015.01.012
29. Holland PM (2014) Death receptor agonist therapies for cancer, which is the right TRAIL? Cytokine Growth Factor Rev 25(2):185–193. doi:10.1016/j.cytogfr.2013.12.009
30. Fouque A, Debure L, Legembre P (2014) The CD95/CD95L signaling pathway: a role in carcinogenesis. Biochim Biophys Acta 1846(1):130–141. doi:10.1016/j.bbcan.2014.04.007
31. Pelekanou V, Kampa M, Kafousi M, Darivianaki K, Sanidas E, Tsiftsis DD, Stathopoulos EN, Tsapis A, Castanas E (2008) Expression of TNF-superfamily members BAFF and APRIL in breast cancer: immunohistochemical study in 52 invasive ductal breast carcinomas. BMC Cancer 8:76. doi:10.1186/1471-2407-8-76
32. Schneider P, Bodmer JL, Thome M, Hofmann K, Holler N, Tschopp J (1997) Characterization of two receptors for TRAIL. FEBS Lett 416(3):329–334
33. Degli-Esposti MA, Smolak PJ, Walczak H, Waugh J, Huang CP, DuBose RF, Goodwin RG, Smith CA (1997) Cloning and characterization of TRAIL-R3, a novel member of the emerging TRAIL receptor family. J Exp Med 186(7):1165–1170
34. Merino D, Lalaoui N, Morizot A, Solary E, Micheau O (2007) TRAIL in cancer therapy: present and future challenges. Expert Opin Ther Targets 11(10):1299–1314. doi:10.1517/14728222.11.10.1299
35. Glenney GW, Wiens GD (2007) Early diversification of the TNF superfamily in teleosts: genomic characterization and expression analysis. J Immunol 178(12):7955–7973
36. Bossen C, Ingold K, Tardivel A, Bodmer JL, Gaide O, Hertig S, Ambrose C, Tschopp J, Schneider P (2006) Interactions of tumor necrosis factor (TNF) and TNF receptor family members in the mouse and human. J Biol Chem 281(20):13964–13971. doi:10.1074/jbc.M601553200
37. Berg MM, Sternberg DW, Hempstead BL, Chao MV (1991) The low-affinity p75 nerve growth factor (NGF) receptor mediates NGF-induced tyrosine phosphorylation. Proc Natl Acad Sci U S A 88(16):7106–7110
38. Rodriguez-Tebar A, Dechant G, Barde YA (1990) Binding of brain-derived neurotrophic factor to the nerve growth factor receptor. Neuron 4(4):487–492
39. Dechant G, Tsoulfas P, Parada LF, Barde YA (1997) The neurotrophin receptor p75 binds neurotrophin-3 on sympathetic neurons with high affinity and specificity. J Neurosci 17(14):5281–5287
40. Nikolaev A, McLaughlin T, O'Leary DD, Tessier-Lavigne M (2009) APP binds DR6 to trigger axon pruning and neuron death via distinct caspases. Nature 457(7232):981–989. doi:10.1038/nature07767. nature07767 [pii]
41. Wang Z, Fan C, Zhou HF, Lu JS, Sun MJ, Song JW, Le Y, Jiang HD, Wang LH, Jiao BH (2014) S5a binds to death receptor-6 to induce THP-1 monocytes to differentiate through the activation of the NF-kappaB pathway. J Cell Sci 127(Pt 15):3257–3268. doi:10.1242/jcs.144105
42. Loetscher H, Pan YC, Lahm HW, Gentz R, Brockhaus M, Tabuchi H, Lesslauer W (1990) Molecular cloning and expression of the human 55 kd tumor necrosis factor receptor. Cell 61(2):351–359
43. Gray PW, Barrett K, Chantry D, Turner M, Feldmann M (1990) Cloning of human tumor necrosis factor (TNF) receptor cDNA and expression of recombinant soluble TNF-binding protein. Proc Natl Acad Sci U S A 87(19):7380–7384
44. Nophar Y, Kemper O, Brakebusch C, Englemann H, Zwang R, Aderka D, Holtmann H, Wallach D (1990) Soluble forms of tumor necrosis factor receptors (TNF-Rs). The cDNA for the type I TNF-R, cloned using amino acid sequence data of its soluble form, encodes both the cell surface and a soluble form of the receptor. EMBO J 9(10):3269–3278
45. Gray PW, Aggarwal BB, Benton CV, Bringman TS, Henzel WJ, Jarrett JA, Leung DW, Moffat B, Ng P, Svedersky LP et al (1984) Cloning and expression of cDNA for human lymphotoxin, a lymphokine with tumour necrosis activity. Nature 312(5996):721–724
46. Shirai T, Yamaguchi H, Ito H, Todd CW, Wallace RB (1985) Cloning and expression in Escherichia coli of the gene for human tumour necrosis factor. Nature 313(6005):803–806

47. Heller RA, Song K, Onasch MA, Fischer WH, Chang D, Ringold GM (1990) Complementary DNA cloning of a receptor for tumor necrosis factor and demonstration of a shed form of the receptor. Proc Natl Acad Sci U S A 87(16):6151–6155
48. Kohno T, Brewer MT, Baker SL, Schwartz PE, King MW, Hale KK, Squires CH, Thompson RC, Vannice JL (1990) A second tumor necrosis factor receptor gene product can shed a naturally occurring tumor necrosis factor inhibitor. Proc Natl Acad Sci U S A 87(21):8331–8335
49. Baens M, Chaffanet M, Cassiman JJ, van den Berghe H, Marynen P (1993) Construction and evaluation of a hncDNA library of human 12p transcribed sequences derived from a somatic cell hybrid. Genomics 16(1):214–218. doi:10.1006/geno.1993.1161
50. Kobayashi Y, Miyamoto D, Asada M, Obinata M, Osawa T (1986) Cloning and expression of human lymphotoxin mRNA derived from a human T cell hybridoma. J Biochem 100(3):727–733
51. Browning JL, Ngam-ek A, Lawton P, DeMarinis J, Tizard R, Chow EP, Hession C, O'Brine-Greco B, Foley SF, Ware CF (1993) Lymphotoxin beta, a novel member of the TNF family that forms a heteromeric complex with lymphotoxin on the cell surface. Cell 72(6):847–856
52. Baum PR, Gayle RB III, Ramsdell F, Srinivasan S, Sorensen RA, Watson ML, Seldin MF, Baker E, Sutherland GR, Clifford KN et al (1994) Molecular characterization of murine and human OX40/OX40 ligand systems: identification of a human OX40 ligand as the HTLV-1-regulated protein gp34. EMBO J 13(17):3992–4001
53. Mallett S, Fossum S, Barclay AN (1990) Characterization of the MRC OX40 antigen of activated CD4 positive T lymphocytes--a molecule related to nerve growth factor receptor. EMBO J 9(4):1063–1068
54. Graf D, Korthauer U, Mages HW, Senger G, Kroczek RA (1992) Cloning of TRAP, a ligand for CD40 on human T cells. Eur J Immunol 22(12):3191–3194. doi:10.1002/eji.1830221226
55. Oehm A, Behrmann I, Falk W, Pawlita M, Maier G, Klas C, Li-Weber M, Richards S, Dhein J, Trauth BC et al (1992) Purification and molecular cloning of the APO-1 cell surface antigen, a member of the tumor necrosis factor/nerve growth factor receptor superfamily. Sequence identity with the Fas antigen. J Biol Chem 267(15):10709–10715
56. Suda T, Takahashi T, Golstein P, Nagata S (1993) Molecular cloning and expression of the Fas ligand, a novel member of the tumor necrosis factor family. Cell 75(6):1169–1178
57. Pitti RM, Marsters SA, Lawrence DA, Roy M, Kischkel FC, Dowd P, Huang A, Donahue CJ, Sherwood SW, Baldwin DT, Godowski PJ, Wood WI, Gurney AL, Hillan KJ, Cohen RL, Goddard AD, Botstein D, Ashkenazi A (1998) Genomic amplification of a decoy receptor for Fas ligand in lung and colon cancer. Nature 396(6712):699–703
58. Mauri DN, Ebner R, Montgomery RI, Kochel KD, Cheung TC, GL Y, Ruben S, Murphy M, Eisenberg RJ, Cohen GH, Spear PG, Ware CF (1998) LIGHT, a new member of the TNF superfamily, and lymphotoxin alpha are ligands for herpesvirus entry mediator. Immunity 8(1):21–30
59. Yu KY, Kwon B, Ni J, Zhai Y, Ebner R, Kwon BS (1999) A newly identified member of tumor necrosis factor receptor superfamily (TR6) suppresses LIGHT-mediated apoptosis. J Biol Chem 274(20):13733–13736
60. Migone TS, Zhang J, Luo X, Zhuang L, Chen C, Hu B, Hong JS, Perry JW, Chen SF, Zhou JX, Cho YH, Ullrich S, Kanakaraj P, Carrell J, Boyd E, Olsen HS, Hu G, Pukac L, Liu D, Ni J, Kim S, Gentz R, Feng P, Moore PA, Ruben SM, Wei P (2002) TL1A is a TNF-like ligand for DR3 and TR6/DcR3 and functions as a T cell costimulator. Immunity 16(3):479–492
61. Wang W, Zhang M, Sun W, Yang S, Su Y, Zhang H, Liu C, Li X, Lin L, Kim S, Okunieff P, Zhang Z, Zhang L (2013) Reduction of decoy receptor 3 enhances TRAIL-mediated apoptosis in pancreatic cancer. PLoS One 8(10):e74272. doi:10.1371/journal.pone.0074272
62. Camerini D, Walz G, Loenen WA, Borst J, Seed B (1991) The T cell activation antigen CD27 is a member of the nerve growth factor/tumor necrosis factor receptor gene family. J Immunol 147(9):3165–3169
63. Goodwin RG, Alderson MR, Smith CA, Armitage RJ, VandenBos T, Jerzy R, Tough TW, Schoenborn MA, Davis-Smith T, Hennen K et al (1993) Molecular and biological charac-

terization of a ligand for CD27 defines a new family of cytokines with homology to tumor necrosis factor. Cell 73(3):447–456
64. Durkop H, Latza U, Hummel M, Eitelbach F, Seed B, Stein H (1992) Molecular cloning and expression of a new member of the nerve growth factor receptor family that is characteristic for Hodgkin's disease. Cell 68(3):421–427
65. Gruss HJ, Herrmann F (1996) CD30 ligand, a member of the TNF ligand superfamily, with growth and activation control CD30+ lymphoid and lymphoma cells. Leuk Lymphoma 20(5-6):397–409. doi:10.3109/10428199609052421
66. Kwon BS, Weissman SM (1989) cDNA sequences of two inducible T-cell genes. Proc Natl Acad Sci U S A 86(6):1963–1967
67. Goodwin RG, Din WS, Davis-Smith T, Anderson DM, Gimpel SD, Sato TA, Maliszewski CR, Brannan CI, Copeland NG, Jenkins NA et al (1993) Molecular cloning of a ligand for the inducible T cell gene 4-1BB: a member of an emerging family of cytokines with homology to tumor necrosis factor. Eur J Immunol 23(10):2631–2641. doi:10.1002/eji.1830231037
68. Pan G, O'Rourke K, Chinnaiyan AM, Gentz R, Ebner R, Ni J, Dixit VM (1997) The receptor for the cytotoxic ligand TRAIL. Science 276(5309):111–113
69. Mongiat M, Ligresti G, Marastoni S, Lorenzon E, Doliana R, Colombatti A (2007) Regulation of the extrinsic apoptotic pathway by the extracellular matrix glycoprotein EMILIN2. Mol Cell Biol 27(20):7176–7187. doi:10.1128/MCB.00696-07
70. MacFarlane M, Ahmad M, Srinivasula SM, Fernandes-Alnemri T, Cohen GM, Alnemri ES (1997) Identification and molecular cloning of two novel receptors for the cytotoxic ligand TRAIL. J Biol Chem 272(41):25417–25420
71. Walczak H, Degli-Esposti MA, Johnson RS, Smolak PJ, Waugh JY, Boiani N, Timour MS, Gerhart MJ, Schooley KA, Smith CA, Goodwin RG, Rauch CT (1997) TRAIL-R2: a novel apoptosis-mediating receptor for TRAIL. EMBO J 16(17):5386–5397
72. Chaudhary PM, Eby M, Jasmin A, Bookwalter A, Murray J, Hood L (1997) Death receptor 5, a new member of the TNFR family, and DR4 induce FADD-dependent apoptosis and activate the NF-kappaB pathway. Immunity 7(6):821–830
73. Nemcovicova I, Benedict CA, Zajonc DM (2013) Structure of human cytomegalovirus UL141 binding to TRAIL-R2 reveals novel, non-canonical death receptor interactions. PLoS Pathog 9(3):e1003224. doi:10.1371/journal.ppat.1003224
74. Smith W, Tomasec P, Aicheler R, Loewendorf A, Nemcovicova I, Wang EC, Stanton RJ, Macauley M, Norris P, Willen L, Ruckova E, Nomoto A, Schneider P, Hahn G, Zajonc DM, Ware CF, Wilkinson GW, Benedict CA (2013) Human cytomegalovirus glycoprotein UL141 targets the TRAIL death receptors to thwart host innate antiviral defenses. Cell Host Microbe 13(3):324–335. doi:10.1016/j.chom.2013.02.003
75. Pan G, Ni J, Wei YF, Yu G, Gentz R, Dixit VM (1997) An antagonist decoy receptor and a death domain-containing receptor for TRAIL. Science 277(5327):815–818
76. Sheridan JP, Marsters SA, Pitti RM, Gurney A, Skubatch M, Baldwin D, Ramakrishnan L, Gray CL, Baker K, Wood WI, Goddard AD, Godowski P, Ashkenazi A (1997) Control of TRAIL-induced apoptosis by a family of signaling and decoy receptors. Science 277(5327):818–821
77. Marsters SA, Sheridan JP, Pitti RM, Huang A, Skubatch M, Baldwin D, Yuan J, Gurney A, Goddard AD, Godowski P, Ashkenazi A (1997) A novel receptor for Apo2L/TRAIL contains a truncated death domain. Curr Biol 7(12):1003–1006
78. Pan G, Ni J, Yu G, Wei YF, Dixit VM (1998) TRUNDD, a new member of the TRAIL receptor family that antagonizes TRAIL signalling. FEBS Lett 424(1-2):41–45
79. Anderson DM, Maraskovsky E, Billingsley WL, Dougall WC, Tometsko ME, Roux ER, Teepe MC, DuBose RF, Cosman D, Galibert L (1997) A homologue of the TNF receptor and its ligand enhance T-cell growth and dendritic-cell function. Nature 390(6656):175–179. doi:10.1038/36593
80. Wong BR, Rho J, Arron J, Robinson E, Orlinick J, Chao M, Kalachikov S, Cayani E, Bartlett FS III, Frankel WN, Lee SY, Choi Y (1997) TRANCE is a novel ligand of the tumor necrosis factor receptor family that activates c-Jun N-terminal kinase in T cells. J Biol Chem 272(40):25190–25194

81. Simonet WS, Lacey DL, Dunstan CR, Kelley M, Chang MS, Luthy R, Nguyen HQ, Wooden S, Bennett L, Boone T, Shimamoto G, DeRose M, Elliott R, Colombero A, Tan HL, Trail G, Sullivan J, Davy E, Bucay N, Renshaw-Gegg L, Hughes TM, Hill D, Pattison W, Campbell P, Sander S, Van G, Tarpley J, Derby P, Lee R, Boyle WJ (1997) Osteoprotegerin: a novel secreted protein involved in the regulation of bone density. Cell 89(2):309–319. S0092-8674(00)80209-3 [pii]
82. Meighan-Mantha RL, Hsu DK, Guo Y, Brown SA, Feng SL, Peifley KA, Alberts GF, Copeland NG, Gilbert DJ, Jenkins NA, Richards CM, Winkles JA (1999) The mitogen-inducible Fn14 gene encodes a type I transmembrane protein that modulates fibroblast adhesion and migration. J Biol Chem 274(46):33166–33176
83. Wiley SR, Cassiano L, Lofton T, Davis-Smith T, Winkles JA, Lindner V, Liu H, Daniel TO, Smith CA, Fanslow WC (2001) A novel TNF receptor family member binds TWEAK and is implicated in angiogenesis. Immunity 15(5):837–846
84. von Bulow GU, Bram RJ (1997) NF-AT activation induced by a CAML-interacting member of the tumor necrosis factor receptor superfamily. Science 278(5335):138–141
85. Hahne M, Kataoka T, Schroter M, Hofmann K, Irmler M, Bodmer JL, Schneider P, Bornand T, Holler N, French LE, Sordat B, Rimoldi D, Tschopp J (1998) APRIL, a new ligand of the tumor necrosis factor family, stimulates tumor cell growth. J Exp Med 188(6):1185–1190
86. Shu HB, Hu WH, Johnson H (1999) TALL-1 is a novel member of the TNF family that is down-regulated by mitogens. J Leukoc Biol 65(5):680–683
87. Thompson JS, Bixler SA, Qian F, Vora K, Scott ML, Cachero TG, Hession C, Schneider P, Sizing ID, Mullen C, Strauch K, Zafari M, Benjamin CD, Tschopp J, Browning JL, Ambrose C (2001) BAFF-R, a newly identified TNF receptor that specifically interacts with BAFF. Science 293(5537):2108–2111. doi:10.1126/science.1061965
88. Mukhopadhyay A, Ni J, Zhai Y, Yu GL, Aggarwal BB (1999) Identification and characterization of a novel cytokine, THANK, a TNF homologue that activates apoptosis, nuclear factor-kappaB, and c-Jun NH2-terminal kinase. J Biol Chem 274(23):15978–15981
89. Schneider P, MacKay F, Steiner V, Hofmann K, Bodmer JL, Holler N, Ambrose C, Lawton P, Bixler S, Acha-Orbea H, Valmori D, Romero P, Werner-Favre C, Zubler RH, Browning JL, Tschopp J (1999) BAFF, a novel ligand of the tumor necrosis factor family, stimulates B cell growth. J Exp Med 189(11):1747–1756
90. Montgomery RI, Warner MS, Lum BJ, Spear PG (1996) Herpes simplex virus-1 entry into cells mediated by a novel member of the TNF/NGF receptor family. Cell 87(3):427–436
91. Watanabe N, Gavrieli M, Sedy JR, Yang J, Fallarino F, Loftin SK, Hurchla MA, Zimmerman N, Sim J, Zang X, Murphy TL, Russell JH, Allison JP, Murphy KM (2003) BTLA is a lymphocyte inhibitory receptor with similarities to CTLA-4 and PD-1. Nat Immunol 4(7):670–679. doi:10.1038/ni944
92. Sedy JR, Gavrieli M, Potter KG, Hurchla MA, Lindsley RC, Hildner K, Scheu S, Pfeffer K, Ware CF, Murphy TL, Murphy KM (2005) B and T lymphocyte attenuator regulates T cell activation through interaction with herpesvirus entry mediator. Nat Immunol 6(1):90–98. doi:10.1038/ni1144
93. Chao MV, Bothwell MA, Ross AH, Koprowski H, Lanahan AA, Buck CR, Sehgal A (1986) Gene transfer and molecular cloning of the human NGF receptor. Science 232(4749):518–521
94. Borsani G, Pizzuti A, Rugarli EI, Falini A, Silani V, Sidoli A, Scarlato G, Baralle FE (1990) cDNA sequence of human beta-NGF. Nucleic Acids Res 18(13):4020
95. Jones KR, Reichardt LF (1990) Molecular cloning of a human gene that is a member of the nerve growth factor family. Proc Natl Acad Sci U S A 87(20):8060–8064
96. Maisonpierre PC, Belluscio L, Squinto S, Ip NY, Furth ME, Lindsay RM, Yancopoulos GD (1990) Neurotrophin-3: a neurotrophic factor related to NGF and BDNF. Science 247(4949 Pt 1):1446–1451
97. Ip NY, Ibanez CF, Nye SH, McClain J, Jones PF, Gies DR, Belluscio L, Le Beau MM, Espinosa R III, Squinto SP et al (1992) Mammalian neurotrophin-4: structure, chromosomal localization, tissue distribution, and receptor specificity. Proc Natl Acad Sci U S A 89(7):3060–3064

98. Laabi Y, Gras MP, Carbonnel F, Brouet JC, Berger R, Larsen CJ, Tsapis A (1992) A new gene, BCM, on chromosome 16 is fused to the interleukin 2 gene by a t(4;16)(q26;p13) translocation in a malignant T cell lymphoma. EMBO J 11(11):3897–3904
99. Nocentini G, Giunchi L, Ronchetti S, Krausz LT, Bartoli A, Moraca R, Migliorati G, Riccardi C (1997) A new member of the tumor necrosis factor/nerve growth factor receptor family inhibits T cell receptor-induced apoptosis. Proc Natl Acad Sci U S A 94(12):6216–6221
100. Kim JD, Choi BK, Bae JS, Lee UH, Han IS, Lee HW, Youn BS, Vinay DS, Kwon BS (2003) Cloning and characterization of GITR ligand. Genes Immun 4(8):564–569. doi:10.1038/sj.gene.6364026
101. Robertson NG, Khetarpal U, Gutierrez-Espeleta GA, Bieber FR, Morton CC (1994) Isolation of novel and known genes from a human fetal cochlear cDNA library using subtractive hybridization and differential screening. Genomics 23(1):42–50. doi:10.1006/geno.1994.1457
102. Sica GL, Zhu G, Tamada K, Liu D, Ni J, Chen L (2001) RELT, a new member of the tumor necrosis factor receptor superfamily, is selectively expressed in hematopoietic tissues and activates transcription factor NF-kappaB. Blood 97(9):2702–2707
103. Pan G, Bauer JH, Haridas V, Wang S, Liu D, Yu G, Vincenz C, Aggarwal BB, Ni J, Dixit VM (1998) Identification and functional characterization of DR6, a novel death domain-containing TNF receptor. FEBS Lett 431(3):351–356
104. Chinnaiyan AM, O'Rourke K, Yu GL, Lyons RH, Garg M, Duan DR, Xing L, Gentz R, Ni J, Dixit VM (1996) Signal transduction by DR3, a death domain-containing receptor related to TNFR-1 and CD95. Science 274(5289):990–992
105. Yan M, Wang LC, Hymowitz SG, Schilbach S, Lee J, Goddard A, de Vos AM, Gao WQ, Dixit VM (2000) Two-amino acid molecular switch in an epithelial morphogen that regulates binding to two distinct receptors. Science 290(5491):523–527
106. Kere J, Srivastava AK, Montonen O, Zonana J, Thomas N, Ferguson B, Munoz F, Morgan D, Clarke A, Baybayan P, Chen EY, Ezer S, Saarialho-Kere U, de la Chapelle A, Schlessinger D (1996) X-linked anhidrotic (hypohidrotic) ectodermal dysplasia is caused by mutation in a novel transmembrane protein. Nat Genet 13(4):409–416. doi:10.1038/ng0895-409
107. De Trez C, Schneider K, Potter K, Droin N, Fulton J, Norris PS, Ha SW, YX F, Murphy T, Murphy KM, Pfeffer K, Benedict CA, Ware CF (2008) The inhibitory HVEM-BTLA pathway counter regulates lymphotoxin receptor signaling to achieve homeostasis of dendritic cells. J Immunol 180(1):238–248
108. Carfi A, Willis SH, Whitbeck JC, Krummenacher C, Cohen GH, Eisenberg RJ, Wiley DC (2001) Herpes simplex virus glycoprotein D bound to the human receptor HveA. Mol Cell 8(1):169–179
109. Terry-Allison T, Montgomery RI, Whitbeck JC, Xu R, Cohen GH, Eisenberg RJ, Spear PG (1998) HveA (herpesvirus entry mediator A), a coreceptor for herpes simplex virus entry, also participates in virus-induced cell fusion. J Virol 72(7):5802–5810
110. Popkin DL, HWt V (2003) Murine cytomegalovirus infection inhibits tumor necrosis factor alpha responses in primary macrophages. J Virol 77(18):10125–10130
111. Seirafian S, Prod'homme V, Sugrue D, Davies J, Fielding C, Tomasec P, Wilkinson GW (2014) Human cytomegalovirus suppresses Fas expression and function. J Gen Virol 95(Pt 4):933–939. doi:10.1099/vir.0.058313-0
112. Di Giovine P, Settembre EC, Bhargava AK, Luftig MA, Lou H, Cohen GH, Eisenberg RJ, Krummenacher C, Carfi A (2011) Structure of herpes simplex virus glycoprotein d bound to the human receptor nectin-1. PLoS Pathog 7(9). doi:10.1371/journal.ppat.1002277. ARTN e1002277
113. Nemcovicova I, Zajonc DM (2014) The structure of cytomegalovirus immune modulator UL141 highlights structural Ig-fold versatility for receptor binding. Acta Crystallogr D Biol Crystallogr 70:851–862. doi:10.1107/S1399004713033750
114. Aoyama E, Kubota S, Khattab HM, Nishida T, Takigawa M (2015) CCN2 enhances RANKL-induced osteoclast differentiation via direct binding to RANK and OPG. Bone 73:242–248. doi:10.1016/j.bone.2014.12.058

115. Tang W, Lu Y, Tian QY, Zhang Y, Guo FJ, Liu GY, Syed NM, Lai Y, Lin EA, Kong L, Su J, Yin F, Ding AH, Zanin-Zhorov A, Dustin ML, Tao J, Craft J, Yin Z, Feng JQ, Abramson SB, XP Y, Liu CJ (2011) The growth factor progranulin binds to TNF receptors and is therapeutic against inflammatory arthritis in mice. Science 332(6028):478–484. doi:10.1126/science.1199214
116. Liu C, Li XX, Gao W, Liu W, Liu DS (2014) Progranulin-derived Atsttrin directly binds to TNFRSF25 (DR3) and inhibits TNF-like ligand 1A (TL1A) activity. PLoS One 9(3):e92743. doi:10.1371/journal.pone.0092743
117. Warzocha K, Bienvenu J, Coiffier B, Salles G (1995) Mechanisms of action of the tumor necrosis factor and lymphotoxin ligand-receptor system. Eur Cytokine Netw 6(2):83–96
118. Browning JL, Miatkowski K, Griffiths DA, Bourdon PR, Hession C, Ambrose CM, Meier W (1996) Preparation and characterization of soluble recombinant heterotrimeric complexes of human lymphotoxins alpha and beta. J Biol Chem 271(15):8618–8626
119. Schuepbach-Mallepell S, Das D, Willen L, Vigolo M, Tardivel A, Lebon L, Kowalczyk-Quintas C, Nys J, Smulski C, Zheng TS, Maskos K, Lammens A, Jiang X, Hess H, Tan SL, Schneider P (2015) Stoichiometry of heteromeric BAFF and APRIL cytokines dictates their receptor binding and signaling properties. J Biol Chem 290(26):16330–16342. doi:10.1074/jbc.M115.661405
120. Lalaoui N, Morle A, Merino D, Jacquemin G, Iessi E, Morizot A, Shirley S, Robert B, Solary E, Garrido C, Micheau O (2011) TRAIL-R4 promotes tumor growth and resistance to apoptosis in cervical carcinoma HeLa cells through AKT. PLoS One 6(5):e19679. doi:10.1371/journal.pone.0019679
121. Lee HW, Lee SH, Lee HW, Ryu YW, Kwon MH, Kim YS (2005) Homomeric and heteromeric interactions of the extracellular domains of death receptors and death decoy receptors. Biochem Biophys Res Commun 330(4):1205–1212
122. Neumann S, Hasenauer J, Pollak N, Scheurich P (2014) Dominant negative effects of tumor necrosis factor (TNF)-related apoptosis-inducing ligand (TRAIL) receptor 4 on TRAIL receptor 1 signaling by formation of heteromeric complexes. J Biol Chem 289:16576–16587. doi:10.1074/jbc.M114.559468
123. Merino D, Lalaoui N, Morizot A, Schneider P, Solary E, Micheau O (2006) Differential inhibition of TRAIL-mediated DR5-DISC formation by decoy receptors 1 and 2. Mol Cell Biol 26(19):7046–7055
124. Schneider P, Thome M, Burns K, Bodmer JL, Hofmann K, Kataoka T, Holler N, Tschopp J (1997) TRAIL receptors 1 (DR4) and 2 (DR5) signal FADD-dependent apoptosis and activate NF-kappaB. Immunity 7(6):831–836
125. Kischkel FC, Lawrence DA, Chuntharapai A, Schow P, Kim KJ, Ashkenazi A (2000) Apo2L/TRAIL-dependent recruitment of endogenous FADD and caspase-8 to death receptors 4 and 5. Immunity 12(6):611–620
126. Yang S, Wang Y, Mei K, Zhang S, Sun X, Ren F, Liu S, Yang Z, Wang X, Qin Z, Chang Z (2015) Tumor necrosis factor receptor 2 (TNFR2).interleukin-17 receptor D (IL-17RD) heteromerization reveals a novel mechanism for NF-kappaB activation. J Biol Chem 290(2):861–871. doi:10.1074/jbc.M114.586560
127. Al-Lamki RS, Mayadas TN (2015) TNF receptors: signaling pathways and contribution to renal dysfunction. Kidney Int 87(2):281–296. doi:10.1038/ki.2014.285
128. Reinehr R, Schliess F, Haussinger D (2003) Hyperosmolarity and CD95L trigger CD95/EGF receptor association and tyrosine phosphorylation of CD95 as prerequisites for CD95 membrane trafficking and DISC formation. FASEB J 17(6):731–733. doi:10.1096/fj.02-0915fje
129. Eberle A, Reinehr R, Becker S, Haussinger D (2005) Fluorescence resonance energy transfer analysis of proapoptotic CD95-EGF receptor interactions in Huh7 cells. Hepatology (Baltimore, MD) 41(2):315–326. doi:10.1002/hep.20564
130. Eberle A, Reinehr R, Becker S, Keitel V, Haussinger D (2007) CD95 tyrosine phosphorylation is required for CD95 oligomerization. Apoptosis 12(4):719–729. doi:10.1007/s10495-006-0003-2

131. Smyth LA, Brady HJ (2005) cMet and Fas receptor interaction inhibits death-inducing signaling complex formation in endothelial cells. Hypertension 46(1):100–106. doi:10.1161/01.HYP.0000167991.82153.16
132. Du W, Uslar L, Sevala S, Shah K (2014) Targeting c-Met receptor overcomes TRAIL-resistance in brain tumors. PLoS One 9(4):e95490. doi:10.1371/journal.pone.0095490
133. Wang X, DeFrances MC, Dai Y, Pediaditakis P, Johnson C, Bell A, Michalopoulos GK, Zarnegar R (2002) A mechanism of cell survival: sequestration of Fas by the HGF receptor Met. Mol Cell 9(2):411–421
134. Shao Z, Browning JL, Lee X, Scott ML, Shulga-Morskaya S, Allaire N, Thill G, Levesque M, Sah D, McCoy JM, Murray B, Jung V, Pepinsky RB, Mi S (2005) TAJ/TROY, an orphan TNF receptor family member, binds Nogo-66 receptor 1 and regulates axonal regeneration. Neuron 45(3):353–359. doi:10.1016/j.neuron.2004.12.050
135. Park JB, Yiu G, Kaneko S, Wang J, Chang J, He XL, Garcia KC, He Z (2005) A TNF receptor family member, TROY, is a coreceptor with Nogo receptor in mediating the inhibitory activity of myelin inhibitors. Neuron 45(3):345–351. doi:10.1016/j.neuron.2004.12.040
136. Hauer J, Puschner S, Ramakrishnan P, Simon U, Bongers M, Federle C, Engelmann H (2005) TNF receptor (TNFR)-associated factor (TRAF) 3 serves as an inhibitor of TRAF2/5-mediated activation of the noncanonical NF-kappaB pathway by TRAF-binding TNFRs. Proc Natl Acad Sci U S A 102(8):2874–2879. doi:10.1073/pnas.0500187102
137. Tartaglia LA, Ayres TM, Wong GH, Goeddel DV (1993) A novel domain within the 55 kd TNF receptor signals cell death. Cell 74(5):845–853. 0092-8674(93)90464-2 [pii]
138. Adam D, Adam-Klages S, Kronke M (1995) Identification of p55 tumor necrosis factor receptor-associated proteins that couple to signaling pathways not initiated by the death domain. J Inflamm 47(1-2):61–66
139. Kim CH, Song YH, Park K, Oh Y, Lee TH (1995) Induction of cell death by myristylated death domain of p55 TNF receptor is not abolished by Iprcg-like point mutation in death domain. J Inflamm 45(4):312–322
140. Huang B, Eberstadt M, Olejniczak ET, Meadows RP, Fesik SW (1996) NMR structure and mutagenesis of the Fas (APO-1/CD95) death domain. Nature 384(6610):638–641. doi:10.1038/384638a0
141. ER MD III, Chui PC, Martelli PF, Dicker DT, El-Deiry WS (2001) Death domain mutagenesis of KILLER/DR5 reveals residues critical for apoptotic signaling. J Biol Chem 276(18):14939–14945
142. Sukits SF, Lin LL, Hsu S, Malakian K, Powers R, GY X (2001) Solution structure of the tumor necrosis factor receptor-1 death domain. J Mol Biol 310(4):895–906. doi:10.1006/jmbi.2001.4790
143. Bodmer JL, Burns K, Schneider P, Hofmann K, Steiner V, Thome M, Bornand T, Hahne M, Schroter M, Becker K, Wilson A, French LE, Browning JL, MacDonald HR, Tschopp J (1997) TRAMP, a novel apoptosis-mediating receptor with sequence homology to tumor necrosis factor receptor 1 and Fas(Apo-1/CD95). Immunity 6(1):79–88
144. Boldin MP, Mett IL, Varfolomeev EE, Chumakov I, Shemer-Avni Y, Camonis JH, Wallach D (1995) Self-association of the "death domains" of the p55 tumor necrosis factor (TNF) receptor and Fas/APO1 prompts signaling for TNF and Fas/APO1 effects. J Biol Chem 270(1):387–391
145. Kitson J, Raven T, Jiang YP, Goeddel DV, Giles KM, Pun KT, Grinham CJ, Brown R, Farrow SN (1996) A death-domain-containing receptor that mediates apoptosis. Nature 384(6607):372–375
146. Boldin MP, Goncharov TM, Goltsev YV, Wallach D (1996) Involvement of MACH, a novel MORT1/FADD-interacting protease, in Fas/APO-1- and TNF receptor-induced cell death. Cell 85(6):803–815
147. Chinnaiyan AM, Tepper CG, Seldin MF, O'Rourke K, Kischkel FC, Hellbardt S, Krammer PH, Peter ME, Dixit VM (1996) FADD/MORT1 is a common mediator of CD95 (Fas/APO-1) and tumor necrosis factor receptor-induced apoptosis. J Biol Chem 271(9):4961–4965

148. Kischkel FC, Hellbardt S, Behrmann I, Germer M, Pawlita M, Krammer PH, Peter ME (1995) Cytotoxicity-dependent APO-1 (Fas/CD95)-associated proteins form a death-inducing signaling complex (DISC) with the receptor. EMBO J 14(22):5579–5588
149. Medema JP, Scaffidi C, Kischkel FC, Shevchenko A, Mann M, Krammer PH, Peter ME (1997) FLICE is activated by association with the CD95 death-inducing signaling complex (DISC). EMBO J 16(10):2794–2804
150. Scaffidi C, Krammer PH, Peter ME (1999) Isolation and analysis of components of CD95 (APO-1/Fas) death-inducing signaling complex. Methods 17(4):287–291
151. Li H, Zhu H, CJ X, Yuan J (1998) Cleavage of BID by caspase 8 mediates the mitochondrial damage in the Fas pathway of apoptosis. Cell 94(4):491–501
152. Desagher S, Osen-Sand A, Nichols A, Eskes R, Montessuit S, Lauper S, Maundrell K, Antonsson B, Martinou JC (1999) Bid-induced conformational change of Bax is responsible for mitochondrial cytochrome c release during apoptosis. J Cell Biol 144(5):891–901
153. Zou H, Li Y, Liu X, Wang X (1999) An APAF-1.cytochrome c multimeric complex is a functional apoptosome that activates procaspase-9. J Biol Chem 274(17):11549–11556
154. Renatus M, Stennicke HR, Scott FL, Liddington RC, Salvesen GS (2001) Dimer formation drives the activation of the cell death protease caspase 9. Proc Natl Acad Sci U S A 98(25):14250–14255
155. Muzio M, Stockwell BR, Stennicke HR, Salvesen GS, Dixit VM (1998) An induced proximity model for caspase-8 activation. J Biol Chem 273(5):2926–2930
156. Micheau O, Thome M, Schneider P, Holler N, Tschopp J, Nicholson DW, Briand C, Grutter MG (2002) The long form of FLIP is an activator of caspase-8 at the Fas death-inducing signaling complex. J Biol Chem 277(47):45162–45171
157. Dickens LS, Boyd RS, Jukes-Jones R, Hughes MA, Robinson GL, Fairall L, Schwabe JW, Cain K, Macfarlane M (2012) A death effector domain chain DISC model reveals a crucial role for caspase-8 chain assembly in mediating apoptotic cell death. Mol Cell 47(2):291–305. doi:10.1016/j.molcel.2012.05.004
158. Schleich K, Warnken U, Fricker N, Ozturk S, Richter P, Kammerer K, Schnolzer M, Krammer PH, Lavrik IN (2012) Stoichiometry of the CD95 death-inducing signaling complex: experimental and modeling evidence for a death effector domain chain model. Mol Cell 47(2):306–319. doi:10.1016/j.molcel.2012.05.006
159. Schleich K, Krammer PH, Lavrik IN (2013) The chains of death: a new view on caspase-8 activation at the DISC. Cell Cycle (Georgetown Tex) 12(2):193–194. doi:10.4161/cc.23464
160. Morle A, Garrido C, Micheau O (2015) Hyperthermia restores apoptosis induced by death receptors through aggregation-induced c-FLIP cytosolic depletion. Cell Death Dis 6:e1633. doi:10.1038/cddis.2015.12
161. Berg D, Lehne M, Muller N, Siegmund D, Munkel S, Sebald W, Pfizenmaier K, Wajant H (2007) Enforced covalent trimerization increases the activity of the TNF ligand family members TRAIL and CD95L. Cell Death Differ 14(12):2021–2034. doi:10.1038/sj.cdd.4402213. 4402213 [pii]
162. Morizot A, Merino D, Lalaoui N, Jacquemin G, Granci V, Iessi E, Lanneau D, Bouyer F, Solary E, Chauffert B, Saas P, Garrido C, Micheau O (2011) Chemotherapy overcomes TRAIL-R4-mediated TRAIL resistance at the DISC level. Cell Death Differ 18(4):700–711. doi:10.1038/cdd.2010.144
163. Beg AA, Baltimore D (1996) An essential role for NF-kappaB in preventing TNF-alpha-induced cell death. Science 274(5288):782–784
164. Polunovsky VA, Wendt CH, Ingbar DH, Peterson MS, Bitterman PB (1994) Induction of endothelial cell apoptosis by TNF alpha: modulation by inhibitors of protein synthesis. Exp Cell Res 214(2):584–594. doi:10.1006/excr.1994.1296
165. Kreuz S, Siegmund D, Scheurich P, Wajant H (2001) NF-kappaB inducers upregulate cFLIP, a cycloheximide-sensitive inhibitor of death receptor signaling. Mol Cell Biol 21(12):3964–3973

166. Micheau O, Lens S, Gaide O, Alevizopoulos K, Tschopp J (2001) NF-kappaB signals induce the expression of c-FLIP. Mol Cell Biol 21(16):5299–5305
167. Yeh WC, de la Pompa JL, McCurrach ME, Shu HB, Elia AJ, Shahinian A, Ng M, Wakeham A, Khoo W, Mitchell K, El-Deiry WS, Lowe SW, Goeddel DV, Mak TW (1998) FADD: essential for embryo development and signaling from some, but not all, inducers of apoptosis. Science 279(5358):1954–1958
168. Harper N, Hughes M, MacFarlane M, Cohen GM (2003) Fas-associated death domain protein and caspase-8 are not recruited to the tumor necrosis factor receptor 1 signaling complex during tumor necrosis factor-induced apoptosis. J Biol Chem 278(28):25534–25541
169. Micheau O, Tschopp J (2003) Induction of TNF receptor I-mediated apoptosis via two sequential signaling complexes. Cell 114(2):181–190
170. Legler DF, Micheau O, Doucey MA, Tschopp J, Bron C (2003) Recruitment of TNF receptor 1 to lipid rafts is essential for TNFalpha-mediated NF-kappaB activation. Immunity 18(5):655–664
171. Ting AT, Pimentel-Muinos FX, Seed B (1996) RIP mediates tumor necrosis factor receptor 1 activation of NF-kappaB but not Fas/APO-1-initiated apoptosis. EMBO J 15(22):6189–6196
172. Hsu H, Shu HB, Pan MG, Goeddel DV (1996) TRADD-TRAF2 and TRADD-FADD interactions define two distinct TNF receptor 1 signal transduction pathways. Cell 84(2):299–308. S0092-8674(00)80984-8 [pii]
173. Hsu H, Xiong J, Goeddel DV (1995) The TNF receptor 1-associated protein TRADD signals cell death and NF-kappa B activation. Cell 81(4):495–504. 0092-8674(95)90070-5 [pii]
174. Shu HB, Takeuchi M, Goeddel DV (1996) The tumor necrosis factor receptor 2 signal transducers TRAF2 and c-IAP1 are components of the tumor necrosis factor receptor 1 signaling complex. Proc Natl Acad Sci U S A 93(24):13973–13978
175. Chhibber-Goel J, Coleman-Vaughan C, Agrawal V, Sawhney N, Hickey E, Powell JC, McCarthy JV (2016) gamma-Secretase activity is required for regulated intramembrane proteolysis of tumor necrosis factor (TNF) receptor 1 and TNF-mediated Pro-apoptotic signaling. J Biol Chem 291(11):5971–5985. doi:10.1074/jbc.M115.679076
176. Wen L, Zhuang L, Luo X, Wei P (2003) TL1A-induced NF-kappaB activation and c-IAP2 production prevent DR3-mediated apoptosis in TF-1 cells. J Biol Chem 278(40):39251–39258. doi:10.1074/jbc.M305833200
177. Ermolaeva MA, Michallet MC, Papadopoulou N, Utermohlen O, Kranidioti K, Kollias G, Tschopp J, Pasparakis M (2008) Function of TRADD in tumor necrosis factor receptor 1 signaling and in TRIF-dependent inflammatory responses. Nat Immunol 9(9):1037–1046. doi:10.1038/ni.1638
178. Pobezinskaya YL, Choksi S, Morgan MJ, Cao X, Liu ZG (2011) The adaptor protein TRADD is essential for TNF-like ligand 1A/death receptor 3 signaling. J Immunol 186(9):5212–5216. doi:10.4049/jimmunol.1002374
179. Thome M, Schneider P, Hofmann K, Fickenscher H, Meinl E, Neipel F, Mattmann C, Burns K, Bodmer JL, Schroter M, Scaffidi C, Krammer PH, Peter ME, Tschopp J (1997) Viral FLICE-inhibitory proteins (FLIPs) prevent apoptosis induced by death receptors. Nature 386(6624):517–521
180. Hu R, Du Q, Yin X, Li J, Wang T, Zhang L (2014) Agonist antibody activates death receptor 6 downstream signaling involving TRADD recruitment. FEBS Lett 588(3):401–407. doi:10.1016/j.febslet.2013.12.010
181. Zeng L, Li T, Xu DC, Liu J, Mao G, Cui MZ, Fu X, Xu X (2012) Death receptor 6 induces apoptosis not through type I or type II pathways, but via a unique mitochondria-dependent pathway by interacting with Bax protein. J Biol Chem 287(34):29125–29133. doi:10.1074/jbc.M112.362038
182. Freidin MM (2001) Antibody to the extracellular domain of the low affinity NGF receptor stimulates p75(NGFR)-mediated apoptosis in cultured sympathetic neurons. J Neurosci Res 64(4):331–340

183. Nichols A, Martinou I, Maundrell K, Martinou JC (1998) The p75 neurotrophin receptor: effects on neuron survival in vitro and interaction with death domain-containing adaptor proteins. Apoptosis 3(4):289–294
184. Wang X, Bauer JH, Li Y, Shao Z, Zetoune FS, Cattaneo E, Vincenz C (2001) Characterization of a p75(NTR) apoptotic signaling pathway using a novel cellular model. J Biol Chem 276(36):33812–33820. doi:10.1074/jbc.M010548200
185. El Yazidi-Belkoura I, Adriaenssens E, Dolle L, Descamps S, Hondermarck H (2003) Tumor necrosis factor receptor-associated death domain protein is involved in the neurotrophin receptor-mediated antiapoptotic activity of nerve growth factor in breast cancer cells. J Biol Chem 278(19):16952–16956. doi:10.1074/jbc.M300631200
186. Della-Bianca V, Rossi F, Armato U, Dal-Pra I, Costantini C, Perini G, Politi V, Della Valle G (2001) Neurotrophin p75 receptor is involved in neuronal damage by prion peptide-(106-126). J Biol Chem 276(42):38929–38933. doi:10.1074/jbc.M107454200
187. Koppinen P, Pispa J, Laurikkala J, Thesleff I, Mikkola ML (2001) Signaling and subcellular localization of the TNF receptor Edar. Exp Cell Res 269(2):180–192. doi:10.1006/excr.2001.5331
188. Tucker AS, Headon DJ, Schneider P, Ferguson BM, Overbeek P, Tschopp J, Sharpe PT (2000) Edar/Eda interactions regulate enamel knot formation in tooth morphogenesis. Development 127(21):4691–4700
189. Kumar A, Eby MT, Sinha S, Jasmin A, Chaudhary PM (2001) The ectodermal dysplasia receptor activates the nuclear factor-kappaB, JNK, and cell death pathways and binds to ectodysplasin A. J Biol Chem 276(4):2668–2677. doi:10.1074/jbc.M008356200
190. Headon DJ, Emmal SA, Ferguson BM, Tucker AS, Justice MJ, Sharpe PT, Zonana J, Overbeek PA (2001) Gene defect in ectodermal dysplasia implicates a death domain adapter in development. Nature 414(6866):913–916. doi:10.1038/414913a
191. Morlon A, Munnich A, Smahi A (2005) TAB2, TRAF6 and TAK1 are involved in NF-kappaB activation induced by the TNF-receptor, Edar and its adaptator Edaradd. Hum Mol Genet 14(23):3751–3757. doi:10.1093/hmg/ddi405
192. Voigt S, Philipp S, Davarnia P, Winoto-Morbach S, Roder C, Arenz C, Trauzold A, Kabelitz D, Schutze S, Kalthoff H, Adam D (2014) TRAIL-induced programmed necrosis as a novel approach to eliminate tumor cells. BMC Cancer 14:74. doi:10.1186/1471-2407-14-74
193. Holler N, Zaru R, Micheau O, Thome M, Attinger A, Valitutti S, Bodmer JL, Schneider P, Seed B, Tschopp J (2000) Fas triggers an alternative, caspase-8-independent cell death pathway using the kinase RIP as effector molecule. Nat Immunol 1(6):489–495
194. Vercammen D, Beyaert R, Denecker G, Goossens V, Van Loo G, Declercq W, Grooten J, Fiers W, Vandenabeele P (1998) Inhibition of caspases increases the sensitivity of L929 cells to necrosis mediated by tumor necrosis factor. J Exp Med 187(9):1477–1485
195. Vercammen D, Brouckaert G, Denecker G, Van de Craen M, Declercq W, Fiers W, Vandenabeele P (1998) Dual signaling of the Fas receptor: initiation of both apoptotic and necrotic cell death pathways. J Exp Med 188(5):919–930
196. Zhang DW, Shao J, Lin J, Zhang N, BJ L, Lin SC, Dong MQ, Han J (2009) RIP3, an energy metabolism regulator that switches TNF-induced cell death from apoptosis to necrosis. Science 325(5938):332–336. doi:10.1126/science.1172308
197. Degterev A, Hitomi J, Germscheid M, Ch'en IL, Korkina O, Teng X, Abbott D, Cuny GD, Yuan C, Wagner G, Hedrick SM, Gerber SA, Lugovskoy A, Yuan J (2008) Identification of RIP1 kinase as a specific cellular target of necrostatins. Nat Chem Biol 4(5):313–321. doi:10.1038/nchembio.83
198. Degterev A, Huang Z, Boyce M, Li Y, Jagtap P, Mizushima N, Cuny GD, Mitchison TJ, Moskowitz MA, Yuan J (2005) Chemical inhibitor of nonapoptotic cell death with therapeutic potential for ischemic brain injury. Nat Chem Biol 1(2):112–119. doi:10.1038/nchembio711
199. Jouan-Lanhouet S, Arshad MI, Piquet-Pellorce C, Martin-Chouly C, Le Moigne-Muller G, Van Herreweghe F, Takahashi N, Sergent O, Lagadic-Gossmann D, Vandenabeele P, Samson M, Dimanche-Boitrel MT (2012) TRAIL induces necroptosis involving RIPK1/

RIPK3-dependent PARP-1 activation. Cell Death Differ 19(12):2003–2014. doi:10.1038/cdd.2012.90
200. Moujalled DM, Cook WD, Okamoto T, Murphy J, Lawlor KE, Vince JE, Vaux DL (2013) TNF can activate RIPK3 and cause programmed necrosis in the absence of RIPK1. Cell Death Dis 4:e465. doi:10.1038/cddis.2012.201
201. Vandenabeele P, Galluzzi L, Vanden Berghe T, Kroemer G (2010) Molecular mechanisms of necroptosis: an ordered cellular explosion. Nat Rev Mol Cell Biol 11(10):700–714. doi:10.1038/nrm2970
202. Singh K, Poteryakhina A, Zheltukhin A, Bhatelia K, Prajapati P, Sripada L, Tomar D, Singh R, Singh AK, Chumakov PM, Singh R (2015) NLRX1 acts as tumor suppressor by regulating TNF-alpha induced apoptosis and metabolism in cancer cells. Biochim Biophys Acta 1853(5):1073–1086. doi:10.1016/j.bbamcr.2015.01.016
203. Munoz-Pinedo C, Ruiz-Ruiz C, Ruiz de Almodovar C, Palacios C, Lopez-Rivas A (2003) Inhibition of glucose metabolism sensitizes tumor cells to death receptor-triggered apoptosis through enhancement of death-inducing signaling complex formation and apical procaspase-8 processing. J Biol Chem 278(15):12759–12768. doi:10.1074/jbc.M212392200
204. Pospisilova J, Vit O, Lorkova L, Klanova M, Zivny J, Klener P, Petrak J (2013) Resistance to TRAIL in mantle cell lymphoma cells is associated with the decreased expression of purine metabolism enzymes. Int J Mol Med 31(5):1273–1279. doi:10.3892/ijmm.2013.1302
205. Qin JZ, Xin H, Nickoloff BJ (2010) Targeting glutamine metabolism sensitizes melanoma cells to TRAIL-induced death. Biochem Biophys Res Commun 398(1):146–152. doi:10.1016/j.bbrc.2010.06.057
206. Degli Esposti M, Ferry G, Masdehors P, Boutin JA, Hickman JA, Dive C (2003) Post-translational modification of Bid has differential effects on its susceptibility to cleavage by caspase 8 or caspase 3. J Biol Chem 278(18):15749–15757. doi:10.1074/jbc.M209208200
207. Alvarado-Kristensson M, Melander F, Leandersson K, Ronnstrand L, Wernstedt C, Andersson T (2004) p38-MAPK signals survival by phosphorylation of caspase-8 and caspase-3 in human neutrophils. J Exp Med 199(4):449–458. doi:10.1084/jem.20031771
208. Desagher S, Osen-Sand A, Montessuit S, Magnenat E, Vilbois F, Hochmann A, Journot L, Antonsson B, Martinou JC (2001) Phosphorylation of bid by casein kinases I and II regulates its cleavage by caspase 8. Mol Cell 8(3):601–611
209. Tsang JL, Jia SH, Parodo J, Plant P, Lodyga M, Charbonney E, Szaszi K, Kapus A, Marshall JC (2016) Tyrosine phosphorylation of caspase-8 abrogates its apoptotic activity and promotes activation of c-Src. PLoS One 11(4):e0153946. doi:10.1371/journal.pone.0153946
210. Dorrie J, Sapala K, Zunino SJ (2002) Interferon-gamma increases the expression of glycosylated CD95 in B-leukemic cells: an inducible model to study the role of glycosylation in CD95-signalling and trafficking. Cytokine 18(2):98–107
211. Klima M, Zajedova J, Doubravska L, Andera L (2009) Functional analysis of the posttranslational modifications of the death receptor 6. Biochim Biophys Acta 1793(10):1579–1587. doi:10.1016/j.bbamcr.2009.07.008
212. Voigt CG, Maurer-Fogy I, Adolf GR (1992) Natural human tumor necrosis factor beta (lymphotoxin). Variable O-glycosylation at Thr7, proteolytic processing, and allelic variation. FEBS Lett 314(1):85–88
213. Browning JL, Dougas I, Ngam-ek A, Bourdon PR, Ehrenfels BN, Miatkowski K, Zafari M, Yampaglia AM, Lawton P, Meier W et al (1995) Characterization of surface lymphotoxin forms. Use of specific monoclonal antibodies and soluble receptors. J Immunol 154(1):33–46
214. Han L, Zhang D, Tao T, Sun X, Liu X, Zhu G, Xu Z, Zhu L, Zhang Y, Liu W, Ke K, Shen A (2015) The role of N-glycan modification of TNFR1 in inflammatory microglia activation. Glycoconj J 32(9):685–693. doi:10.1007/s10719-015-9619-1
215. Wagner KW, Punnoose EA, Januario T, Lawrence DA, Pitti RM, Lancaster K, Lee D, von Goetz M, Yee SF, Totpal K, Huw L, Katta V, Cavet G, Hymowitz SG, Amler L, Ashkenazi A (2007) Death-receptor O-glycosylation controls tumor-cell sensitivity to the proapoptotic ligand Apo2L/TRAIL. Nat Med 13(9):1070–1077. doi:10.1038/nm1627. nm1627 [pii]

216. Ward-Kavanagh LK, Lin WW, Sedy JR, Ware CF (2016) The TNF receptor superfamily in co-stimulating and co-inhibitory responses. Immunity 44(5):1005–1019. doi:10.1016/j.immuni.2016.04.019
217. Tschopp J, Irmler M, Thome M (1998) Inhibition of fas death signals by FLIPs. Curr Opin Immunol 10(5):552–558
218. Bertin J, Armstrong RC, Ottilie S, Martin DA, Wang Y, Banks S, Wang GH, Senkevich TG, Alnemri ES, Moss B, Lenardo MJ, Tomaselli KJ, Cohen JI (1997) Death effector domain-containing herpesvirus and poxvirus proteins inhibit both Fas- and TNFR1-induced apoptosis. Proc Natl Acad Sci U S A 94(4):1172–1176
219. Irmler M, Thome M, Hahne M, Schneider P, Hofmann K, Steiner V, Bodmer JL, Schroter M, Burns K, Mattmann C, Rimoldi D, French LE, Tschopp J (1997) Inhibition of death receptor signals by cellular FLIP. Nature 388(6638):190–195
220. Silke J, Hartland EL (2013) Masters, marionettes and modulators: intersection of pathogen virulence factors and mammalian death receptor signaling. Curr Opin Immunol 25(4):436–440. doi:10.1016/j.coi.2013.05.011
221. Benedict CA (2003) Viruses and the TNF-related cytokines, an evolving battle. Cytokine Growth Factor Rev 14(3-4):349–357
222. Peitsch MC, Jongeneel CV (1993) A 3-D model for the CD40 ligand predicts that it is a compact trimer similar to the tumor necrosis factors. Int Immunol 5(2):233–238
223. Schuchmann M, Hess S, Bufler P, Brakebusch C, Wallach D, Porter A, Riethmuller G, Engelmann H (1995) Functional discrepancies between tumor necrosis factor and lymphotoxin alpha explained by trimer stability and distinct receptor interactions. Eur J Immunol 25(8):2183–2189. doi:10.1002/eji.1830250810
224. Smith RA, Baglioni C (1987) The active form of tumor necrosis factor is a trimer. J Biol Chem 262(15):6951–6954
225. Granger GA, Laserna EC, Kolb WP, Chapman F (1973) Human lymphotoxin: purification and some properties. Proc Natl Acad Sci U S A 70(1):27–30
226. Lum L, Wong BR, Josien R, Becherer JD, Erdjument-Bromage H, Schlondorff J, Tempst P, Choi Y, Blobel CP (1999) Evidence for a role of a tumor necrosis factor-alpha (TNF-alpha)-converting enzyme-like protease in shedding of TRANCE, a TNF family member involved in osteoclastogenesis and dendritic cell survival. J Biol Chem 274(19):13613–13618
227. Moss ML, Jin SL, Becherer JD, Bickett DM, Burkhart W, Chen WJ, Hassler D, Leesnitzer MT, McGeehan G, Milla M, Moyer M, Rocque W, Seaton T, Schoenen F, Warner J, Willard D (1997) Structural features and biochemical properties of TNF-alpha converting enzyme (TACE). J Neuroimmunol 72(2):127–129
228. Elomaa O, Pulkkinen K, Hannelius U, Mikkola M, Saarialho-Kere U, Kere J (2001) Ectodysplasin is released by proteolytic shedding and binds to the EDAR protein. Hum Mol Genet 10(9):953–962
229. Fourie AM, Coles F, Moreno V, Karlsson L (2003) Catalytic activity of ADAM8, ADAM15, and MDC-L (ADAM28) on synthetic peptide substrates and in ectodomain cleavage of CD23. J Biol Chem 278(33):30469–30477. doi:10.1074/jbc.M213157200
230. Yamamoto A, Nagamuta M, Usami H, Sugawara Y, Watanabe N, Niitsu Y, Urushizaki I (1986) Release of tumor necrosis factor (TNF) into mouse peritoneal fluids by OK-432, a streptococcal preparation. Immunopharmacology 11(2):79–86
231. Rebuffini E, Zuccarino L, Grecchi E, Carinci F, Merulla VE (2012) Picibanil (OK-432) in the treatment of head and neck lymphangiomas in children. Dent Res J (Isfahan) 9(Suppl 2):S192–S196. doi:10.4103/1735-3327.109752
232. Cal S, Lopez-Otin C (2015) ADAMTS proteases and cancer. Matrix Biol 44-46:77–85. doi:10.1016/j.matbio.2015.01.013
233. Owen-Schaub LB, Angelo LS, Radinsky R, Ware CF, Gesner TG, Bartos DP (1995) Soluble Fas/APO-1 in tumor cells: a potential regulator of apoptosis? Cancer Lett 94(1):1–8
234. Tanaka M, Suda T, Takahashi T, Nagata S (1995) Expression of the functional soluble form of human fas ligand in activated lymphocytes. EMBO J 14(6):1129–1135

235. Liabakk NB, Sundan A, Torp S, Aukrust P, Froland SS, Espevik T (2002) Development, characterization and use of monoclonal antibodies against sTRAIL: measurement of sTRAIL by ELISA. J Immunol Methods 259(1-2):119–128
236. Graf D, Muller S, Korthauer U, van Kooten C, Weise C, Kroczek RA (1995) A soluble form of TRAP (CD40 ligand) is rapidly released after T cell activation. Eur J Immunol 25(6):1749–1754. doi:10.1002/eji.1830250639
237. Salih HR, Schmetzer HM, Burke C, Starling GC, Dunn R, Pelka-Fleischer R, Nuessler V, Kiener PA (2001) Soluble CD137 (4-1BB) ligand is released following leukocyte activation and is found in sera of patients with hematological malignancies. J Immunol 167(7):4059–4066
238. Knight AK, Radigan L, Marron T, Langs A, Zhang L, Cunningham-Rundles C (2007) High serum levels of BAFF, APRIL, and TACI in common variable immunodeficiency. Clin Immunol 124(2):182–189. doi:10.1016/j.clim.2007.04.012
239. Morel Y, Schiano de Colella JM, Harrop J, Deen KC, Holmes SD, Wattam TA, Khandekar SS, Truneh A, Sweet RW, Gastaut JA, Olive D, Costello RT (2000) Reciprocal expression of the TNF family receptor herpes virus entry mediator and its ligand LIGHT on activated T cells: LIGHT down-regulates its own receptor. J Immunol 165(8):4397–4404
240. Chicheportiche Y, Bourdon PR, Xu H, Hsu YM, Scott H, Hession C, Garcia I, Browning JL (1997) TWEAK, a new secreted ligand in the tumor necrosis factor family that weakly induces apoptosis. J Biol Chem 272(51):32401–32410
241. Baxter FO, Came PJ, Abell K, Kedjouar B, Huth M, Rajewsky K, Pasparakis M, Watson CJ (2006) IKKbeta/2 induces TWEAK and apoptosis in mammary epithelial cells. Development 133(17):3485–3494. doi:10.1242/dev.02502
242. Meyer T, Amaya M, Desai H, Robles-Carrillo L, Hatfield M, Francis JL, Amirkhosravi A (2010) Human platelets contain and release TWEAK. Platelets 21(7):571–574. doi:10.3109/09537104.2010.512403
243. Kanamaru F, Iwai H, Ikeda T, Nakajima A, Ishikawa I, Azuma M (2004) Expression of membrane-bound and soluble receptor activator of NF-kappaB ligand (RANKL) in human T cells. Immunol Lett 94(3):239–246. doi:10.1016/j.imlet.2004.05.010
244. Muck C, Herndler-Brandstetter D, Micutkova L, Grubeck-Loebenstein B, Jansen-Durr P (2010) Two functionally distinct isoforms of TL1A (TNFSF15) generated by differential ectodomain shedding. J Gerontol A Biol Sci Med Sci 65(11):1165–1180. doi:10.1093/gerona/glq129
245. Gearing AJ, Beckett P, Christodoulou M, Churchill M, Clements J, Davidson AH, Drummond AH, Galloway WA, Gilbert R, Gordon JL et al (1994) Processing of tumour necrosis factor-alpha precursor by metalloproteinases. Nature 370(6490):555–557. doi:10.1038/370555a0
246. Kayagaki N, Kawasaki A, Ebata T, Ohmoto H, Ikeda S, Inoue S, Yoshino K, Okumura K, Yagita H (1995) Metalloproteinase-mediated release of human Fas ligand. J Exp Med 182(6):1777–1783
247. Kawakubo T, Okamoto K, Iwata J, Shin M, Okamoto Y, Yasukochi A, Nakayama KI, Kadowaki T, Tsukuba T, Yamamoto K (2007) Cathepsin E prevents tumor growth and metastasis by catalyzing the proteolytic release of soluble TRAIL from tumor cell surface. Cancer Res 67(22):10869–10878. doi:10.1158/0008-5472.CAN-07-2048
248. Lopez-Fraga M, Fernandez R, Albar JP, Hahne M (2001) Biologically active APRIL is secreted following intracellular processing in the Golgi apparatus by furin convertase. EMBO Rep 2(10):945–951. doi:10.1093/embo-reports/kve198
249. Bjornberg F, Lantz M, Gullberg U (1995) Metalloproteases and serineproteases are involved in the cleavage of the two tumour necrosis factor (TNF) receptors to soluble forms in the myeloid cell lines U-937 and THP-1. Scand J Immunol 42(4):418–424
250. Kagawa K, Nakano A, Miki H, Oda A, Amou H, Takeuchi K, Nakamura S, Harada T, Fujii S, Yata K, Ozaki S, Matsumoto T, Abe M (2012) Inhibition of TACE activity enhances the susceptibility of myeloma cells to TRAIL. PLoS One 7(2):e31594. doi:10.1371/journal.pone.0031594

251. Hansen HP, Dietrich S, Kisseleva T, Mokros T, Mentlein R, Lange HH, Murphy G, Lemke H (2000) CD30 shedding from Karpas 299 lymphoma cells is mediated by TNF-alpha-converting enzyme. J Immunol 165(12):6703–6709
252. Nemoto E, Tada H, Shimauchi H (2002) Disruption of CD40/CD40 ligand interaction with cleavage of CD40 on human gingival fibroblasts by human leukocyte elastase resulting in down-regulation of chemokine production. J Leukoc Biol 72(3):538–545
253. Contin C, Pitard V, Itai T, Nagata S, Moreau JF, Dechanet-Merville J (2003) Membrane-anchored CD40 is processed by the tumor necrosis factor-alpha-converting enzyme. Implications for CD40 signaling. J Biol Chem 278(35):32801–32809. doi:10.1074/jbc.M209993200
254. Nielsen MA, Andersen T, Etzerodt A, Kragstrup TW, Rasmussen TK, Stengaard-Pedersen K, Hetland ML, Horslev-Petersen K, Junker P, Ostergaard M, Hvid M, Moestrup SK, Deleuran B (2016) A disintegrin and metalloprotease-17 and galectin-9 are important regulators of local 4-1BB activity and disease outcome in rheumatoid arthritis. Rheumatology (Oxford). doi:10.1093/rheumatology/kew237
255. Bell JH, Herrera AH, Li Y, Walcheck B (2007) Role of ADAM17 in the ectodomain shedding of TNF-alpha and its receptors by neutrophils and macrophages. J Leukoc Biol 82(1):173–176
256. Bartsch JW, Wildeboer D, Koller G, Naus S, Rittger A, Moss ML, Minai Y, Jockusch H (2010) Tumor necrosis factor-alpha (TNF-alpha) regulates shedding of TNF-alpha receptor 1 by the metalloprotease-disintegrin ADAM8: evidence for a protease-regulated feedback loop in neuroprotection. J Neurosci 30(36):12210–12218
257. Zhou Y, Liu X, Xu L, Tseng H, Cao Y, Jiang J, Ciccarelli BT, Yang G, Patterson CJ, Hunter ZR, Treon SP (2011) Matrix metalloproteinase-8 is overexpressed in Waldenstrom's macroglobulinemia cells, and specific inhibition of this metalloproteinase blocks release of soluble CD27. Clin Lymphoma Myeloma Leuk 11(1):172–175. doi:10.3816/CLML.2011.n.041
258. Eichenauer DA, Simhadri VL, von Strandmann EP, Ludwig A, Matthews V, Reiners KS, von Tresckow B, Saftig P, Rose-John S, Engert A, Hansen HP (2007) ADAM10 inhibition of human CD30 shedding increases specificity of targeted immunotherapy in vitro. Cancer Res 67(1):332–338. doi:10.1158/0008-5472.CAN-06-2470
259. Strand S, Vollmer P, van den Abeelen L, Gottfried D, Alla V, Heid H, Kuball J, Theobald M, Galle PR, Strand D (2004) Cleavage of CD95 by matrix metalloproteinase-7 induces apoptosis resistance in tumour cells. Oncogene 23(20):3732–3736. doi:10.1038/sj.onc.1207387
260. Tanikawa C, Ri C, Kumar V, Nakamura Y, Matsuda K (2010) Crosstalk of EDA-A2/XEDAR in the p53 signaling pathway. Mol Cancer Res 8(6):855–863. doi:10.1158/1541-7786.MCR-09-0484
261. Vicario A, Kisiswa L, Tann JY, Kelly CE, Ibanez CF (2015) Neuron-type-specific signaling by the p75NTR death receptor is regulated by differential proteolytic cleavage. J Cell Sci 128(8):1507–1517. doi:10.1242/jcs.161745
262. Laurent SA, Hoffmann FS, Kuhn PH, Cheng Q, Chu Y, Schmidt-Supprian M, Hauck SM, Schuh E, Krumbholz M, Rubsamen H, Wanngren J, Khademi M, Olsson T, Alexander T, Hiepe F, Pfister HW, Weber F, Jenne D, Wekerle H, Hohlfeld R, Lichtenthaler SF, Meinl E (2015) gamma-Secretase directly sheds the survival receptor BCMA from plasma cells. Nat Commun 6:7333. doi:10.1038/ncomms8333
263. Zhao Y, Jin M, Ma J, Zhang S, Li W, Chen Y, Zhou Y, Tao H, Liu Y, Wang L, Han H, Niu G, Tao H, Liu C, Gao B (2013) Inhibition effect of enteropeptidase on RANKL-RANK signalling by cleavage of RANK. FEBS Lett 587(18):2958–2964. doi:10.1016/j.febslet.2013.08.005
264. Michaelson JS, Cho S, Browning B, Zheng TS, Lincecum JM, Wang MZ, Hsu YM, Burkly LC (2005) Tweak induces mammary epithelial branching morphogenesis. Oncogene 24(16):2613–2624. doi:10.1038/sj.onc.1208208
265. Trebing J, Arana JA, Salzmann S, Wajant H (2014) Analyzing the signaling capabilities of soluble and membrane TWEAK. Methods Mol Biol 1155:31–45. doi:10.1007/978-1-4939-0669-7_4

266. Carmona Arana JA, Seher A, Neumann M, Lang I, Siegmund D, Wajant H (2014) TNF receptor-associated factor 1 is a major target of soluble TWEAK. Front Immunol 5:63. doi:10.3389/fimmu.2014.00063
267. Grell M (1995) Tumor necrosis factor (TNF) receptors in cellular signaling of soluble and membrane-expressed TNF. J Inflamm 47(1-2):8–17
268. Ardestani S, Li B, Deskins DL, Wu H, Massion PP, Young PP (2013) Membrane versus soluble isoforms of TNF-alpha exert opposing effects on tumor growth and survival of tumor-associated myeloid cells. Cancer Res 73(13):3938–3950. doi:10.1158/0008-5472.CAN-13-0002
269. Schneider P, Holler N, Bodmer JL, Hahne M, Frei K, Fontana A, Tschopp J (1998) Conversion of membrane-bound Fas(CD95) ligand to its soluble form is associated with downregulation of its proapoptotic activity and loss of liver toxicity. J Exp Med 187(8):1205–1213
270. Grell M, Douni E, Wajant H, Lohden M, Clauss M, Maxeiner B, Georgopoulos S, Lesslauer W, Kollias G, Pfizenmaier K, Scheurich P (1995) The transmembrane form of tumor necrosis factor is the prime activating ligand of the 80 kDa tumor necrosis factor receptor. Cell 83(5):793–802
271. Cheng J, Zhou T, Liu C, Shapiro JP, Brauer MJ, Kiefer MC, Barr PJ, Mountz JD (1994) Protection from Fas-mediated apoptosis by a soluble form of the Fas molecule. Science 263(5154):1759–1762
272. Poissonnier A, Sanseau D, Le Gallo M, Malleter M, Levoin N, Viel R, Morere L, Penna A, Blanco P, Dupuy A, Poizeau F, Fautrel A, Seneschal J, Jouan F, Ritz J, Forcade E, Rioux N, Contin-Bordes C, Ducret T, Vacher AM, Barrow PA, Flynn RJ, Vacher P, Legembre P (2016) CD95-mediated calcium signaling promotes T helper 17 trafficking to inflamed organs in lupus-prone mice. Immunity 45(1):209–223. doi:10.1016/j.immuni.2016.06.028
273. Barnhart BC, Legembre P, Pietras E, Bubici C, Franzoso G, Peter ME (2004) CD95 ligand induces motility and invasiveness of apoptosis-resistant tumor cells. EMBO J 23(15):3175–3185. doi:10.1038/sj.emboj.7600325
274. Lee JK, Sayers TJ, Back TC, Wigginton JM, Wiltrout RH (2003) Lack of FasL-mediated killing leads to in vivo tumor promotion in mouse Lewis lung cancer. Apoptosis 8(2):151–160
275. Chen L, Park SM, Tumanov AV, Hau A, Sawada K, Feig C, Turner JR, Fu YX, Romero IL, Lengyel E, Peter ME (2010) CD95 promotes tumour growth. Nature 465(7297):492–496. doi:10.1038/nature09075
276. Malleter M, Tauzin S, Bessede A, Castellano R, Goubard A, Godey F, Leveque J, Jezequel P, Campion L, Campone M, Ducret T, MacGrogan G, Debure L, Collette Y, Vacher P, Legembre P (2013) CD95L cell surface cleavage triggers a prometastatic signaling pathway in triple-negative breast cancer. Cancer Res 73(22):6711–6721. doi:10.1158/0008-5472.CAN-13-1794
277. Tauzin S, Chaigne-Delalande B, Selva E, Khadra N, Daburon S, Contin-Bordes C, Blanco P, Le Seyec J, Ducret T, Counillon L, Moreau JF, Hofman P, Vacher P, Legembre P (2011) The naturally processed CD95L elicits a c-yes/calcium/PI3K-driven cell migration pathway. PLoS Biol 9(6):e1001090. doi:10.1371/journal.pbio.1001090
278. Smyth MJ, Cretney E, Takeda K, Wiltrout RH, Sedger LM, Kayagaki N, Yagita H, Okumura K (2001) Tumor necrosis factor-related apoptosis-inducing ligand (TRAIL) contributes to interferon gamma-dependent natural killer cell protection from tumor metastasis. J Exp Med 193(6):661–670
279. Takeda K, Hayakawa Y, Smyth MJ, Kayagaki N, Yamaguchi N, Kakuta S, Iwakura Y, Yagita H, Okumura K (2001) Involvement of tumor necrosis factor-related apoptosis-inducing ligand in surveillance of tumor metastasis by liver natural killer cells. Nat Med 7(1):94–100
280. Cretney E, Takeda K, Yagita H, Glaccum M, Peschon JJ, Smyth MJ (2002) Increased susceptibility to tumor initiation and metastasis in TNF-related apoptosis-inducing ligand-deficient mice. J Immunol 168(3):1356–1361
281. Somasekharan SP, Koc M, Morizot A, Micheau O, Sorensen PH, Gaide O, Andera L, Martinou JC (2013) TRAIL promotes membrane blebbing, detachment and migration of

cells displaying a dysfunctional intrinsic pathway of apoptosis. Apoptosis 18(3):324–336. doi:10.1007/s10495-012-0782-6
282. Trauzold A, Siegmund D, Schniewind B, Sipos B, Egberts J, Zorenkov D, Emme D, Roder C, Kalthoff H, Wajant H (2006) TRAIL promotes metastasis of human pancreatic ductal adenocarcinoma. Oncogene 25(56):7434–7439
283. Takahashi K, Takeda K, Saiki I, Irimura T, Hayakawa Y (2013) Functional roles of tumor necrosis factor-related apoptosis-inducing ligand-DR5 interaction in B16F10 cells by activating the nuclear factor-kappaB pathway to induce metastatic potential. Cancer Sci 104(5):558–562. doi:10.1111/cas.12112
284. Fritsche H, Heilmann T, Tower RJ, Hauser C, von Au A, El-Sheikh D, Campbell GM, Alp G, Schewe D, Hubner S, Tiwari S, Kownatzki D, Boretius S, Adam D, Jonat W, Becker T, Gluer CC, Zoller M, Kalthoff H, Schem C, Trauzold A (2015) TRAIL-R2 promotes skeletal metastasis in a breast cancer xenograft mouse model. Oncotarget 6(11):9502–9516
285. von Karstedt S, Conti A, Nobis M, Montinaro A, Hartwig T, Lemke J, Legler K, Annewanter F, Campbell AD, Taraborrelli L, Grosse-Wilde A, Coy JF, El-Bahrawy MA, Bergmann F, Koschny R, Werner J, Ganten TM, Schweiger T, Hoetzenecker K, Kenessey I, Hegedus B, Bergmann M, Hauser C, Egberts JH, Becker T, Rocken C, Kalthoff H, Trauzold A, Anderson KI, Sansom OJ, Walczak H (2015) Cancer cell-autonomous TRAIL-R signaling promotes KRAS-driven cancer progression, invasion, and metastasis. Cancer Cell 27(4):561–573. doi:10.1016/j.ccell.2015.02.014
286. Utsumi T, Takeshige T, Tanaka K, Takami K, Kira Y, Klostergaard J, Ishisaka R (2001) Transmembrane TNF (pro-TNF) is palmitoylated. FEBS Lett 500(1-2):1–6
287. Feig C, Tchikov V, Schutze S, Peter ME (2007) Palmitoylation of CD95 facilitates formation of SDS-stable receptor aggregates that initiate apoptosis signaling. EMBO J 26(1):221–231. doi:10.1038/sj.emboj.7601460
288. Rossin A, Derouet M, Abdel-Sater F, Hueber AO (2009) Palmitoylation of the TRAIL receptor DR4 confers an efficient TRAIL-induced cell death signalling. Biochem J 419(1):185–192, 182 p following 192 doi:10.1042/BJ20081212. BJ20081212 [pii]
289. Underwood CK, Reid K, May LM, Bartlett PF, Coulson EJ (2008) Palmitoylation of the C-terminal fragment of p75(NTR) regulates death signaling and is required for subsequent cleavage by gamma-secretase. Mol Cell Neurosci 37(2):346–358. doi:10.1016/j.mcn.2007.10.005
290. Stevenson FT, Bursten SL, Locksley RM, Lovett DH (1992) Myristyl acylation of the tumor necrosis factor alpha precursor on specific lysine residues. J Exp Med 176(4):1053–1062
291. Poggi M, Kara I, Brunel JM, Landrier JF, Govers R, Bonardo B, Fluhrer R, Haass C, Alessi MC, Peiretti F (2013) Palmitoylation of TNF alpha is involved in the regulation of TNF receptor 1 signalling. Biochim Biophys Acta 1833(3):602–612. doi:10.1016/j.bbamcr.2012.11.009
292. Jiang H, Zhang X, Lin H (2016) Lysine fatty acylation promotes lysosomal targeting of TNF-alpha. Sci Rep 6:24371. doi:10.1038/srep24371
293. Jiang H, Khan S, Wang Y, Charron G, He B, Sebastian C, Du J, Kim R, Ge E, Mostoslavsky R, Hang HC, Hao Q, Lin H (2013) SIRT6 regulates TNF-alpha secretion through hydrolysis of long-chain fatty acyl lysine. Nature 496(7443):110–113. doi:10.1038/nature12038
294. Chakrabandhu K, Herincs Z, Huault S, Dost B, Peng L, Conchonaud F, Marguet D, He HT, Hueber AO (2007) Palmitoylation is required for efficient Fas cell death signaling. EMBO J 26(1):209–220. doi:10.1038/sj.emboj.7601456. 7601456 [pii]
295. Gajate C, Mollinedo F (2015) Lipid rafts and raft-mediated supramolecular entities in the regulation of CD95 death receptor apoptotic signaling. Apoptosis 20(5):584–606. doi:10.1007/s10495-015-1104-6
296. Rossin A, Durivault J, Chakhtoura-Feghali T, Lounnas N, Gagnoux-Palacios L, Hueber AO (2015) Fas palmitoylation by the palmitoyl acyltransferase DHHC7 regulates Fas stability. Cell Death Differ 22(4):643–653. doi:10.1038/cdd.2014.153
297. Vesa J, Kruttgen A, Cosgaya JM, Shooter EM (2000) Palmitoylation of the p75 neurotrophin receptor has no effect on its interaction with TrkA or on TrkA-mediated

down-regulation of cell adhesion molecules. J Neurosci Res 62(2):225–233. doi:10.1002/1097-4547(20001015)62:2<225::AID-JNR7>3.0.CO;2-9

298. Leon-Bollotte L, Subramaniam S, Cauvard O, Plenchette-Colas S, Paul C, Godard C, Martinez-Ruiz A, Legembre P, Jeannin JF, Bettaieb A (2011) S-nitrosylation of the death receptor fas promotes fas ligand-mediated apoptosis in cancer cells. Gastroenterology 140 (7):2009-2018., 2018 e2001-2004 doi:10.1053/j.gastro.2011.02.053
299. Tang Z, Bauer JA, Morrison B, Lindner DJ (2006) Nitrosylcobalamin promotes cell death via S nitrosylation of Apo2L/TRAIL receptor DR4. Mol Cell Biol 26(15):5588–5594. doi:10.1128/MCB.00199-06
300. Stamler JS, Simon DI, Osborne JA, Mullins ME, Jaraki O, Michel T, Singel DJ, Loscalzo J (1992) S-nitrosylation of proteins with nitric oxide: synthesis and characterization of biologically active compounds. Proc Natl Acad Sci U S A 89(1):444–448
301. Li S, Zhang L, Yao Q, Li L, Dong N, Rong J, Gao W, Ding X, Sun L, Chen X, Chen S, Shao F (2013) Pathogen blocks host death receptor signalling by arginine GlcNAcylation of death domains. Nature 501(7466):242–246. doi:10.1038/nature12436
302. Pearson JS, Giogha C, Ong SY, Kennedy CL, Kelly M, Robinson KS, Lung TW, Mansell A, Riedmaier P, Oates CV, Zaid A, Muhlen S, Crepin VF, Marches O, Ang CS, Williamson NA, O'Reilly LA, Bankovacki A, Nachbur U, Infusini G, Webb AI, Silke J, Strasser A, Frankel G, Hartland EL (2013) A type III effector antagonizes death receptor signalling during bacterial gut infection. Nature 501(7466):247–251. doi:10.1038/nature12524
303. Varki A, Sharon N (2009) Historical Background and Overview. In: Varki A, Cummings RD, Esko JD et al (eds) Essentials of glycobiology, 2nd edn. Cold Spring Harbor Laboratory Press, Cold Spring Harbor, NY
304. Stanley P, Schachter H, Taniguchi N (2009) N-Glycans. In: Varki A, Cummings RD, Esko JD et al (eds) Essentials of glycobiology, 2nd edn. Cold Spring Harbor Laboratory Press, Cold Spring Harbor, NY
305. Brockhausen I, Schachter H, Stanley P (2009) O-GalNAc glycans. In: Varki A, Cummings RD, Esko JD et al (eds) Essentials of glycobiology, 2nd edn. Cold Spring Harbor Laboratory Press, Cold Spring Harbor, NY
306. Chauhan JS, Rao A, Raghava GP (2013) In silico platform for prediction of N-, O- and C-glycosites in eukaryotic protein sequences. PLoS One 8(6):e67008. doi:10.1371/journal.pone.0067008
307. Jue DM, Sherry B, Luedke C, Manogue KR, Cerami A (1990) Processing of newly synthesized cachectin/tumor necrosis factor in endotoxin-stimulated macrophages. Biochemistry 29(36):8371–8377
308. Aggarwal BB, Henzel WJ, Moffat B, Kohr WJ, Harkins RN (1985) Primary structure of human lymphotoxin derived from 1788 lymphoblastoid cell line. J Biol Chem 260(4):2334–2344
309. Kofler G, Gottfried I, Benjamin D, Tschachler E (1992) Size heterogeneity of human lymphotoxin is due to O-linked glycosylation. Lymphokine Cytokine Res 11(1):9–14
310. Corti A, Merli S, Bagnasco L, D'Ambrosio F, Marino M, Cassani G (1995) Identification of two forms (31-33 and 48 kD) of the urinary soluble p55 tumor necrosis factor receptor that are differentially N- and O-glycosylated. J Interferon Cytokine Res 15(2):143–152. doi:10.1089/jir.1995.15.143
311. Corti A, D'Ambrosio F, Marino M, Merli S, Cassani G (1995) Identification of differentially glycosylated forms of the soluble p75 tumor necrosis factor (TNF) receptor in human urine. Eur Cytokine Netw 6(1):29–35
312. Zola H, Fusco M, Ridings J, Flego LR, Weedon HM, Nicholson I, Organ N, Roberton DM, Macardle PJ (1996) The Fas antigen (CD95) on human lymphoid cells: epitope analysis with ten antibodies. Tissue Antigens 48(5):519–530
313. Monlauzeur L, Breuza L, Le Bivic A (1998) Putative O-glycosylation sites and a membrane anchor are necessary for apical delivery of the human neurotrophin receptor in Caco-2 cells. J Biol Chem 273(46):30263–30270
314. Breuza L, Garcia M, Delgrossi MH, Le Bivic A (2002) Role of the membrane-proximal O-glycosylation site in sorting of the human receptor for neurotrophins to the apical membrane of MDCK cells. Exp Cell Res 273(2):178–186. doi:10.1006/excr.2001.5442

315. Shatnyeva OM, Kubarenko AV, Weber CE, Pappa A, Schwartz-Albiez R, Weber AN, Krammer PH, Lavrik IN (2011) Modulation of the CD95-induced apoptosis: the role of CD95 N-glycosylation. PLoS One 6(5):e19927. doi:10.1371/journal.pone.0019927
316. Dufour F, Rattier T, Shirley S, Picarda G, Constatinescu AA, Morlé A, Zakaria AB, Marcion G, Causse S, Szegezdi E, Zajonc DM, Seigneuric R, Guichard G, Picaud F, Herlem G, Garrido C, Schneider P, Benedict CA, Micheau O (2017) N-glycosylation of mouse TRAIL-R and human TRAIL-R1 enhances TRAIL-induced death. Cell Death Differ 24(3):500–510
317. Yoshida T, Shiraishi T, Horinaka M, Wakada M, Sakai T (2007) Glycosylation modulates TRAIL-R1/death receptor 4 protein: different regulations of two pro-apoptotic receptors for TRAIL by tunicamycin. Oncol Rep 18(5):1239–1242
318. Lichtenstein RG, Rabinovich GA (2013) Glycobiology of cell death: when glycans and lectins govern cell fate. Cell Death Differ 20(8):976–986. doi:10.1038/cdd.2013.50
319. Peter ME, Hellbardt S, Schwartz-Albiez R, Westendorp MO, Walczak H, Moldenhauer G, Grell M, Krammer PH (1995) Cell surface sialylation plays a role in modulating sensitivity towards APO-1-mediated apoptotic cell death. Cell Death Differ 2(3):163–171
320. Keppler OT, Peter ME, Hinderlich S, Moldenhauer G, Stehling P, Schmitz I, Schwartz-Albiez R, Reutter W, Pawlita M (1999) Differential sialylation of cell surface glycoconjugates in a human B lymphoma cell line regulates susceptibility for CD95 (APO-1/Fas)-mediated apoptosis and for infection by a lymphotropic virus. Glycobiology 9(6):557–569
321. Swindall AF, Bellis SL (2011) Sialylation of the Fas death receptor by ST6Gal-I provides protection against Fas-mediated apoptosis in colon carcinoma cells. J Biol Chem 286(26):22982–22990. doi:10.1074/jbc.M110.211375
322. Liu Z, Swindall AF, Kesterson RA, Schoeb TR, Bullard DC, Bellis SL (2011) ST6Gal-I regulates macrophage apoptosis via alpha2-6 sialylation of the TNFR1 death receptor. J Biol Chem 286(45):39654–39662. doi:10.1074/jbc.M111.276063
323. Moriwaki K, Noda K, Furukawa Y, Ohshima K, Uchiyama A, Nakagawa T, Taniguchi N, Daigo Y, Nakamura Y, Hayashi N, Miyoshi E (2009) Deficiency of GMDS leads to escape from NK cell-mediated tumor surveillance through modulation of TRAIL signaling. Gastroenterology 137(1):188–198, 198 e181–182. doi:10.1053/j.gastro.2009.04.002
324. Moriwaki K, Shinzaki S, Miyoshi E (2011) GDP-mannose-4,6-dehydratase (GMDS) deficiency renders colon cancer cells resistant to tumor necrosis factor-related apoptosis-inducing ligand (TRAIL) receptor- and CD95-mediated apoptosis by inhibiting complex II formation. J Biol Chem 286(50):43123–43133. doi:10.1074/jbc.M111.262741
325. Lee YJ, Song YK, Song JJ, Siervo-Sassi RR, Kim HR, Li L, Spitz DR, Lokshin A, Kim JH (2003) Reconstitution of galectin-3 alters glutathione content and potentiates TRAIL-induced cytotoxicity by dephosphorylation of Akt. Exp Cell Res 288(1):21–34
326. Oka N, Nakahara S, Takenaka Y, Fukumori T, Hogan V, Kanayama HO, Yanagawa T, Raz A (2005) Galectin-3 inhibits tumor necrosis factor-related apoptosis-inducing ligand-induced apoptosis by activating Akt in human bladder carcinoma cells. Cancer Res 65(17):7546–7553. doi:10.1158/0008-5472.CAN-05-1197
327. Lin CI, Whang EE, Abramson MA, Donner DB, Bertagnolli MM, Moore FD Jr, Ruan DT (2009) Galectin-3 regulates apoptosis and doxorubicin chemoresistance in papillary thyroid cancer cells. Biochem Biophys Res Commun 379(2):626–631. doi:10.1016/j.bbrc.2008.12.153
328. Fukumori T, Takenaka Y, Oka N, Yoshii T, Hogan V, Inohara H, Kanayama HO, Kim HR, Raz A (2004) Endogenous galectin-3 determines the routing of CD95 apoptotic signaling pathways. Cancer Res 64(10):3376–3379. doi:10.1158/0008-5472.CAN-04-0336
329. Mazurek N, Jie Sun Y, Feng Liu K, Gilcrease MZ, Schober W, Nangia-Makker P, Raz A, Bresalier RS (2007) Phosphorylated galectin-3 mediates tumor necrosis factor-related apoptosis-inducing ligand (TRAIL) signaling by regulating PTEN in human breast carcinoma cells. J Biol Chem 282(29):21337–21348
330. Mazurek N, Byrd JC, Sun Y, Ueno S, Bresalier RS (2011) A galectin-3 sequence polymorphism confers TRAIL sensitivity to human breast cancer cells. Cancer 117(19):4375–4380. doi:10.1002/cncr.26078

331. Mazurek N, Byrd JC, Sun Y, Hafley M, Ramirez K, Burks J, Bresalier RS (2012) Cell-surface galectin-3 confers resistance to TRAIL by impeding trafficking of death receptors in metastatic colon adenocarcinoma cells. Cell Death Differ 19(3):523–533. doi:10.1038/cdd.2011.123
332. Brandt B, Buchse T, Abou-Eladab EF, Tiedge M, Krause E, Jeschke U, Walzel H (2008) Galectin-1 induced activation of the apoptotic death-receptor pathway in human Jurkat T lymphocytes. Histochem Cell Biol 129(5):599–609. doi:10.1007/s00418-008-0395-x
333. Madireddi S, Eun SY, Lee SW, Nemcovicova I, Mehta AK, Zajonc DM, Nishi N, Niki T, Hirashima M, Croft M (2014) Galectin-9 controls the therapeutic activity of 4-1BB-targeting antibodies. J Exp Med 211(7):1433–1448. doi:10.1084/jem.20132687
334. Boscher C, Dennis JW, Nabi IR (2011) Glycosylation, galectins and cellular signaling. Curr Opin Cell Biol 23(4):383–392. doi:10.1016/j.ceb.2011.05.001
335. Stowell SR, Arthur CM, Mehta P, Slanina KA, Blixt O, Leffler H, Smith DF, Cummings RD (2008) Galectin-1, -2, and -3 exhibit differential recognition of sialylated glycans and blood group antigens. J Biol Chem 283(15):10109–10123. doi:10.1074/jbc.M709545200
336. de Oliveira JT, de Matos AJ, Santos AL, Pinto R, Gomes J, Hespanhol V, Chammas R, Manninen A, Bernardes ES, Albuquerque Reis C, Rutteman G, Gartner F (2011) Sialylation regulates galectin-3/ligand interplay during mammary tumour progression--a case of targeted uncloaking. Int J Dev Biol 55(7-9):823–834. doi:10.1387/ijdb.113359jt
337. McDonald AG, Hayes JM, Davey GP (2016) Metabolic flux control in glycosylation. Curr Opin Struct Biol 40:97–103. doi:10.1016/j.sbi.2016.08.007
338. Heegaard PM (1992) Changes in serum glycoprotein glycosylation during experimental inflammation in mice are general, unrelated to protein type, and opposite changes in man and rat: studies on mouse serum alpha 1-acid glycoprotein, alpha 1-esterase, and alpha 1-protease inhibitor. Inflammation 16(6):631–644
339. Rombouts Y, Jonasdottir HS, Hipgrave Ederveen AL, Reiding KR, Jansen BC, Freysdottir J, Hardardottir I, Ioan-Facsinay A, Giera M, Wuhrer M (2016) Acute phase inflammation is characterized by rapid changes in plasma/peritoneal fluid N-glycosylation in mice. Glycoconj J 33(3):457–470. doi:10.1007/s10719-015-9648-9
340. Turner GA (1992) N-glycosylation of serum proteins in disease and its investigation using lectins. Clin Chim Acta 208(3):149–171
341. Rak JW, Basolo F, Elliott JW, Russo J, Miller FR (1991) Cell surface glycosylation changes accompanying immortalization and transformation of normal human mammary epithelial cells. Cancer Lett 57(1):27–36. 0304-3835(91)90059-Q [pii]

Chapter 12
System Modeling of Receptor-Induced Apoptosis

François Bertaux, Dirk Drasdo, and Grégory Batt

Abstract Receptor-induced apoptosis is a complex signal transduction pathway involving numerous protein–protein interactions and post-translational modifications. The response to death receptor stimulation varies significantly from one cell line to another and even from one cell to another within a given cell line. In this context, it is often difficult to assess whether the molecular mechanisms identified so far are sufficient to explain the rich quantitative observations now available, and to detect possible gaps in our understanding. This is precisely where computational systems biology approaches may contribute. In this chapter, we review studies done in this direction, focusing on those that provided a significant insight on the functioning of this complex pathway by tightly integrating experimental and computational approaches.

Keywords Computational systems biology • Signal transduction models • Receptor-induced apoptosis • Modeling cell types • Modeling phenotypic heterogeneity

---

F. Bertaux (✉)
INRIA Paris, 2 rue Simone Iff, 75589, Paris cedex 12, France

Department of Mathematics, Imperial College London, London SW7 2AZ, UK

Inria Saclay – Ile-de-France, 91120 Palaiseau, France
e-mail: f.bertaux@imperial.ac.uk

D. Drasdo
INRIA Paris, 2 rue Simone Iff, 75589, Paris cedex 12, France

G. Batt (✉)
Inria Saclay – Ile-de-France, 91120 Palaiseau, France
e-mail: Gregory.Batt@inria.fr

O. Micheau (ed.), *TRAIL, Fas Ligand, TNF and TLR3 in Cancer*, Resistance to Targeted Anti-Cancer Therapeutics, DOI 10.1007/978-3-319-56805-8_12

12.1 Introduction

Apoptosis is a form of programmed cell death conserved among metazoans playing a central role in development and involved in many diseases. Notably, most successful nonsurgical cancer therapies eventually result in the activation of apoptosis in cancer cells [1]. Apoptosis can be triggered internally (via an "intrinsic" pathway) following DNA damage or other intrinsic stimuli, or externally (via an "extrinsic" pathway) following the binding of "death" ligands to "death" receptors. Receptor-induced apoptosis raised therapeutical interest as anticancer strategy for at least two reasons. Firstly it can be highly selective for certain cell types, ideally targeting only cancer cells. Secondly it does not require a functional p53 protein, which is frequently mutated in tumor cells, providing resistance to chemotherapeutic drugs relying on the DNA damage response. Several death ligand–receptor pairs exist. While TNFα (and its receptors TNFRs) and CD95L (and its receptor CD95) were discovered first, TRAIL (and its receptors DRs) has the highest selectivity towards cancer cells [2]. From a largest perspective, the latter is also a reference system illustrating how complex circuits involving graded and competing molecular signals can generate binary decisions. Because of its high interest, both for systems biology and therapeutics, tremendous research efforts have been done to better understand its functioning [3–8].

The control and regulation of apoptosis involve many genes whose products mediate numerous protein–protein interactions, post-translational modifications, transcriptional regulations, etc., yielding a highly complex picture. The sensitivity of cells to a given death ligand stimulation is multifactorial, and the effect of genetic perturbations on cell survival is highly context-dependent. As a result, the interpretation of results obtained on a specific cell line and for a few genetic perturbations or conditions is delicate and cannot be readily generalized. The system model paradigm is well suited to deal with this complexity. Computational approaches attempt to integrate known mechanisms and interactions into mathematical models, whose predictions can be used to propose new experiments for model validation. When applied to apoptosis, system level modeling, which started approximately 15 years ago, was indeed instrumental in improving our understanding of this complex process. This was achieved by tightly integrating data of increasing quality and by increasing the scope and/or level of details of models. Excellent reviews discuss these modeling works [9–15].

Despite these achievements, important fundamental questions remain to be answered, especially on the role of phenotypic heterogeneity and how it impacts the response to, as well as how it is changed by, treatments by death ligands [16]. Why do isogenic cells respond differently to the same amount of death ligand? Indeed, it is often the case that not all treated cells die, and when cells die, their death times are very heterogeneous. How different from dying cells are surviving cells before treatment (i.e., *why* cells survive)? How different are surviving cells from what they were just before treatment (i.e., who *are* survivors)? Can these differences explain the decreased efficiency of subsequent treatments (i.e., *what* make cells more resistant)? Importantly, the two last questions, while critical for understanding the efficiency of treatments, are starting to be addressed only since very recently [17, 18]. Here, we review the contributions of system modeling studies to our understanding of receptor-induced apoptosis with a specific focus towards those important questions. We do not aim to exhaustively describe all the modeling work done on receptor-induced apoptosis. Rather, we describe a few key studies that are highly illustrative of how the system modeling approaches can provide decisive insights.

12.2 Modeling the Biochemistry of Receptor-Induced Apoptosis

12.2.1 Early Efforts: From Known Players and Reactions to a System Model

Many proteins playing a key role in receptor-induced apoptosis are known since decades, together with a qualitative picture of how they interact, either to convey external death signals to promote the activation of the core executioners of apoptosis or on the contrary to act as "inhibitors" or "blockers" of death signalling. Figure 12.1 provides a schematic overview of apoptotic pathways.

Despite this qualitative knowledge, how precisely cell response emerges from protein interactions in different cell lines and in response to stimulations of different strengths was not well understood. This led Fussenegger and colleagues [19], and later Eissing and colleagues [20], to quantitatively interpret such qualitative schemes and translate them into mathematical models describing the kinetics of the underlying biochemical reactions using the simplest quantitative mathematical framework, ordinary differential equations (ODEs). Assuming specific values for parameters (reaction rate constants and protein initial concentrations) and specific initial conditions (initial protein concentrations), these models can be used to simulate the temporal evolution of molecular species concentrations.

These early studies did not quantitatively compared simulation results to data. Their explanatory power was therefore not well established. Still, by studying how simulated cell behaviors depend on the different parameters, these models provided interesting qualitative insights on the structure of the pathways, that is, on the molecular implementation of receptor-induced apoptosis. For example, Eissing and colleagues rightfully concluded from their model that there must be a caspase-8 inhibitor to allow for both (1) fast kinetics of apoptosis at sufficient stimulation levels and (2) the existence of a threshold stimuli intensity below which apoptosis is not triggered [20].

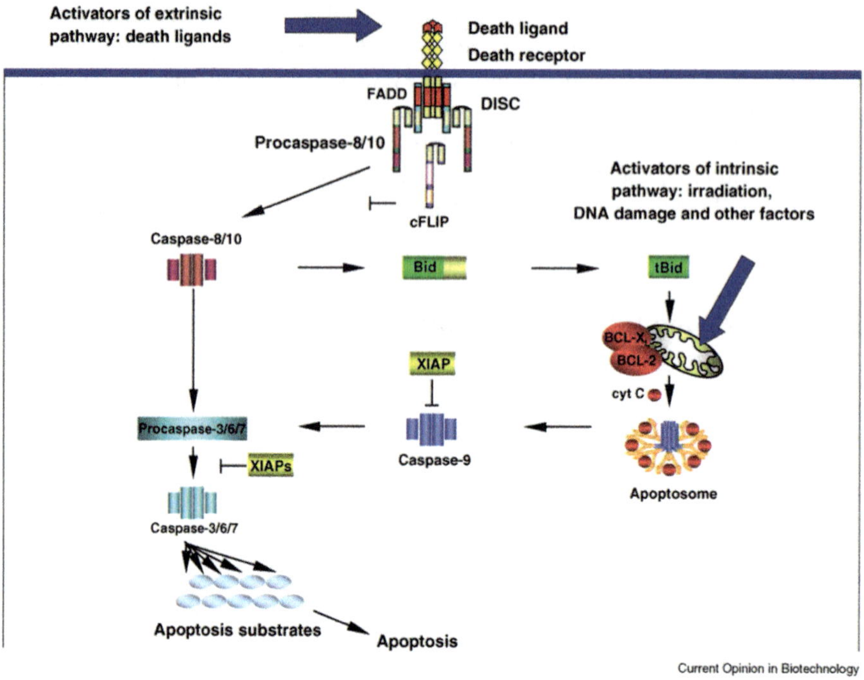

Fig. 12.1 Schematic representation of extrinsic and intrinsic apoptosis pathways at the molecular level. Only the main actors and interactions are represented. Death ligands bind their cognate receptors and promote assembly of DISCs complexes that can lead to the activation of the critical initiator caspases caspase-8/10. Initiator caspases can activate effector caspases either directly or by promoting the activation of the mitochondrial apoptosis pathway via Bid. This realizes a connection with the intrinsic apoptosis pathway, also activating the mitochondrial pathway and eventually activating effector caspases. Reprinted from [11], with permission from Elsevier

12.2.2 Tight Integration of Kinetic Modeling and Quantitative Experimental Data Revealed Key Mechanistic Features of Receptor-Induced Apoptosis

After those early efforts, several groups employed approaches that integrated more tightly the construction and analysis of ODE models of receptor-induced apoptosis with experimental data. These approaches have been particularly fruitful. Indeed, they revealed several key mechanistic features of receptor-induced apoptosis.

A pioneering work for the systems biology of apoptosis is the study of CD-95 induced apoptosis by Bentele et al. [21]. The authors constructed an ODE-based kinetic model combining mechanistic and "black box" reactions. Their initial model contains 41 species, 50 unknown parameters and is notably detailed regarding reactions taking place at the death-inducing signalling complex (DISC): the requirement for the recruitment of two pro-caspase-8 molecules for their activation, as well as the competitive recruitment of cFLIP, were detailed. In order to reduce the risks of overfitting and detect parameter non-identifiability, the authors used a sensitivity analysis approach to reduce model complexity before testing the model against data. In order to test the model, they obtained quantitative data characterizing the kinetics of caspase activation for several stimulation strengths. The data consisted in quantitative western blots corresponding to protein concentrations averaged over the cell population. The model predicted a threshold for ligand concentration below which no death should be seen, and this prediction was validated experimentally. In the model, the existence of this threshold is caused by cFLIP, which incorporates into newly assembled DISCs and thus blocks pro-caspase-8 processing. Hence, downstream death signalling only occurs for stimulation doses high enough to enable the assembly of a sufficient number of DISCs, capable of overcoming this blockade. By using an inhibitor of protein synthesis (cycloheximide, abbr. CHX) and exploiting differences in protein half-lives (cFLIP is short-lived whereas pro-caspase-8 is long-lived), they decreased cFLIP levels while preserving pro-caspase-8 levels and observed the predicted significant decrease of the threshold needed to obtain cell death.

One main limitation of the approach by Bentele and colleagues is the use of population-level measurements for quantifying caspase activation. It was already known that the kinetics of caspase activation was different in different cells. More precisely, single-cell reporters for probing cytochrome c release [22] and effector caspase activation [23] revealed that these events are rapid and relatively invariant in terms of duration and intensity from one cell to another and for different stimulus, whereas their initiation times are highly variable. An important, although often implicit assumption in kinetic models of biochemical pathways is that they represent reactions taking place in individual cells: an enzyme in one cell does not catalyze reactions in another cell. Therefore, in the presence of heterogeneity it is not appropriate to reason in terms of population-averaged quantities. Single-cell reporters enabling to measure the abundance or activity of biochemical species with live-cell imaging are therefore appealing tools to test and interrogate on a proper footing kinetic models. And indeed, single-cell reporters in combination with kinetic modeling revealed a number of key mechanistic features of receptor-induced apoptosis.

The first study integrating kinetic modeling with such single-cell data investigated apoptosis induced by staurosporine [24]. Although staurosporine does not induce apoptosis via death receptors, it triggers MOMP (mitochondrial outer membrane permeabilization) and then a rapid, all-or-none effector caspase activation. These molecular events form the downstream part of both extrinsic and intrinsic apoptosis pathways. The authors focused on the events directly following MOMP, using realistic kinetics of cytochrome c and Smac release and apoptosome formation as inputs to their model, which then predicted effector caspase activation kinetics. The amount of XIAP was found to be a key factor in the kinetics of effector caspase activation following MOMP. Interestingly, the model predicted the existence of a small range of XIAP concentrations for which MOMP is followed by a slow and partial effector caspase activation, a prediction that was then confirmed experimentally.

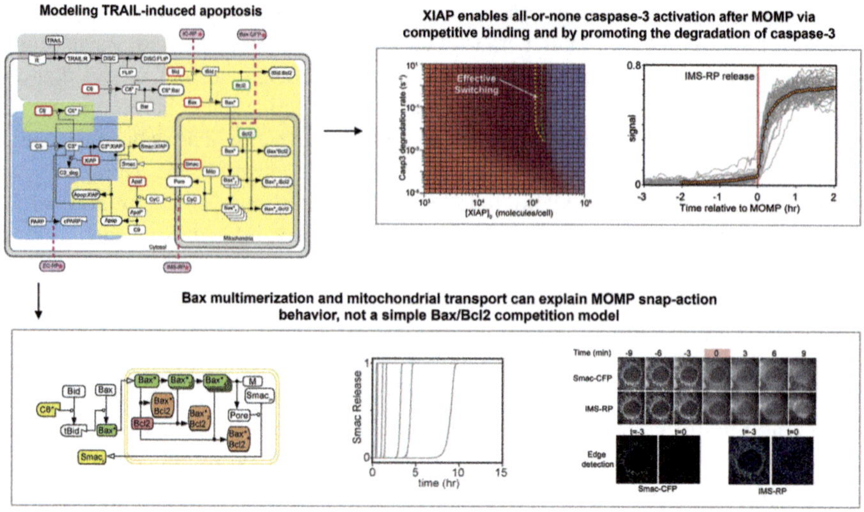

Fig. 12.2 Key mechanistic features of apoptosis revealed by integrated kinetic modeling and single-cell experiments. A relatively complete model of TRAIL-induced apoptosis by Albeck and colleagues developed in combination with new single-cell reporters for initiator caspase activity and MOMP allowed new mechanistic insights [25]. For example, XIAP control of caspase-3 activity during the variable pre-MOMP delay does not rely solely on competitive binding but also on its ability to promote caspase-3 proteasomal degradation (*right*). Another mechanistic insight relates to the role of network topology in generating snap-action behavior at the level of MOMP (*bottom*). Bax multimerization and mitochondrial transport can explain observed behavior, as opposed to a simple competition model between activated Bax and Bcl2. Figure elements reproduced from [25, 26]

Albeck and colleagues were the first to integrate, in a single model, initiator caspase activation (via TRAIL binding to death receptors), MOMP regulation and effector caspase activation [25]. The model featured 58 species (native protein and protein complexes) and 70 parameters (Fig. 12.2, top left). Instrumental in their work was the development of a single-cell reporter for initiator caspase activity [26], which showed that this activity slowly rises at a variable rate between cells during the pre-MOMP period, and that despite this increasing activity, no significant effector caspase activity is observed; the latter arises suddenly and completely following MOMP (Fig. 12.2, top right). The model revealed that XIAP enables this all-or-none switching behavior not only by competitive binding of caspase 3, but also by promoting its degradation via the proteasome (Fig. 12.2, top center). Another mechanistic insight brought by this model relates to the role of network topology in generating snap-action behavior at the level of MOMP (Fig. 12.2, bottom): Bax multimerization and mitochondrial transport can quantitatively explain the observed behavior despite the presence of Bcl2, whereas a simple competition model between activated Bax and Bcl2 could not.

Other remarkable works relying on such an integrated approach of quantitative experiments with kinetic modeling include the investigation of the activation of NF-κB signalling in parallel to death signalling in response to CD95-L exposure [27].

12.3 Modeling Populations of Individual Cells: The Role of Heterogeneity in Protein Levels

The previous studies shed light on how snap-action behaviors at the level of MOMP and effector caspase activation enable a tightly constrained all-or-none control over apoptosis commitment. Such an all-or-none control is probably beneficial at the organism level, because partial effector caspase activation is genotoxic and could result in potential harmful mutations. But why different cells from the same cell line submitted to the same stimulus in the same conditions trigger MOMP after a highly variable delay from one another? Also, in most studies discussed so far, cells were co-treated with the protein synthesis inhibitor cycloheximide (CHX). Blocking protein synthesis is interesting to disentangle the influence of signal transduction pathways from the influence of downstream genetic regulations. However, in these conditions, all cells eventually die, whereas in normal conditions, a fraction of the cell population often survives, a property of vital importance in the context of therapy. What are the origins of fractional killing? Are the mechanisms responsible for MOMP timing variability in treatments with CHX also involved in fractional killing without CHX?

An important study from the Sorger group brought key insights into these questions [28]. Using live-cell microscopy, the authors followed the fate of individual HeLa cells after exposure to TRAIL + CHX or TRAIL alone treatments. In both conditions, a significant variability was observed, in death times for TRAIL + CHX treatments, and in cell fate and death times for TRAIL alone treatments. Importantly, to investigate the role of differences in cell state that exist across cells at the time of treatment in determining cell fate and death times, they recorded normal cell proliferation for a duration of about one cell cycle before applying the treatment in order to identify (1) pairs of cells that are sisters and (2) how much time elapsed between their division and treatment. Such lineage information was exquisitely insightful (note that similar experimental observations were made earlier by Rehm et al. [29] and later by Bhola and Simons [30]). First, in the TRAIL + CHX treatment, recently divided sister cells displayed a strong correlation in their death time, despite the high overall variability of death time among cells. This established that (1) death time variability is caused by preexisting differences, conserved at cell division; and (2) in presence of CHX, TRAIL signalling is almost entirely deterministic (but again, depends on preexisting differences). In other words, because one could accurately predict the fate of one recently divided cell by observing the fate of its sister, there is no significant randomness in the signalling reactions taking place between TRAIL + CHX exposure and apoptosis commitment.

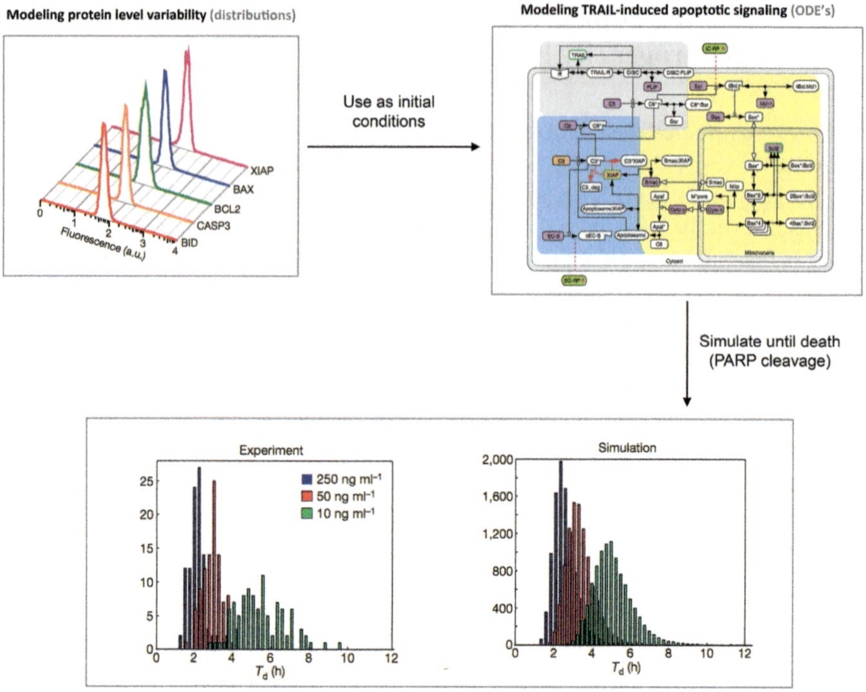

Fig. 12.3 Initial variability in protein levels explains variability in the timing of death. Spencer and colleagues combined a previously proposed ODE model of TRAIL-induced apoptosis signalling with the use of distributions for the initial values of proteins levels as could be measured by immunochemistry and flow cytometry to represent the heterogeneity in protein levels existing in cell populations [28]. Then they recorded the variability in the timing of death for different doses of TRAIL and in presence or absence of cycloheximide within the in silico cell population. The resulting distributions closely resemble the distributions obtained from experimental data. Figure elements reproduced from [28]

This led Spencer and colleagues to the hypothesis that differences in *initial levels* for proteins involved in TRAIL apoptotic signalling are the main determinants of cell fate variability. Mathematical modeling was used to test further this hypothesis (Fig. 12.3). They relied on the same kinetic ODE model (with minor modifications) of the protein–protein reactions mediating TRAIL apoptotic signalling as in their previous study [25]. However, instead of using a single population-averaged value for the initial level of each protein in the pathway, they created an in silico cell population by sampling many times protein levels from *distributions*, meant to reproduce the natural variability in protein levels within a population of HeLa cells (some of those distributions were actually measured experimentally using immunofluorescence and flow cytometry). Good agreement between model predictions and data for TRAIL + CHX treatments was then obtained (Fig. 12.3), therefore supporting that in these conditions initial variability in protein levels are the main determinants of the observed death time variability.

Additionally, when considering pairs of sister cells born long before TRAIL + CHX treatments, the correlation between their death times continuously decreases, showing that the cell determinants setting this death time fluctuate over time with a timescale of the order of a cell cycle. Notably, protein levels in human cells have been shown to fluctuate with similar time scales [31]. It is therefore probable that the natural slow fluctuations of protein levels are responsible for the decorrelation of sister cell fates after their division. For TRAIL alone treatments, a similar effect is seen, but firstly the correlation for recently divided cells is reduced compared to TRAIL + CHX treatments, and secondly this correlation decreases markedly faster with sister cells' age. Because the primary effect of CHX is to block protein synthesis, this also strongly suggests that cell fate variability in TRAIL-induced apoptosis originates from synthesis-induced fluctuations in protein levels.

Note that by nature, the model used by Sorger and colleagues cannot account for the sister cell data, a limitation inherent to all deterministic models in which cell-to-cell differences are *static*, that is, cell-to-cell differences are modeled by distributions of values for initial protein concentrations or for time-invariant parameters. Such models do not explain how cell-to-cell variability can be *generated*, which is indispensable if reestablishment of cell-to-cell variability after TRAIL application should be understood. A prime candidate for the (re)generation of cell heterogeneity is stochastic protein fluctuations that are missed out in the previous approach. Note also that no attempt to reproduce cell fate variability data in TRAIL alone treatments, a critical observation, was made. One can cite two reasons. Firstly, the model was trained against TRAIL + CHX data, removing the influence of many parameters constraining protein production. Secondly, fractional killing was thought to result mostly from the activation of survival pathways and these pathways were not included in the model.

Among the other modeling studies investigating cell-to-cell variability in receptor-induced apoptosis, it is worth mentioning the work by Toivonen and colleagues [32]. These authors extended the model of CD-95L induced apoptosis from [21] with variable synthesis and degradation rates for the short-lived protein c-FLIP, and their analysis predicted c-FLIP targeted degradation as being a fundamental determinant of death receptor responses, in agreement with experimental observations.

12.4 Modeling Different Cell Lines and Their Different Sensitivities to Receptor-Induced Apoptosis

From the discussion in the previous section, we see that differences in protein levels could be a main determinant of cell fate differences. Thus, knowing the expression levels of the proteins involved in extrinsic apoptosis in a given cell line could help predicting its sensitivity to different death ligand stimulations. Stated differently, we adopt here the viewpoint in which cell lines do not differ by the *topology* of their pathways but rather by the *levels* or more specifically by the *distributions* of the proteins involved in these pathways. This idea motivated another study by the

Sorger group [33]. Using their previous model as a reference for the rates of biochemical reactions of extrinsic apoptosis, they studied the biochemical basis of the Type I/Type II behaviors. Type I (II) behavior refers to cells that do not require (do require) MOMP to commit to apoptosis after death ligand stimulation. As a consequence, a strong overexpression of Bcl2 proteins renders cells resistant to death ligand stimulation only in type II cells.

The authors could successfully classify the Type I/II behavior of a set of cell lines solely based on the expression levels of the proteins involved in apoptotic signal transduction. Their approach was based on direct finite-time Lyapunov exponent (DLE) analysis, which measures the influence of changes in initial protein concentration on the future states of the system. More precisely, when computing DLEs for different initial conditions, they obtained a narrow region of high DLE values, i.e., a region where small changes in initial conditions lead to large deviations in cell state after stimulation, separating two large regions having comparatively low DLE values (Fig. 12.4, bottom left). When positioning cell lines on this space based on

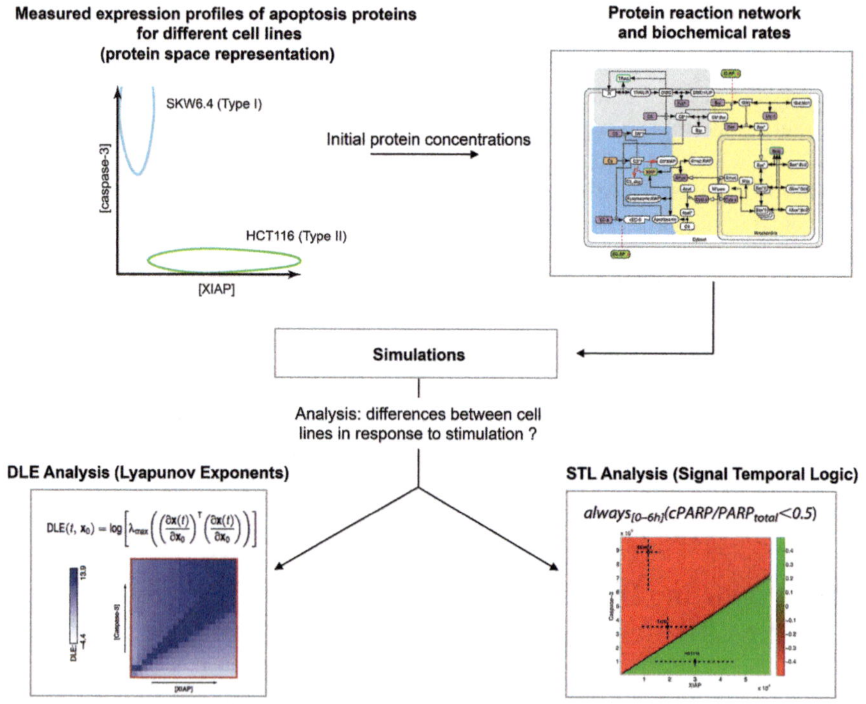

Fig. 12.4 Simulating the differential sensitivity of cancer cell lines to receptor-induced apoptosis. Different cell lines express extrinsic apoptosis proteins at different levels (leading to different distributions of single-cell level expression), and those differences a priori impact on their response to receptor stimulation. Aldridge and colleagues [33] used Lyapunov exponent analysis to study and demonstrated its ability to classify and compare different cell lines. Stoma and colleagues [34] proposed an alternative to Lyapunov exponents, Signal Temporal Logic (STL), that allows to formally encode behavioral differences as measured by various experimental assays. Figure elements reproduced from [33, 34]

measured expression levels, they found that Type I and Type II cell lines were on opposite sides of the high-DLE region, while cell lines exhibiting mixed behaviors were close to it.

One limitation of the DLE analysis is that the DLE is a number that is difficult to interpret. It reflects a sensitivity of the future states to the initial conditions, but it does not give information about what is perturbed in the states. In addition, one has to choose a time horizon to compute DLEs, which might have a strong influence on the results. We have therefore proposed another approach, based on Signal Temporal Logic (STL) instead of DLE [34]. Temporal logics are flexible property specification languages that allow describing expected features of behaviors. Experimentally observed behaviors are explicitly encoded in STL. This approach allowed us to discover that the notion of Type I and Type II has limits, as there exist several interpretations of being a Type I or a Type II cell which are not equivalent (Fig. 12.4, bottom right).

The idea that differences in protein expression levels between cell lines could predict differences in response to death ligand stimulation from a mechanistic model of extrinsic apoptosis was also used in other studies [35]. Recently, a similar approach has been applied to patient-derived cell lines to predict their sensitivity to treatment [36], although here they use statistical modeling (rather than mechanistic modeling) to map expression profiles to sensitivity.

12.5 Modeling Fluctuations of Protein Levels to Extend the Temporal Scope of Existing Models

Until now, the modeling approaches we have discussed represent the naturally arising differences in protein levels between individual cells of a given cell line by static distributions, and such distributions are then used as initial conditions for deterministic models of extrinsic apoptosis signalling (see Sect. 12.3). In particular, one of the most important mechanisms that generate these distributions, the burstiness of gene expression and therefore the stochastic nature of protein turnover, is not accounted for in the above-mentioned models. Whether such fluctuations are responsible for the observed decrease of the correlation of death times of sister cells with their age at treatment as discussed in Sect. 12.3 is an interesting question. Not accounting for protein fluctuations fundamentally limits the temporal scope of a given protein–protein interaction model, even if its kinetic parameters are appropriately constrained. With this approach, we addressed the question of what *are* surviving cells after treatment, and hence what will be their resistance to future treatment applications (Fig. 12.5, top) [18]. It relies on modeling stochastic gene expression (stochastic switches of the promoter between an active and an inactive transcriptional state, and stochastic production and degradation of the mRNA) and protein turnover for *all* (native) proteins appearing in the model. As a result, protein levels slowly fluctuate in each individual cell such that, overall, the distributions of the

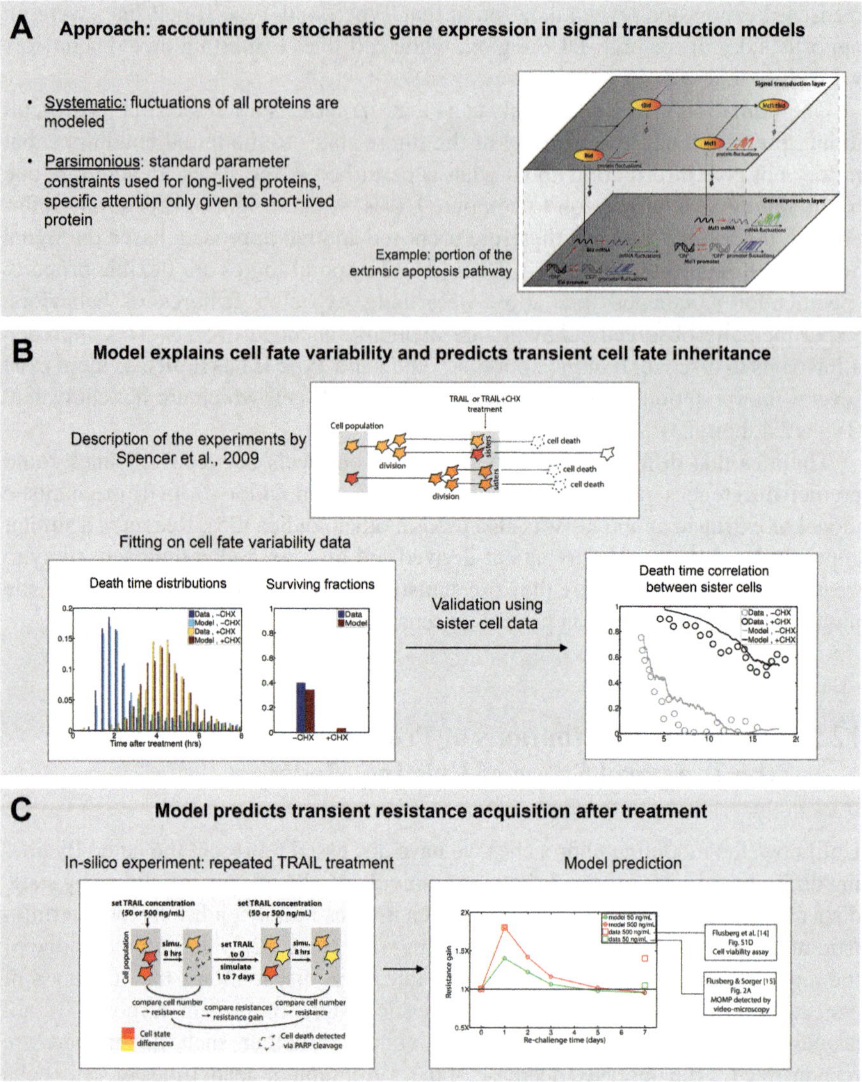

Fig. 12.5 Systematic, parsimonious modeling of stochastic gene expression together with TRAIL apoptotic signalling explains fractional killing and predicts transient cell fate inheritance and transient resistance acquisition. (**a**) Schematic description of the modeling approach. (**b**) Results of the approach when applied to model and data of Spencer and colleagues [28]. (**c**) Simulation of consecutive TRAIL treatments reproduces the observed transient resistance acquisition [18]. Figure elements reproduced from [18]

protein concentrations in the whole cell population are the ones observed in [28]. This means that the naturally occurring cell-to-cell variability, previously accounted by predetermined distributions for initial protein concentrations, is now an emerging property of the model.

While such model extension a priori introduces many unknown parameters, we found that using simple constraints from the literature on parameter values one readily obtains good approximations of protein fluctuations for most proteins. Only short-lived proteins necessitate particular attention. This finding is a cornerstone of the approach, as it allows to strongly reduce the number of unconstrained parameters, facilitating exploration of the parameter space and reducing the risks of overfitting. We applied this modeling approach to extend the model of TRAIL-induced apoptosis used by Spencer and colleagues. Among the 17 native proteins appearing in the model, only gene expression parameters for Flip and Mcl1 (known to be very short-lived at both the mRNA and protein levels) were used for fitting the data, while standard parameter constraints were used for all others. The model could quantitatively fit cell death distributions and cell survival fractions for both TRAIL + CHX and TRAIL alone treatments (Fig. 12.5, middle, left). Moreover, sister cell data (decrease in their death time correlation as they age) that have not been used to fit our model could be predicted (Fig. 12.5, middle, right), thus validating the approach.

The finding that cell survival does not require TRAIL-induced activation of survival pathways, but can occur solely from the interplay of stochastic gene expression, fast turnover of certain anti-apoptotic proteins, Flip and Mcl1, and rapid degradation of activated forms challenges the classical view about the role of survival pathways in response to TRAIL [37]. While it does not mean that survival pathways do not play a role in cell survival after TRAIL exposure, our results strongly suggest that they are not the sole contributors to cell survival.

Finally, because the model can predict changes in cell states (i.e., cell protein content) of the population caused by a first treatment as well as the recovery of cells to their normal states (i.e., initial protein distributions) after treatment based on stochastic gene expression and protein turnover, the efficiency of a second treatment as a function of the time between treatments could be investigated. In agreement with data, simulations showed a marked but transient increase of the population resistance after a treatment (Fig. 12.5, bottom). We therefore provide a simple mechanistic explanation to the observed reversible resistance of cells to repeated treatments.

12.6 Conclusions and Perspectives

In this chapter, we survey how system modeling of receptor-induced apoptosis has been instrumental in improving our understanding of this process at several levels: the molecular level, the level of cellular decisions between life and death, and the level of cell populations exhibiting various degrees of resistance as a function of their protein expression profiles or their treatment history.

More precisely, ordinary differential equations models recapitulating known reactions between proteins during apoptosis signalling are useful when compared to short-term (a few hours) population data about protein level and state kinetics (Sect. 12.2). They allow verifying that the structure of known reactions is compatible with what is experimentally observed and can provide estimates of the associated biochemical rates (although parameter non-identifiability often prevents the obtention of unique estimates). Comparing model predictions with population data has fundamental limitations, and comparison to single-cell data (obtained by means of cell-level reporters for well-defined biochemical activities or events) is a priori more meaningful. Indeed, in the context of receptor-induced apoptosis, it has revealed important kinetic features regarding MOMP regulation and effector caspase activation (Sect. 12.2).

Still, there are two difficulties arising when comparing ODE models of protein–protein reactions with such single-cell data. First, protein synthesis, which is noisy and hence generates differences from cell to cell, can have an impact on signalling dynamics at the protein level. This effect can only be temporally mitigated by using protein synthesis inhibitors like cycloheximide. Second, model predictions depend on initial conditions, such as the prestimulation levels of the protein involved in receptor-induced signalling. We have seen that most of the variability in death timing following TRAIL (and cycloheximide) treatment can be explained when realistic random distributions of initial protein levels are used as initial conditions for an ODE model of TRAIL-induced apoptosis signalling (Sect. 12.3). This result is important as it demonstrates that TRAIL-induced apoptosis signalling is not intrinsically noisy, and that cell state (i.e., the levels of apoptosis proteins) differences at treatment time are a major determinant of cell fate variability. Indeed, we have seen that the protein expression profiles of different cell lines can inform about their sensitivity to extrinsic death stimulation when used as initial conditions of a single (i.e., the same for all cell lines) ODE model of apoptotic signalling (Sect. 12.4).

However, while cell fate is almost fully determined by cell state at treatment time when protein synthesis is blocked, it is only partially the case in normal treatment conditions, in which survival of a fraction of the population is often observed. Indeed, protein synthesis can interact with receptor-induced signalling and steer cell fate in one direction or another. In Sect. 12.5, we see how systematic but parameter-parsimonious modeling of stochastic gene expression within ODE models of signal transduction dynamics can explain important observations on the dynamics of cell-to-cell variability in TRAIL-induced apoptosis. This approach allows extending the temporal scope of ODE models of receptor-induced apoptosis. This is required to investigate the response of cell populations to multiple treatments separated in time, for which resistance acquisition is very often observed. An important prediction of such models is that transient resistance acquisition can occurs in the absence of stimulus-induced pro-survival transcriptional activity.

Despite those promising advances, many questions remain without clear answers. For example, while the important role in cell survival of the targeted degradation of many pro- and anti-apoptotic proteins is increasingly recognized [38], accurate estimates of the corresponding rates are not available, and to which extent those rates fluctuate in single cells and vary from cell to cell is not known. Experiments using proteasome inhibitors are difficult to interpret because they have a global (but not necessarily identical) effect on all degradation rates. More targeted approaches (for example using specific single-cell reporters) could be very useful to better understand the role of targeted degradation in receptor-induced apoptosis.

While current models of receptor-induced apoptosis can be quite large (up to 100 species and reactions), they are often omitting structural details either because those details are not understood very well or because a simplifying representation is deliberately preferred. For example, the ligand-induced receptor clustering at cell surface, the processing of caspase-8 at the DISC, the role of the different Flip isoforms in that processing, and the interactions of all MOMP regulators at the mitochondrial surface are generally significantly simplified. Such simplified representations can be accurate and therefore sufficient to address many questions. Still, to test and improve our molecular-level understanding of receptor-induced apoptosis, more detailed mechanisms can be introduced into existing models, and model predictions can be compared to new data generated with adequate tools (such as relevant single-cell reporters). Without the "right" data, increasing model complexity is probably vain.

Finally, while mathematical models of receptor-induced apoptosis start to address the question of long-term behavior of cell populations repeatedly treated by death receptor agonists, the amount and quality of corresponding experimental data is very scarce. Most in vitro studies still only measure the efficiency of one-time treatment to model cell lines, and repeated treatments are only seen in mouse xenografts studies, in which time points and measurements are limited, and many effects related to the in vivo context can affect the response. Quantitative population dynamics data (i.e., cell proliferation and death rate as a function of time) for cell lines cultured in vitro and submitted to repeated treatments could prove very useful to better understand resistance acquisition, and to map it to molecular mechanisms with the aid of mathematical models. Also, the potential impact of spatial organization of the cells in tumors may generate further inhomogeneities that are not captured by models disregarding space, and hence a full understanding will eventually have to explore the possible effects of space.

Acknowledgments This work was supported by the research grants Syne2arti ANR-10-COSINUS-007 and Investissements d'Avenir Iceberg ANR-IABI-3096 from the French National Research Agency.

References

1. Hassan M, Watari H, AbuAlmaaty A, Ohba Y, Sakuragi N (2014) Apoptosis and molecular targeting therapy in cancer. Biomed Res Int 2014:150823–150845
2. Johnstone RW, Frew AJ, Smyth MJ (2008) The TRAIL apoptotic pathway in cancer onset, progression and therapy. Nat Rev Cancer 8:782–798. doi:10.1038/nrc2465

3. Ashkenazi A, Dixit VM (1999) Apoptosis control by death and decoy receptors. Curr Opin Cell Biol 11:255–260. doi:10.1016/S0955-0674(99)80034-9
4. Kimberley FC, Screaton GR (2004) Following a TRAIL: update on a ligand and its five receptors. Cell Res 14:359–372
5. Ashkenazi A (2008) Directing cancer cells to self-destruct with pro-apoptotic receptor agonists. Nat Rev Drug Discov 7:1001–1012
6. Taylor RC, Cullen SP, Martin SJ (2008) Apoptosis: controlled demolition at the cellular level. Nat Rev Mol Cell Biol 9:231–241
7. Youle RJ, Strasser A (2008) The BCL-2 protein family: opposing activities that mediate cell death. Nat Rev Mol Cell Biol 9:47–59
8. Wiezorek J, Holland P, Graves J (2010) Death receptor agonists as a targeted therapy for cancer. Clin Cancer Res 16:1701–1708
9. Bentele M, Eils R (2005) Systems biology of apoptosis. In: Alberghina L, Westerhoff HV (eds) Systems biology (Stevenage). Springer, Berlin/Heidelberg, pp 349–372
10. Bialik S, Zalckvar E, Ber Y, Rubinstein AD, Kimchi A (2010) Systems biology analysis of programmed cell death. Trends Biochem Sci 35:556–564
11. Lavrik IN (2010) Systems biology of apoptosis signaling networks. Curr Opin Biotechnol 21:551–555
12. Spencer SL, Sorger PK (2011) Measuring and modeling apoptosis in single cells. Cell 144:926–939
13. Schleich K, Lavrik IN (2013) Mathematical modeling of apoptosis. Cell Commun Signal 11:44
14. Huber HJ, McKiernan RG, Prehn JHM (2014) Harnessing system models of cell death signalling for cytotoxic chemotherapy: towards personalised medicine approaches? J Mol Med 92:227–237
15. Lavrik IN (2014) Systems biology of death receptor networks: live and let die. Cell Death Dis 5:e1259
16. Flusberg D, Sorger PK (2015) Surviving apoptosis: life-death signaling in single cells. Trends Cell Biol 25(8):446–458
17. Flusberg DA, Roux J, Spencer SL, Sorger PK (2013) Cells surviving fractional killing by TRAIL exhibit transient but sustainable resistance and inflammatory phenotypes. Mol Biol Cell 24:2186–2200
18. Bertaux F, Stoma S, Drasdo D, Batt G (2014) Modeling dynamics of cell-to-cell variability in TRAIL-induced apoptosis explains fractional killing and predicts reversible resistance. PLoS Comput Biol 10:e1003893. doi:10.1371/journal.pcbi.1003893
19. Fussenegger M, Bailey JE, Varner J (2000) A mathematical model of caspase function in apoptosis. Nat Biotechnol 18:768–774. doi:10.1038/77589
20. Eissing T, Conzelmann H, Gilles ED, Allgöwer F, Bullinger E, Scheurich P (2004) Bistability analyses of a caspase activation model for receptor-induced apoptosis. J Biol Chem 279:36892–36897. doi:10.1074/jbc.M404893200
21. Bentele M, Lavrik I, Ulrich M, Stösser S, Heermann DW, Kalthoff H, Krammer PH, Eils R (2004) Mathematical modeling reveals threshold mechanism in CD95-induced apoptosis. J Cell Biol 166:839–851
22. Goldstein JC, Waterhouse NJ, Juin P, Evan GI, Green DR (2000) The coordinate release of cytochrome c during apoptosis is rapid, complete and kinetically invariant. Nat Cell Biol 2:156–162
23. Tyas L, Brophy VA, Pope A, Rivett AJ, Tavare JM (2000) Rapid caspase-3 activation during apoptosis revealed using fluorescence-resonance energy transfer. EMBO Rep 1:266–270
24. Rehm M, Huber HJ, Dussmann H, Prehn JHM (2006) Systems analysis of effector caspase activation and its control by X-linked inhibitor of apoptosis protein. EMBO J 25:4338–4349
25. Albeck JG, Burke JM, Spencer SL, Lauffenburger DA, Sorger PK (2008) Modeling a snap-action, variable-delay switch controlling extrinsic cell death. PLoS Biol 6:2831–2852. doi:10.1371/journal.pbio.0060299

26. Albeck JG, Burke JM, Aldridge BB, Zhang M, DA L, Sorger PK (2008) Quantitative analysis of pathways controlling extrinsic apoptosis in single cells. Mol Cell 30:11–25. doi:10.1016/j.molcel.2008.02.012
27. Neumann L, Pforr C, Beaudouin J, Pappa A, Fricker N, Krammer PH, Lavrik IN, Eils R (2010) Dynamics within the CD95 death-inducing signaling complex decide life and death of cells. Mol Syst Biol 6:352. doi:10.1038/msb.2010.6
28. Spencer SL, Gaudet S, Albeck JG, Burke JM, Sorger PK (2009) Non-genetic origins of cell-to-cell variability in TRAIL-induced apoptosis. Nature 459:428–432. doi:10.1038/nature08012
29. Rehm M, Huber HJ, Hellwig CT, Anguissola S, Dussmann H, Prehn JHM (2009) Dynamics of outer mitochondrial membrane permeabilization during apoptosis. Cell Death Differ 16:613–623
30. Bhola PD, Simon SM (2009) Determinism and divergence of apoptosis susceptibility in mammalian cells. J Cell Sci 122:4296–4302. doi:10.1242/jcs.055590
31. Sigal A, Milo R, Cohen A, Geva-Zatorsky N, Klein Y, Liron Y, Rosenfeld N, Danon T, Perzov N, Alon U (2006) Variability and memory of protein levels in human cells. Nature 444:643–646. doi:10.1038/nature05316
32. Toivonen HT, Meinander A, Asaoka T, Westerlund M, Pettersson F, Mikhailov A, Eriksson JE, Saxén H (2011) Modeling reveals that dynamic regulation of c-FLIP levels determines cell-to-cell distribution of CD95-mediated apoptosis. J Biol Chem 286:18375–18382
33. Aldridge BB, Gaudet S, DA L, Sorger PK (2011) Lyapunov exponents and phase diagrams reveal multi-factorial control over TRAIL-induced apoptosis. Mol Syst Biol 7:1–21. doi:10.1038/msb.2011.85
34. Stoma S, Donzé A, Bertaux F, Maler O, Batt G (2013) STL-based analysis of TRAIL-induced apoptosis challenges the notion of type I/type II cell line classification. PLoS Comput Biol 9:e1003056. doi:10.1371/journal.pcbi.1003056
35. Schmid J, Dussmann H, Boukes GJ, Flanagan L, Lindner AU, O'Connor CL, Rehm M, Prehn JHM, Huber HJ (2012) Systems analysis of cancer cell heterogeneity in caspase-dependent apoptosis subsequent to mitochondrial outer membrane permeabilization. J Biol Chem 287:41546–41559
36. Passante E, Wurstle ML, Hellwig CT, Leverkus M, Rehm M (2013) Systems analysis of apoptosis protein expression allows the case-specific prediction of cell death responsiveness of melanoma cells. Cell Death Differ 20:1521–1531
37. Falschlehner C, Emmerich CH, Gerlach B, Walczak H (2007) TRAIL signalling: decisions between life and death. Int J Biochem Cell Biol 39:1462–1475. doi:10.1016/j.biocel.2007.02.007
38. Roux J, Hafner M, Bandara S, Sims JJ, Hudson H, Chai D, Sorger PK (2015) Fractional killing arises from cell-to-cell variability in overcoming a caspase activity threshold. Mol Syst Biol 11:803

Index

O. Micheau (ed.), *TRAIL, Fas Ligand, TNF and TLR3 in Cancer*, Resistance to Targeted Anti-Cancer Therapeutics, DOI 10.1007/978-3-319-56805-8

Printed by Printforce, the Netherlands